HEALTH COMMUNICATION
IN PRACTICE

A Case Study Approach

LEA'S COMMUNICATION SERIES

Jennings Bryant/Dolf Zillmann, General Editors

Selected Titles in Applied Communication
(Teresa L. Thompson, Advisory Editor) include:

For a complete list of titles in LEA's Communication Series, please contact Lawrence Erlbaum Associates, Publishers, at www.erlbaum.com.

HEALTH COMMUNICATION IN PRACTICE

A Case Study Approach

Edited by

Eileen Berlin Ray
Cleveland State University

LEA

LAWRENCE ERLBAUM ASSOCIATES, PUBLISHERS

2005 Mahwah, New Jersey London

Senior Acquisitions Editor:	Linda Bathgate
Assistant Editor:	Karin Wittig Bates
Cover Design:	Kathryn Houghtaling Lacey
Textbook Production Manager:	Paul Smolenski
Full-Service Compositor:	TechBooks
Text and Cover Printer:	Hamilton Printing Company

This book was typeset in 10/12 pt. Times, Italic, Bold, Bold Italic. The heads were typeset in Americana, and Americana Bold Italic.

Lawrence Erlbaum Associates, Inc., Publishers
10 Industrial Avenue
Mahwah, New Jersey 07430
www.erlbaum.com

Library of Congress Cataloging-in-Publication Data

Health communication in practice : a case study approach / edited by Eileen
Berlin Ray.
    p. ; cm.—(LEA's communication series)
  Includes bibliographical references and index.
  ISBN 0-8058-4757-X (hardcover : alk. paper)—ISBN 0-8058-4758-8 (pbk. : alk. paper)
  1. Communication in medicine—Case studies. 2. Communication in public health—Case studies.
3. Physician and patient—Case studies.
  [DNLM: 1. Professional-Patient Relations. 2. Communication. 3. Patient Care—Case Reports.
4. Patient Care—psychology. W 62 H4343 2005] I. Ray, Eileen Berlin. II. Series.
  R118.H433 2005
  610.69′6—dc22

                                               2004024823

Printed in the United States of America
10 9 8 7 6 5 4 3 2 1

To my father,

N. Paul Berlin

1922–2003

Who taught me to stand up for what I believe in even when he disagreed,
to take responsibility and apologize for mistakes made,
and that there isn't much that a hug and a corny joke can't make better.

Contents

Introduction

In 1993, when Lawrence Erlbaum Associates published *Case Studies in Health Communication* (Ray, 1993), it was perhaps the second case studies book in the communication discipline (following Sypher, 1990) and the first in health communication. Since then, there have been several more that take a case studies approach, focusing on contexts such as interpersonal communication (Braithwaite & Wood, 2000), organizational communication (Keyton & Shockley-Zalabak, 2004), and communication and disenfranchisement (Ray, 1996). The fact that this genre is now commonly used in various communication classes speaks to its utility and importance as a pedagogical tool.

Case studies provide an important instructional aid in the classroom. They bring academic material to life, make it relevant to students so that concepts and theories stay with them after the class ends, and help students to examine and challenge their ways of doing things. Case studies are valuable in health communication as students read cases about, for example, communication that resulted in good or poor health outcomes, persons with disabilities communicating their needs and desires, the impact of managed care, and how public health campaigns are developed and evaluated. Cases may instigate dialogue outside the classroom. Discussing issues such as advance directives or organ donation can be softened when couched in the context of a case, enabling families and friends to talk about these sensitive topics. Good case studies integrate theory and practice in a way that makes it barely noticeable and almost painless to students.

We learn a great deal about the health care system and health communication when we are forced to confront it in a time of crisis. When the crisis is over, we reflect on decisions we made, interactions we had, information we sought, and what we might have done differently. We have a newfound wealth of knowledge about the health care system. Although hindsight is 20/20, it would have been especially helpful to have some of that information at the beginning, rather than at the end, of a health care crisis. Case studies can provide some of this insight up front. By reading about others' experiences, we are more attuned to questions to ask, support to seek, when and how to assert ourselves, and how we can communicate most effectively. In this sense, case studies are both descriptive and prescriptive.

Health Communication in Practice: A Case Study Approach offers several additions to the 1993 text. First, authors include members of the medical community as well as communication scholars. This combination adds to the richness and reality of the situations presented in the cases. Second, there is a list of relevant concepts and their definitions at the end of each case. This was added as a result of feedback from my students who read drafts of the cases. Third, topics reflect changes in health communication issues over the past 10 years. Although some cover themes that are also found in the 1993 volume (e.g., persons with disabilities, the elderly, job stress and burnout among hospital staff, and information dissemination), the new cases provide a different and updated perspective. Some of the new topics in this volume include delivering bad news, genetic testing, intercultural communication, grieving families, and international health campaigns. As you will see in the following overview, this volume covers a plethora of health communication issues.

OVERVIEW OF THE CASES

The organization of the case studies in this volume is somewhat arbitrary, offering instructors one way (my way) of framing the cases. Several themes run throughout many of the cases, such as the social construction of identity and the renegotiating of this identity and relational roles during and following a health crisis, stigma and its management, provider–recipient communication, the importance of formal and informal social support, and the role of patient activism in our health care. My goal was to include cases that cover a range of topics that can be organized to fit a variety of pedagogic strategies. The following overview provides a brief description of these cases.

Part I is distinguished by its dominant focus on provider–recipient communication and its importance to subsequent diagnosis and treatment. The first two cases (Cegala and Thompson & Gillotti) focus on doctor–patient communication in terms of making the diagnosis and then communicating diagnosis and treatment options to the patient. In Chapter 1, Cegala presents actual discourse between a physician and patient in the first three minutes of their interview. These first three minutes are critical for the patient's treatment. Most decisions about diagnosis and treatment are made based on what patients tell their physicians about their medical condition, which takes place during history-taking when they report their symptoms. In addition to affecting the accuracy of a patient's diagnosis, incorrect treatment can lead to malpractice suits. Whereas Cegala's case focuses on the dyadic communication leading to the provider's assessment, Thompson and Gillotti (Chapter 2) focus on the impact of the provider's delivery of bad news to a patient. Through observing other doctors and experiences within her own family, Christie, a medical resident, observes a range of methods, some much better than others, to balance giving bad news and providing support to patients. It is clear that the timing of the news, the source delivering it, and the medium used impact what patients and their family members hear and process. Given that they must make decisions about treatment based on this information, its effective delivery is crucial. In Chapter 3 (Babrow & Dinn), we depart from the physician–patient dyad to the relationship between a physical therapist and patient. We meet Charlie, a 68-year-old retired farmer who is recovering from a life-altering stroke. We see the intersection of his physical and emotional recovery, not only for Charlie but for his wife and daughters as well. This is exacerbated by their lack of communication about their feelings and frustrations with Charlie's health issues. Lack of communication is also central in Charlie's relationship with his physical therapist. Their poor communication results in very different perceptions of how much progress has been made. The assessment of progress is critical because the physical therapist is legally bound to only work with patients as long as they are making satisfactory progress. When the therapist stops therapy, Charlie suffers an emotional setback as well. There are no easy answers here, but the complexities of life-altering health events and the impact of communication, or lack of it, are painfully clear.

Chapters 4 and 5 emphasize the patient's role as activist. In Chapter 4, Sharf, Haidet, and Kroll discuss the concept of narrative and its importance in shaping how patients respond to both the experience of serious illness and the quality of the patient–physician relationship. Joanne, a 34-year-old woman, tells her story of attempting to manage her treatment for diabetes. She works hard to balance accepting guidance from her doctor and controlling her own treatment. This case provides an exemplar for how we can develop partnerships with our doctors and the importance of perceiving ourselves as active participants in control of our health care. Chapter 5 continues the issue of patients taking an active role in their health care. Cline and Young explore the impact of direct-to-consumer advertising (DTCA) on doctor–patient relationships. With more than $2 billion spent on DTCA in 2002, we have become inundated with media messages encouraging us to ask our doctors for particular prescriptions. Although both proponents and opponents agree that DTCA is changing the health care relationship from a traditional paternalistic model toward a participatory model, they do not agree about the consequences of this change. This case provides a debate of the issue among five doctors, each representing different perspectives, as they discuss their treatment of patients who seek prescriptions based on consumer advertising.

Part II focuses on issues in decision making. Chapter 6 (Bylund & Imes) juxtaposes two scenarios, childbirth and prostate cancer. Both underscore the importance of examining the medical, relational, and personal contexts and their impact on decision making. An understanding of the interaction among the medical context, the relational context between the patient and care provider, and each person's personal context, including input from family and friends, is essential to appreciate the complexities of health-related decision making. O'Hair, Thompson, and Sparks (Chapter 7) use the Cancer Survivorship and Agency Model (CSAM) as an explanatory mechanism for determining how and why certain decisions are made about medical care. The model is made up of four somewhat sequential stages. We follow Ann Benton, a 64-year-old woman diagnosed with pancreatic cancer, as she moves from shock to uncertainty to empowerment to agency and see how the CSAM provides a framework for understanding the decisions she makes regarding her treatment. In Chapter 8, Edgar, Satterfield, and Whaley provide scenarios using diabetes to exemplify many of the issues and variables to be considered (e.g., audience/culture, message content, and structure) in designing messages to explain illness. We meet 15-year-old Victor after his diagnosis of type 2 diabetes and observe how his doctor explains his illness and treatment to him. We also meet Charlene, 44, a Lakota Sioux woman, who is diagnosed with a prediabetic condition. When Charlene returns to her family home, she meets Mary, a community health representative, who explains the disease using stories and metaphors that Charlene can easily understand and relate to. The importance of tailoring health messages is continued in Chapter 9 by Kopfman and E. B. Ray. This time, we see the adaptation of medical information to young children and the importance of language and metaphors to encourage their compliance with prescribed regimens. We also consider how these explanations may change when communicating health information to siblings or peers. The case also brings forth the different opinions adults have about what type and how much information is appropriate for children to know about their own and others' illnesses.

Part III focuses on issues in social identity; how people, as a result of various events in their lives, must redefine who they are and renegotiate their relationships. In Chapter 10 (Silk), we meet Henry, 33, who survived a head-on collision with another motor vehicle and suffered traumatic brain injury. As a result, Henry has had difficulty with short-term memory and behavioral control, was paralyzed from the waist down, and needs assistance with his adult daily living skills. He has been living at a rehabilitation center, and this case focuses on a meeting with his treatment team and parents. This case underscores not only the importance of the communication among the team members and among them, Henry, and his parents, but also how their verbal and nonverbal communication impacts Henry as he attempts to redefine his identity as a person with disabilities. In Chapter 11 (Murray-Johnson & McGrew), we follow 22-year-old Sandra through her counseling sessions with Karen at a battered women's shelter. Through the use of communication accommodation, Karen is able to help Sandra make different decisions, regain self-esteem, and shift her identity from passive victim to strong survivor. Chapter 12 (Rintamaki & Brashers) deals with how people manage the stigma of HIV in their social encounters. People with HIV have to decide if disclosing their health status to others is worth the risk. What impact is this disclosure likely to have on how they are perceived and on the relationship? By observing a small support group of people living with HIV, this case highlights these dilemmas and provides examples of strategies people employ to manage HIV stigma. Through the breast cancer narratives of four very different women, Ford and Christmon (Chapter 13), examine how each woman's story becomes a mechanism for "explaining" the experience of breast cancer to herself and to others. Through the communicative act of telling their stories, the women provide insight into how they try to make sense of their illness by reflecting on their experiences and renegotiating their identities with the significant others in their lives. In Chapter 14, Braithwaite and Japp deal with issues of identity and stigma for people with visible and invisible disabilities. Others may not accommodate to a person with an invisible disability because they may forget the person is not completely healthy or may not know or believe they are really disabled. For the person with the disability, managing the communication problems can be as difficult as the physical challenges. Support groups can help those with invisible disabilities by providing a forum to share experiences and information with similar others.

Part IV focuses on communication dynamics within families and with health care providers through some of life's unexpected health situations. Parrott and Weiner (Chapter 15) consider communication issues related to genetic counseling and sharing information among family members. The difficulties occur when a family member is discovered to have an inherited gene that has potentially serious health implications. Ethical issues regarding decisions by family members to be tested, how that information is used, and long-term concerns are highlighted. In addition to the immediate health concern, the authors also raise issues of potential problems if positive results become part of a person's medical record. In Chapter 16, Carol Mills and her husband welcome a child with trisomy 21 into their family. Their positive perspective is challenged by people in the medical and therapeutic communities. Mills recounts some of the major medical and therapy provider interactions she and her husband have experienced as the parents of a child with trisomy 21, as well as the experiences of several of their friends. Some of these experiences are joyous, others are infuriating, and still others are heartbreaking. For the parents of a child with special needs, these interactions carry great importance and power, and impact them from diagnosis on. Chapter 17 (Hullett) describes The Center, a support center specifically designed to help grieving families. They tailor their services to the specific needs of their members according to the ways in which grief affects family members of varying ages. In this case, we observe support groups for adults, teens, and children as each attempts to deal with their grief. Not all are successful; marriages end, children hide their grief in drugs or alcohol. But for those who are able to talk about their emotions in this safe environment, there is a high likelihood that they will successfully grieve their loss and move on. In Chapter 18, Flint, Query, and Parrish introduce us to the Gonzalez family, an Hispanic family dealing with Alzheimer's disease (AD). Hispanics are twice as likely to develop AD than Caucasians by the age of 90. Cultural norms include not talking about illness, rejecting formal outside assistance and relying instead on family members as caregivers and the only means of social support. In this case, secrecy surrounds the illnesses and deaths of two family members, both victims of AD. The case explores what happens when this information is disclosed and the implications for family relationships, support, and health care decisions.

As we age, many of us will have to move from independent living to more and more dependence on others. We may move in with family or to a retirement village, an assisted living facility, or a nursing home. For many, the physical changes are compounded by psychological difficulties adapting to these new environments. In Chapter 19 (Pitts, Krieger, & Nussbaum), we meet Kris, a remarkably articulate 92-year-old widower who has moved from independently living with his wife to their living together in assisted living until her death, to his permanent relocation to an intensive nursing care room. Although the community in which Kris resides prides itself on maintaining the dignity of its residents, offering an independent lifestyle, and providing opportunities for social engagement, Kris reveals his personal struggle to create and sustain relationships and accept that he must now depend greatly on others for daily assistance.

Part V focuses on issues in the delivery of health care. Health care delivery has changed dramatically with the proliferation of managed care. The shift from a service to business model has forced hospitals to stay competitive by reducing costs at all levels. National trends such as hospital overcrowding and nursing shortages add to an increasingly difficult work environment. The impact is felt most strongly by care providers and ultimately affect patient care. In Chapter 20 (Apker), we follow Rob, a 35-year-old registered nurse at a 900-bed city hospital that relies heavily on Medicare and Medicaid funding for patient health care costs. We watch Rob struggle to meet his personal standards of nursing in the face of stresses caused by the realities of budget cuts, staff shortages, and reduced patient stays. We see additional health care delivery differences caused by racial and socioeconomic disparities. These demographics impact access to health care, insurance coverage, and treatment. In Chapter 21, G. B. Ray addresses these issues through the prenatal care of Angela and Jeffrey, an African American couple pregnant with their first child. Their excitement of becoming new parents becomes overshadowed by the realities of escalating health care needs and costs. They are also faced with a paternalistic, dogmatic communication style from their care provider once he is aware of their financial situation. The couple works hard to meet their current and future health needs, but the stresses of paying for this care and interacting with their doctor casts a negative pall over their relationship during what should be a joyous time in their lives. In Chapter 22 (Angelelli & Geist-Martin), we observe communication breakdown and miscommunication when a third party is involved. In this case, the patient and nurse must use an interpreter as they discuss prenatal testing. The triadic communication is further complicated by differences in language, health care beliefs and practices, and reliance on the interpreter to accurately reflect these cultural differences. For the health care provider, the interpreter keeps the patient on track; for the patient, the interpreter is a co-conversationalist.

Chapter 23 (Murphy, Eisenberg, Sutcliffe, & Schenkel) focuses on the communication among hospital emergency department members as they try to find and correct errors before they escalate into a crisis. The authors follow a single detailed case, a "near miss" regarding a serious head trauma. They describe the events of that day using three different sense-making frames to show how different kinds of information led to a deceptively straightforward set of individual and organizational actions that almost had an adverse effect on the patient. Lammers, Lindholm, and Hazeu (Chapter 24) go beyond a specific illness episode and examine hidden communication—the exchanges and relationships between hospitals, doctors, clinics, and governmental regulators. This case concerns a successful and popular physician who practiced neonatal medicine as a member of a multispecialty medical group. The authors focus on the organizational, economic, and regulatory context and emphasize the formal rules that constrain communication between providers and nonproviders other than patients, such as administrators, managers, and contract officers. In Chapter 25 (du Pré), we see an example of health care delivery that works. Faced with a health care system in which staff morale was low, patients were not satisfied with their care, and staff turnover was high, the leaders transformed the hospital's culture. The result was an organization named by *Fortune* magazine as one of the 100 best companies to work for in the United States in 2002 and 2003 and one that consistently ranks among the top 1% of hospitals in the United States in patient satisfaction. This case examines how this metamorphosis was accomplished through organizational members' use of communication to establish heroes and villains, shared values, rituals and ceremonies, and active communication networks.

Finally, Part VI highlights issues related to health campaigns designed to disseminate health-related information and change behaviors. Lederman and Stewart (Chapter 26) focus on college drinking norms. The image of heavy drinking among college students is created and reinforced through the media and students sharing their "war stories." After more than a decade of study, however, researchers at Rutgers University found that while the majority of students did not drink dangerously, a high proportion of first-year students did. This case follows the development, implementation, and evaluation of a campaign to educate first-year students about the real drinking norms on their campus. In Chapter 27, Beck uses Michael J. Fox's disclosure of Parkinson's disease (PD) to analyze how someone famous constructs his narrative to protect his private life while being in the public spotlight. When people suffer illness or injury, they, their families, and concerned others are faced with reorienting their lives to incorporate these challenges. This is further complicated when the afflicted person is in the public spotlight. Fox shifts his identity from primarily an actor to an activist. For a celebrity, the process of enacting a preferred social self in light of an emergent health issue can be complicated. Fox has the opportunity to use his celebrity to further the cause of PD and does so through magazine articles, television interviews, and testifying before a Senate subcommittee. In doing so, he tries to navigate the difficult terrain of his private life and public persona, especially because his celebrity status enables him to raise public awareness and millions of dollars for research of PD.

Witte's case study (Chapter 28) shows how a fear appeal theory was used in Ethiopia to design both research and an entertainment education program. Using the Extended Parallel Process Model (EPPM) theory as a framework, formative research was used to develop a 26-week radio serial drama to promote family planning. The case describes the Ethiopian context and research project, the EPPM, and the results of the research. Chapter 29 (Kreps) describes a unique health communication research initiative sponsored by the National Cancer Institute. It was designed to learn how to communicate effectively through new communication technologies with several hard-to-reach groups of people in the United States. Called the Digital Divide Pilot Projects, they developed and tested new strategies for providing different poor and underserved groups of people with access to current and accurate information about cancer prevention, control, and treatment. Kreps describes four pilot projects and the new community strategies each developed for providing these groups with access to relevant computer-based information about cancer.

As you can see from the descriptions, these cases include many topics, populations, contexts, and issues. The contributors to this volume are scholars and practitioners who bring their expertise to each case and bring to life obvious and subtle complexities across positive and negative examples of health communication. The cases tackle timely topics, are insightful, and add to our corpus of materials for teaching health communication.

ACKNOWLEDGMENTS

There are many people to thank for making this book a reality. First, I was fortunate to work with an outstanding group of contributors. They worked hard, responded quickly to my feedback, and kept their sense of humor. They were committed to this project from the beginning, and their enthusiasm never waned. Second, I want to thank my husband, George, and our children, Bryan and Lesley, for their constant support, love, and laughs. Third, I am extremely grateful to Linda Bathgate and Karin Wittig Bates at Lawrence Erlbaum Associates for their support throughout this project. All of these people reminded me so many times, in so many ways, that we were all in this together. I am very fortunate to have them in my personal and professional life as my friends and colleagues.

REFERENCES

Braithwaite, D. O., & Wood, J. T. (Eds.). (2000). *Case studies in interpersonal communication: Processes and problems.* Belmont, CA: Wadsworth.

Keyton, J., & Shockley-Zalabak, P. (Ed.). (2004). *Case studies for organizational communication: Understanding communication processes.* Los Angeles, CA: Roxbury.

Ray, E. B. (Ed.). (1993). *Case studies in health communication.* Hillsdale, NJ: Lawrence Erlbaum Associates.

Ray, E. B. (Ed.). (1996). *Case studies in communication and disenfranchisement: Applications to social health issues.* Mahwah, NJ: Lawrence Erlbaum Associates.

Sypher, B. D. (Ed.). (1990). *Case studies in organizational communication.* New York: Guilford.

List of Contributors

Claudia V. Angelelli, Ph.D.
Department of Spanish and Portuguese
San Diego State University
San Diego, CA 92182

Julie A. Apker, Ph.D.
Department of Communication
Western Michigan University
Kalamazoo, MI 49008-5318

Austin S. Babrow, Ph.D.
Department of Communication
Purdue University
West Lafayette, IN 47907

Christina S. Beck, Ph.D.
School of Communication Studies
Ohio University
Athens, OH 45701

Dawn O. Braithwaite, Ph.D.
Department of Communication Studies
University of Nebraska-Lincoln
Lincoln, NE 68588

Dale E. Brashers, Ph.D.
Department of Speech Communication
University of Illinois at Urbana-Champaign
Urbana, IL 61801

Carma L. Bylund, Ph.D.
Center for Education Research and
    Evaluation
Department of Sociomedical Sciences
Columbia University Medical Center
New York, NY 10032

Donald J. Cegala, Ph.D.
School of Journalism and Communication
Department of Family Medicine
Ohio State University
Columbus, OH 43210

Brigitte Cobbs Christmon, M.A.
Department of Communication
Western Michigan University
Kalamazoo, MI 49008

Rebecca J. Welch Cline, Ph.D.
Barbara Ann Karmanos Cancer Institute
Hudson Webber Cancer Research Center
Wayne State University
Detroit, MI 48201

David O'Connor Dinn, P.T.
Department of Communication
Purdue University
West Lafayette, IN 47907

Athena du Pré, Ph.D.
Department of Communication Arts
University of West Florida
Pensacola, FL 32514

Timothy M. Edgar, Ph.D.
Department of Marketing Communication
Emerson College
Boston, MA 02116

Eric M. Eisenberg, Ph.D.
Department of Communication
University of South Florida
Tampa, FL 33620

Lyle J. Flint, Ph.D.
Department of Communication Studies
Ball State University
Muncie, IN 47306

Leigh Arden Ford, Ph.D.
Department of Communication
Western Michigan University
Kalamazoo, MI 49008

Patricia Geist-Martin, Ph.D.
School of Communication
San Diego State University
San Diego, CA 92182

Catherine M. Gillotti, Ph.D.
Department of Communications
    and Creative Arts
Purdue University, Calumet
Hammond, IN 46323

Paul Haidet, M.D.
Department of Medicine
Baylor College of Medicine and Houston
    Center for Quality of Care and Utilization
    Studies
Houston, TX 77030

Heidi M. Hazeu, M.A.
Department of Speech Communication
University of Illinois at Urbana-Champaign
Urbana, IL 61801

Craig R. Hullett, Ph.D.
Department of Communication Arts
University of Wisconsin-Madison
Madison, WI 53706

Rebecca S. Imes, M.A.
Department of Communication Studies
University of Iowa
Iowa City, IA 52242

Phyllis Japp, Ph.D.
Department of Communication Studies
University of Nebraska-Lincoln
Lincoln, NE 68588

Jenifer E. Kopfman, Ph.D.
School of Communication
Cleveland State University
Cleveland, OH 44115

Gary L. Kreps, Ph.D.
Department of Communication
George Mason University
Fairfax, VA 22030

Janice L. Krieger, M.A.
Department of Communication Arts
    and Sciences
The Pennsylvania State University
University Park, PA 16802

Tony L. Kroll, M.A.
Department of Communication
Texas A&M University and Houston Center
    for Quality of Care and Utilization Studies
College Station, TX 77843

John C. Lammers, Ph.D.
Department of Speech Communication
University of Illinois at Urbana-Champaign
Urbana, IL 61801

Linda C. Lederman, Ph.D.
Center for Communication and Health Issues
School of Communication, Information and
    Library Studies
Rutgers University
New Brunswick, NJ 08901

Kristin A. Lindholm, M.A.
Department of Speech Communication
University of Illinois at Urbana-Champaign
Urbana, IL 61801

Cat McGrew, M.A.
School of Communication
Ohio State University
Columbus, OH 43210

Carol Bishop Mills, Ph.D.
Department of Communication Studies
University of Alabama-Birmingham
Birmingham, AL 35294

Alexandra G. Murphy, Ph.D.
Department of Communication
DePaul University
Chicago, IL 60614

Lisa Murray-Johnson, Ph.D.
School of Communication
Ohio State University
Columbus, OH 43210

Jon F. Nussbaum, Ph.D.
Department of Communication Arts
    and Sciences
Pennsylvania State University
University Park, PA 16802

Dan O'Hair, Ph.D.
Department of Communication
University of Oklahoma
Norman, OK 73019

Alyssa Parrish, M.A.
School of Communication
University of Houston
Houston, TX 77204

Roxanne L. Parrott, Ph.D.
Department of Communication Arts
    and Sciences
Pennsylvania State University
University Park, PA 16802

Margaret J. Pitts, M.A.
Department of Communication Arts
    and Sciences
Pennsylvania State University
University Park, PA 16802

Jim L. Query, Jr., Ph.D.
School of Communication
University of Houston
Houston, TX 77204

Eileen Berlin Ray, Ph.D.
School of Communication
Cleveland State University
Cleveland, OH 44115

George B. Ray, Ph.D.
School of Communication
Cleveland State University
Cleveland, OH 44115

Lance S. Rintamaki, Ph.D.
Midwest Center for Health Services
    and Policy Research
Hines VA Hospital
Hines, IL 60141

Dawn W. Satterfield, Ph.D.
Centers for Disease Control and Prevention
Division of Diabetes Translation
Atlanta, GA 30341

Steven Schenkel, M.D.
University of Michigan Medical School
1500 East Medical Center Drive
Ann Arbor, MI 48109

Barbara F. Sharf, Ph.D.
Department of Communication
Texas A&M University
College Station, TX 77843

Kami J. Silk, Ph.D.
Department of Communication
Michigan State University
E. Lansing, MI 48824

Lisa Sparks, Ph.D.
Department of Communication
George Mason University
Fairfax, VA, 22030

Lea P. Stewart, Ph.D.
School of Communication, Information
    and Library Studies
Rutgers University
New Brunswick, NJ 08901

Kathleen M. Sutcliffe, Ph.D.
University of Michigan Business School
701 Tappan Street
Ann Arbor, MI 48109

Sharlene R. Thompson, M.A.
Department of Communication
University of Oklahoma
Norman, OK 73019

Teresa L. Thompson, Ph.D.
Department of Communication
University of Dayton
Dayton, OH 45469

Judith Weiner, M.A.
Department of Communication Arts
    and Sciences
Pennsylvania State University
University Park, PA 16802

Bryan B. Whaley, Ph.D.
Department of Communication
    Studies
University of San Francisco
San Francisco, CA 94117

Kim Witte, Ph.D.
Center for Communication Programs
Johns Hopkins University
1485 Sylvan Glen
Okemos, MI 48864

Henry N. Young, Ph.D.
Center for Health Services Research
    in Primary Care
University of California, Davis
Davis, CA 95616

HEALTH COMMUNICATION IN PRACTICE

A Case Study Approach

I

Issues in Provider–Recipient Communication

1

The First Three Minutes

Donald J. Cegala
Ohio State University

Mr. Smith has been experiencing lower back pain for a few weeks and finally decided to see his primary care physician because the pain was getting to be more than he could tolerate. Following is the first part of his interview with his doctor:

1 *Doc:* Well, good morning Mr. Smith. How are you today?

2 *Pat:* Not too bad. How are you?

3 *Doc:* I'm fine, thanks. What can I do for you today?

4 *Pat:* Well, Dr. Jones I've been having this terrible pain in my back. It just, I can't
5   even . . .

6 *Doc:* Back pain. Exactly where is the pain?

7 *Pat:* Right here (pointing to the left side, lower back).

8 *Doc:* Does it hurt any place else?

9 *Pat:* Not in my back, but I do have a pain in the back of my leg, all the way down
10   to

11 *Doc:* Mm, I see. How long have you had this back pain?

12 *Pat:* Oh, about two weeks I think. It just

13 *Doc:* Did you do anything to bring it on, like lifting a heavy object or anything like
14   that?

15 *Pat:* No not that I can remember. I was just sitting in a chair and all of a sudden I
16   started feeling this pain in my back and

17 *Doc:* Is the pain sharp or dull?

18 *Pat:* Oh, real sharp. Like a knife.

19 *Doc:* And is the pain steady or intermittent?

20 *Pat:* It's pretty much constant.

21 *Doc:* Anything make it feel better or worse?

22 *Pat:* Well, almost nothing makes it feel better—I've taken lots of aspirin but that
23   doesn't seem to help much. Sitting definitely makes it worse, at least more so

24   than walking. But, I'm having a hard time walking too and with all that's
25   going on I just can't
26 *Doc:*   How much aspirin have you been taking? Have you been taking anything else
27   with it?
28 *Pat:*   Let's see I think I've been taking about . . . . . .

PHYSICIAN–PATIENT COMMUNICATION

Scholars have been studying physician–patient communication for at least 30 years. There is an enormous literature on many aspects of how physicians and patients communicate, as well as considerable research on communication skills training for physicians and patients. Among other things, this work has led to the development of various models of physician–patient communication. Over the last 50 years, these models have evolved from paternalistic approaches in which the physician is characterized as a benevolent all-knowing father figure directing a passive patient to more current views in which the physician–patient relationship is defined by mutuality and partnership. Although there is some evidence that actual physician–patient relationships have changed over the years to reflect many features of scholars' models, there is also scholarly and anecdotal evidence indicating that there is considerable discrepancy between actual physician–patient communication and current ideal models based on mutuality and partnership (Braddock, Edwards, Hasenberg, Laidley, & Levinson, 1999). In short, there is yet much work for both physicians and patients to do to bring significant change and improvement to the quality of physician–patient communication.

The goal of this case is to draw attention to ways of changing and improving the first three minutes of physician–patient interviews. This is an important goal, as research shows that most of what goes wrong in a medical interview is often keyed to what happens or does not happen at the beginning rather than the middle or end of the interview. Even so, improving the first three minutes of medical interviews is only a first step. However, because of space constraints, only issues relevant to the first three minutes of the interview will be addressed here.

KEY PHYSICIAN SKILLS

In this section, the literature on physician–patient communication is used to characterize what is good and poor communication on the physician's part in the aforementioned snippet.

Dr. Jones did well in greeting the patient by using his name and being friendly (assuming that his nonverbal communication matched the text, e.g., he smiled and perhaps touched or shook hands with Mr. Smith). There is just one small point where Dr. Jones could improve. In line 1, he said, "How are you today?" It is good that Dr. Jones asked the patient how he was feeling, but the specific wording of his statement is a bit too broad. For example, one could easily imagine a moderate-to-long reply from Mr. Smith that had little or nothing to do with the medical reason(s) for his making the appointment. Thus, Dr. Jones' statement invites a potentially moderate-to-long response from Mr. Smith that might be time-consuming and not directly relevant to the business at hand. A better opening statement might be something like, "Good morning, Mr. Smith. It's nice to see you again."

Dr. Jones interrupted the patient several times (lines 5/6, 10/11, 12/13, 16/17, 25/26). The timing of these interruptions potentially has a significant impact on the course and even outcomes of the interview. For example, in 1984, Howard Beckman and Richard Frankel published what is now considered a classic study of the first few minutes of physician–patient interviews (Beckman & Frankel, 1984). The results of their work were so dramatic that, 15 years later, their study was replicated and published in a leading medical journal with similar findings (Marvel, Epstein, Flowers, & Beckman, 1999). Both of these studies found that in most medical interviews, patients were interrupted within just 18 to 23 seconds after the interview began. Moreover, the majority of interruptions occurred on the patient's first expressed complaint, and only a very small percentage of patients (about 2%) ever completed their agenda (i.e., why they were there) once they were interrupted.

The true significance of these findings is probably not immediately apparent to most people because their implications are tied to other research about physician–patient communication that may not be widely known to the general public. For example, in our modern, highly technological society, it is easy to think of medical care in terms of sophisticated tests, marvelous surgical procedures, and high-tech machines like computed tomography and positron-emission tomography scanners. But the fact of the matter is that most decisions about diagnosis and treatment (such as deciding to order a test or procedure) are made on the basis of what patients report to physicians about their medical conditions. Indeed, research shows that up to about 80% of such medical decision making is based on information the patient provides during history-taking and reporting of symptoms. Accordingly, anything that prevents patients from completely expressing their agenda during medical interviews can potentially jeopardize the accuracy of diagnosis and treatment plans, and, ultimately, patients' health and safety, to say nothing of the potential for malpractice suits and other factors that contribute to escalating health care costs.

There are additional reasons the results of these studies are so important. It was found that physicians tended to interrupt patients on hearing their first expressed concern. Research shows that the first expressed concern often may not be the most medically important matter or even the primary reason the patient came in to see the physician. When physicians immediately begin asking closed questions[1] about the first expressed concern, they risk taking the interview down a narrow path that may miss the real reasons a patient made the appointment. Thus, if physicians use an interview style like the one illustrated previously, they may not determine the patient's real reason for the appointment or may only learn of it at the very end of the interview.

Yet, there are potential serious problems with this interview style, even if the patient's first expressed concern *is* most medically important and *is* the primary reason for the patient making the appointment. Note how Dr. Jones conducts the interview on hearing that Mr. Smith is experiencing back pain at line 6. Dr. Jones' questions are not only closed, they are biomedically focused, that is, they are directed to the physical causes and systems involved in the patient's likely medical problem. Although biomedical information is essential to an accurate diagnosis and treatment plan, it is often not the only essential information relevant to accurate medical decision making. Patients, especially those with chronic conditions, often not only have a physical ailment but also have life experiences associated with the disease. Some people say this is the difference between a disease and an illness. If a physician only gathers information about the patient's disease without also understanding the broader context of the patient's medical problem, the chances are that vitally important information will be missed and the accuracy of the physician's diagnosis and treatment plan can be seriously jeopardized.

Dr. Jones' questions reflect how most physicians are trained in medical school. The questions are designed to elicit specific information about the patient's symptoms so that the physician can determine a diagnosis and treatment plan. Thus, the purpose of closed, biomedically focused questions is well intended, but there is a more appropriate place in the interview for asking such questions. At this point, in the very beginning of the interview, it is more important to determine the patient's complete agenda. Once all of the reasons for the patient's visit are identified, the physician can better determine (with the patient's agreement) which agenda items are most important to address and then can begin doing so in greater detail.

If we consider the critique of Dr. Jones' communication and the discussion of research findings underlying the critique, what might a "corrected" dialogue look like?

1 *Doc:*   Well, good morning Mr. Smith, it's nice to see you again.
2 *Pat:*   Hi doctor Jones. It's good to see you too.
3 *Doc:*   What's on your agenda today?
4 *Pat:*   Dr. Jones I've been having this terrible pain in my back. It just . . . I can't
5   seem to get it to settle down. It just hurts a lot.
6 *Doc:*   I see. What else can you tell me?
7 *Pat:*   Well, let's see. It started about two weeks ago. I was just sitting at my desk
8   and all of a sudden I got this shooting pain in my back and it's been hurting
9   ever since.
10 *Doc:* Um hum (2 second pause)
11 *Pat:* And, well my leg hurts too. I have this sharp pain running all the way down
12   the back of my left leg. I've been taking lots of aspirin, but that doesn't seem
13   to help much.
14 *Doc:* Help *much*?
15 *Pat:* It seems to ease the pain somewhat, but I've been taking so much that I think
16   it's starting to bother my stomach. Besides it doesn't suppress the pain enough
17   for me to do my regular activities. It's just been awful the last few weeks. I
18   can't sit at my desk and work for more than 20 minutes at a time because it
19   hurts so much. I'm losing a lot of work time and my productivity has fallen
20   drastically. If I don't get rid of this pain soon, I'm afraid I'll never catch up
21   with my work. I've got too much to do to put up with this.
22 *Doc:* I see. Anything else you can tell me?
23 *Pat:* I don't think so, that's about it.
24 *Doc:* Are there any other things you wanted to discuss today besides your back
25   pain?
26 *Pat:* No, that is the main thing.
27 *Doc:* Sure there's nothing else, nothing else at all?
28 *Pat:* Well not as far as additional complaints, but I am really worried about this
29   back. My father had back problems when he was about my age and I saw him
30   suffer for years. He finally got back surgery and his pain was even worse
31   after the surgery. Eventually he had to quit work and go on disability. He
32   was just plain miserable. I'm really worried that the same thing is about to
33   happen to me. I just can't afford for that to happen.
34 *Doc:* OK, let me make sure I have heard everything correctly so far. You have
35   been in a lot of pain for about two weeks. In addition to pain in your back,
36   you have pain all the way down the back of your left leg. You have been
37   taking aspirin, but it doesn't help much, and you think that the amount of
38   aspirin you've been taking may be upsetting your stomach. Your pain is
39   disrupting your work schedule because sitting is very uncomfortable. You are
40   concerned about losing needed work time, and you are worried that you may
41   have back problems similar to your father's. Does that pretty much sum up
42   the situation, or did I leave out something?
43 *Pat:* No, you have summarized all of the key points correctly.
44 *Doc:* OK, I will need to ask you some more questions about your pain and examine
45   you. But, before doing that I want to be sure there isn't anything else that
46   comes to mind that you want to share at this point. Anything at all?
47 *Pat:* No, that's it.

Dr. Jone's interviewing style changed in significant ways to reflect the research findings discussed earlier. For one thing, Dr. Jones did not immediately begin asking closed, biomedically focused questions on hearing that Mr. Smith was experiencing back pain. Instead, Dr. Jones began with an open question that encouraged Mr. Smith to talk (line 6). Then, at line 10, Dr. Jones used a continuer and silence to encourage Mr. Smith to continue with his story. At line 14, Dr. Jones simply repeated a key term in Mr. Smith's previous turn to urge him to talk more about the effects of taking aspirin. In two subsequent turns (lines 22 and 27), Dr. Jones asked open questions to see if there was anything else Mr. Smith wanted to add. At lines 34 to 42, Dr. Jones summarized all of the key information Mr. Smith provided, including his worries about missing work and a family history of back pain. Finally, Dr. Jones assured Mr. Smith that he would soon attend to his back problem by asking more questions and doing an examination, but before doing so, he wanted to be sure there wasn't something else Mr. Smith wanted to say.

This is a very different interview style than illustrated in the first snippet. Not only did Dr. Jones' communication style change, but so did Mr. Smith's. Mr. Smith not only provided much of the same detail about his back pain that he did in the first snippet, he also provided additional specifics, such as side effects from taking aspirin, the amount of time he can sit before being overcome with pain, his anxiety about losing work time and feeling pressure to resolve his pain before he falls too far behind, and his worries about his father's experiences and the fear of that happening to him. Overall, by using a patient-centered style of communicating Dr. Jones obtained far more information about Mr. Smith's illness than was elicited using the doctor-centered style in the first snippet. Not only did he obtain more information, but the quality of the information was significantly better. For example, by understanding Mr. Smith's fears about him ending up like his father, Dr. Jones can address those concerns after the examination. He might, for example, find that Mr. Jones' problem is muscular and not disc-related, and therefore he does not need surgery. Or, if surgery is indicated, Dr. Jones can explain that surgical procedures and overall treatment of back pain have improved dramatically since his father had back surgery. In short, Dr. Jones can find ways to reassure Mr. Smith and help to ease his anxiety and fears, which incidentally are probably adding to Mr. Smith's physical ailment.

Normally, when using this patient-centered interview style, a physician would need to negotiate an agenda for the appointment because often patients want to discuss more items than a typical 15-minute appointment can accommodate. In this instance, that was not necessary because Mr. Smith had only one complaint. Unfortunately, there is not enough space to consider what should happen during the rest of Mr. Smith's interview. Suffice it to say, immediately following the first 3 minutes, Dr. Jones would need to explore Mr. Smith's condition in greater detail. Ultimately, he would ask closed questions to clarify points and to explore areas that Mr. Smith had not mentioned, but Dr. Jones should continue to seek information in a patient-centered style, allowing Mr. Smith to tell his story as completely as possible. After the examination, Dr. Jones should urge Mr. Smith to be involved as much possible in discussion about the diagnosis of his problem and what can be done for it, and Dr. Jones should be as clear and informative as possible about the diagnosis and prognosis of the problem and possible treatment options for addressing it.

Before turning briefly to patient communication responsibilities, it may be useful to close this section by addressing an important additional matter regarding the first and second snippets. It has been suggested that the interviewing style illustrated in snippet two is more communicatively effective and results in better health care than the style characterized in snippet one. However, it is also clear that snippet two is noticeably longer than snippet one, in fact about 34% longer. Anyone familiar with issues about escalating health costs recognizes that increasing demands on physicians' time contributes to rising health care costs. Thus, it is fair to ask whether a more open interview style will contribute to escalating health care costs. The simple answer is "no." Remember that only the first 3 minutes of the medical interview have been considered, and only one case has been illustrated. What a physician does communicatively during the first 3 minutes of the interview has a significant impact on the rest of the appointment. Indeed, the investment of an additional minute or so, if that is even needed, can make a difference in several minutes later on in the interview. Most of the research on physician and patient communication skills training indicates that patient-centered interviewing on the physician's part and active participation on the patient's part does not significantly increase the length of medical interviews, especially once the relevant communication skills have been mastered.

PATIENT COMMUNICATION RESPONSIBILITIES

So far, the focus has been on what physicians can do communicatively to improve medical interviews during the first 3 minutes. As already suggested, there is considerably more that can be said about how physicians should communicate during the rest of the interview. However, like any communication event, the process and outcomes of physician–patient encounters are a function of what *both* physicians and patients communicatively contribute to the event.

Clearly, Mr. Smith's discourse style changed from the first to the second snippet, but most of that is attributable to the change in the physician's discourse style. There is some literature on the effects of patient communication skills training that suggests how patients can contribute to more effective medical interviews (Anderson & Sharpe, 1991; Cegala & Lenzmeier Broz, 2003). This literature was not addressed here because the most significant patient contributions to medical interviews usually occur after the first three minutes, specifically during the history-taking stage (immediately following the first three minutes) and during the postexamination stage. The three key patient communication competencies for these stages of the interview are: (a) providing detailed information about family history, current symptoms, and psychosocial experiences (e.g., problems, anxieties, or worries related to home, work, and/or social environments); (b) asking questions about diagnosis, prognosis, tests and procedures, and treatment options; and (c) expressing opinions and concerns about such matters as treatment plans. The following Web site contains specific information and guidelines about patient communication skills: http://patcom.jcomm.ohio-state.edu. The reader is urged to access the Web site and consider what patients' communicative responsibilities are and how they can best help to improve physician–patient communication. In doing so, keep in mind the basic principle expressed earlier: The process and effects of all interpersonal communication are functions of the participants' communicative contributions. Thus, when considering ways to improve physician–patient communication, one must consider the discourse moves of each participant and how those implied meanings affect the conversational partner and the definition of the situation at hand.

RELEVANT CONCEPTS

Biomedical: The physical causes and systems involved in a patient's medical problem. This is in contrast to social and psychological aspects of illness.

Disease vs. illness: A disease is the physically based aspect of a medical problem, such as the biological causes of diabetes or high blood pressure. An illness is concerned with how the patient lives with a disease, that is, how the disease affects the quality of life along psychological and social lines.

Open vs. closed questions: Open questions do not imply a specific answer; instead, they allow the respondent to elaborate as desired in formulating a reply to the question, such as: What was your childhood like? Closed questions prompt brief, specific replies, such as: What is your age?

Patient-centered interview style: This is a communication style that reflects patients perspectives on their illnesses. It includes allowing patients to tell their stories without interruption, using open-ended questions, gathering information about the patient's views of the illness and what can be done to treat it, and in general engaging the patient in a partnership characterized by information exchange and negotiation.

Patient communication skills: These are communication tactics that patients use during a medical interview. They include such moves as asking questions, providing detailed information about symptoms and history, verifying understanding of information that is given to them, expressing concerns, and offering opinions.

DISCUSSION QUESTIONS

1. How would you characterize the first physician–patient interaction based on your experience as a patient? Would you say it was typical? If so, why? If not, what is different here?

2. Why is it so important for physicians to use the type of interview style discussed here in the first 3 minutes? What kinds of things can go wrong during the first 3 minutes? How might these events impact on the rest of the interview?

3. Under what circumstances might a physician interrupting a patient or a patient interrupting a physician be viewed positively, or at least not negatively? What aspects of the communication situation are likely to influence participants' views?

4. One of the key communication skills a physician needs is to gather information about the patient's symptoms and, in general, the patient's medical problem. How do open and closed questions relate to the physician's information gathering? Are closed questions necessarily ineffective, or are there places in the interview where they are useful? Are open questions necessarily always preferred, or are there instances where open questions might be ineffective?

5. What communication responsibilities do patients have in a typical medical interview? Why are these communication skills important to the effectiveness of the interview?

ENDNOTE

[1]Closed questions project to brief, structured answers. For example, the question, How old are you? projects to an answer like "25." This is in contrast to open questions that do not restrict the amount of detail the responder provides in answering the question, such as, "Can you tell me about what it was like when you were growing up?"

REFERENCES/SUGGESTED READINGS

Anderson, L. A., & Sharpe, P. A. (1991). Improving patient and provider communication: A synthesis and review of communication interventions. *Patient Education and Counseling, 17*, 99–134.

Beckman, H., & Frankel, R. (1984). The effect of physician behavior on the collection of data. *Annals of Internal Medicine, 101*, 692–696.

Braddock, C. H., III, Edwards, K. A., Hasenberg, N. M., Laidley, T. L., & Levinson, W. (1999). Informed decision making in outpatient practice: Time to get back to basics. *Journal of the American Medical Association, 282*, 2313–2320.

Cegala, D. J., & Lenzmeier Broz, S. (2003). Provider and patient communication skills training. In A. Dorsey, T. L. Thompson, K. Miller, & R. Parrott (Eds.), *Handbook of health communication* (pp. 95–119). Mahwah, NJ: Lawrence Erlbaum Associates.

Emanuel, E. J., & Emanuel, L. L. (1992). Four models of the physician-patient relationship. *Journal of the American Medical Association, 267,* 2221–2226.

Marvel, M. K., Epstein, R. M., Flowers, K., & Beckman, H. B. (1999). Soliciting the patient's agenda: Have we improved? *Journal of the American Medical Association, 281,* 283–287.

Silverman, J., Kurtz, S., & Draper, J. (1998). *Skills for communicating with patients.* Abingdon, UK: Radcliff Medical Press.

Additional Resources

Buckman, R., Baile, W. F., & Korsch, B. (1999). Communication skills in clinical practice. *Communication: The basics (Tape 1).* Toronto, CA: Medical Audio Visual Communications.

Smith, R. C. (2002). *Patient-centered interviewing: An evidence-based method (Tape 1).* East Lansing, MI: Instructional Media Center, Michigan State University. http://patcom.jcomm.ohio-state.edu

2

Staying Out of the Line of Fire: A Medical Student Learns About Bad News Delivery

Teresa L. Thompson
University of Dayton

Catherine Gillotti
Purdue University, Calumet

Sitting in her first med school class, Christie glanced around at all the other students who were positioned near her. She wondered what had prompted them to attempt the arduous process of becoming physicians. Probably different reasons for different people, many of them subsumed under the umbrella of "helping people" in one way or another, she suspected. She thought back to the day in high school when she had decided to become a doctor. She and her mother had been sitting at the kitchen table, chatting about the dance to which she had gone the night before, when her older brother, Matt, had called. She remembered her mother almost shouting into the phone, in frustration.

> *Matt:* Hi Mom.
> *Mom:* Hi Matt. Are you okay? You don't sound like yourself.
> *Matt:* No. Not really, I just got some bad news. I didn't tell you and Dad about it before now because I didn't want to worry you.
> *Mom:* Tell us what?
> *Matt:* I had some tests run by my family physician because I was getting light-headed and feeling some chest pain.
> *Mom:* Matt, why didn't you tell us?
> *Matt* (in frustration): I told you, I didn't want to worry you.
> *Mom:* What tests did he order?
> *Matt:* He did an EKG.
> *Mom:* What did the results show?
> *Matt:* Well, Dr. Shaker's medical assistant (MA) called me today.
> *Mom:* A medical assistant called? When did you go to the doctor?
> *Matt:* I had the tests done last Monday. Anyway, I couldn't get anything out of this person other than that I now need to see a cardiologist.
> *Mom:* Did you get a chance to talk to Dr. Shaker?
> *Matt:* No, they said that he was unavailable because it's Saturday.

Mom: What did the MA say?

Matt: She said that the test results showed some abnormalities and that I would need to see a cardiologist in the coming weeks. I asked to speak to the doctor. He wasn't available. And then I asked her to be more specific about what 'abnormalities' there were. She said that she could not interpret the results, but was told to call me with the news. I told her sarcastically that didn't help me much.

Mom: This is not how it's supposed to be done, Matt. I can tell you as a triage nurse for more than 25 years that we would *never* call a patient on the weekend with any kind of news that might be perceived as bad unless it were an emergency.

Matt: Do you think I need to go to the ER?

Mom: No. The MA would have instructed you to do so if it were an emergency. But are you having any symptoms?

Matt: No. I feel fine except for not knowing what any of this means.

Mom (sighing with relief): Come on over, Matt, and we can talk more.

His mother collapsed at the table with her head in her hands.

Matt came over later that day, and they all sat around in frustration, complaining about how this potentially bad news had been delivered and speculating about whether there was cause for worry. Christie's mom kept pointing out that Matt should have received the news from his physician, not from the MA, and should not have received a call at home on a Saturday, when he couldn't get any additional information. Although they felt great concern about Matt's condition and prognosis, they felt equally great frustration about the lack of information they had at this point and the inability to acquire more. Christie remembered thinking, "When I become a doctor, I'm going to make sure that news like this is given to people in a way that doesn't make a bad situation even worse!" Although she had been thinking about medicine for some time, that was the first time she recalled saying to herself, "When I become a doctor...."

Matt's subsequent visit to the cardiologist resulted in yet more bad news. On Monday, Matt called his primary care physician's office, who scheduled an appointment with a highly recommended local cardiologist. Matt had to wait several days to see this doctor—several days that were characterized by much anxiety and uncertainty. The doctor seemed to be a good one, however, so the family was hopeful that more information would shortly be forthcoming. The cardiologist, Dr. Schmitz, scheduled a series of tests for Matt, including a thallium stress test, an EKG, and some blood work. After these results came in, a heart cathertization was scheduled. Still feeling as if they had no idea of the extent of Matt's problems, the family waited anxiously outside the room in which the procedure was being conducted, hoping for some information. Matt's wife, Emily, was invited inside the recovery room after the procedure, while the remainder of the family continued to wait outside. Matt was still groggy from the catheterization, so Emily tried to focus on understanding the diagnosis and treatment plan. But she had difficulty doing so, as Dr. Schmitz told her a lot of things very quickly. It appeared that Matt didn't have any blockages to the heart, which was good news. Matt's mother was relieved because Matt was so young, and she knew all too well after being a nurse that the more invasive the procedure, the harder the recovery. In Matt's case, the heart itself looked enlarged. "It's his weight," Dr. Schmitz, said, "His heart looks like a Volkswagen engine that been pulling a Mac truck!" That analogy, of course, alarmed Emily. Dr. Schmitz ignored the alarmed look on Emily's face and went on to tell her about several different kinds of medication that Matt should take, how he should change his diet, the kind of exercise routine he should undertake, that his cholesterol and blood pressure were too high, and on and on. Then he added, "If he doesn't get this under control, his heart may just give out." Matt understood very little of this following the procedure, except the last statement, and Emily felt so shaken up by the news that she, too, could process only limited bits of the information.

Whereas the rest of the family was both worried about Matt and critical of how the doctors had handled the whole bad-news delivery process, Christie's older brother, George, had a different attitude. "I think doctors should just be blunt—just tell everybody the truth whenever they know anything. Don't worry about being tactful or nice about it—I'd just want to know as much as possible as soon as possible. I don't care how they say it."

"Easy for you to say now," replied Christie's mom, "while you're healthy and strong. See if you feel that way if you're lying on some table, half out of it, and told that you're likely to die!"

These experiences stayed in Christie's mind. Although delivering bad news more effectively was not the only reason she had decided to become a doctor, it remained an important one for her. She was determined to try to learn what she could during her med school years so that, when the time came, she didn't devastate or overwhelm families in the way that her's had been affected by the delivery of the news about Matt's heart problems. As Christie continued her medical school career, she found opportunity after opportunity to first observe and then practice bad-news delivery. For the most part, she did not find models for delivering bad news very helpful. Her observations of practicing physicians included seeing the elderly Dr. Gumperz tell a middle-aged man, after surgery, "Well, Phil, you've only got one kidney, but it's a big kidney!" She saw a cardiologist go out to the waiting family of a patient who had just died on the operating table and heard the physician tell the family, "I'm afraid that things aren't going very well," only to come back shortly and tell them that the patient had indeed died.

Christie was explicitly taught by most of her instructors to maintain emotional distance from her patients and *not* to show emotions toward them. One attending physician, with whom she did rounds on a regular basis during her first year of residency, harped on this point all the time, "You can't afford to get emotionally involved with your patients. You can't care for them, or you'll burn yourself out. You have to keep yourself distant from them. Don't let yourself care. Don't act like you care." Not showing emotions, however, resulted in a cold, unfeeling practice of medicine and communication of bad news to patients, and Christie rejected that approach. She felt that there are some times when you stop being a doctor and start being a person. She felt even more convicted about this when she read an ethnography about medical school students written by an author named Fred Hafferty (1989). She was halfway through the book when she phoned her mom for their weekly check-in call.

    Mom: Hi, Christie! How are you doing?

    Christie: I'm doing well, but I'm tired as usual.

    Mom: Are you getting enough rest?

    Christie: Mom, you know what the life of a resident is like. You get to sleep 10 minutes here and 10 minutes there.

    Mom: Well, I just hate to hear that you are over-worked and over-stressed. Besides, it's my right to worry about you—that's what mothers do. (They both laughed.)

    Christie: Well, I suppose it is your God-given right. Hey mom, I have to tell you about this book I'm reading.

    Mom: Yeah?

    Christie: It is called *Into the Valley.* The author, Hafferty, followed a class of medical students through an entire year of study. He focused on their perceptions of their anatomy class and interviewed the students about their feelings about working on cadavers. Some of the students admitted having waking hallucinations about their cadavers. They talked about seeing them in public places.

Mom: Well, I remember you complaining about the smell of formaldehyde during the year you had anatomy, but I don't remember you talking about seeing your cadaver walking around campus.

Christie: No, I didn't hallucinate about them but some of my classmates said they did. It was hard getting used to working on our cadavers. Most of us named them. Anyway, one student whom Hafferty interviewed actually said that if he saw a dead animal and a dead body on the side of the road, he would want to treat them the same. Can you believe he actually said that on the record?

Mom: Well, yes I can. I have worked with some really pompous and cold-hearted physicians over the years. Then again, I have worked with some really compassionate and empathetic ones as well.

Christie: That's true, Mom. You probably have worked with dozens of physicians like this over the years. I promise you, though, I won't become that kind of unfeeling physician.

Mom: I could never imagine you being that detached.

Christie: I can't imagine wanting to continue to practice medicine if I don't connect with my patients on a human level.

Mom: What did the author conclude from this study?

Christie: Well, I'm only halfway through the book, but he claims that physicians are socialized to dehumanize patients because technically their first patient is a cadaver.

Mom: What do you think of that?

Christie: Well, as a resident I would say that not all physicians dehumanize their patients. At the same time, his point is well taken because our professors in medical school stress not becoming too attached to our patients. Well, Mom, I guess I should get back to it. Thanks for the check-in.

Mom: You know I love hearing from you. Thanks for calling. Get plenty of rest, Christie. You'll be a better doctor for it.

Christie: I will. Give my love to everyone and talk to you soon.

Mom: I love you, too. Have a good week.

Some doctors Christie observed tried to deliver bad news in a way that didn't devastate families or patients, but ended up doing as much harm as good through inappropriate attempts at reassurance. Christie had never realized how disconfirming reassurance could be until she saw Dr. Eviston, a new attending at the hospital, try to be overly encouraging and jolly when she told a patient about her breast cancer, "All right, Lynn, you've got breast cancer. But we'll lick this! Don't you worry. Everything's just fine!" It then hit her that acting like something wasn't really bad when it was indeed bad disconfirms the patient's feelings and experiences of reality.

Christie also discovered some other things related to the use of language and other problems in bad-news delivery as she spent more time around health care.

Christie: You know, Mom, I can't believe how some of these doctors I work with use such ambiguous and euphemistic language with patients. I heard one physician tell a patient that their "loved one had gone on to a better place" instead of saying that she had indeed died.

Mom: Well, maybe the doctor was trying to soften the blow.

Christie: Well there is being compassionate, but there's something to be said for being up-front and factual. And then there was the time that Dr. Goetz told a man his diagnosis of inoperable cancer by asking him if he had his affairs in order?

Mom: That is definitely evasive.

Christie: I think the worst experience I have seen of good news that sounded like bad news was a urologist who had just performed a dilatation on a 24 year old woman. She had feelings of urgency and pressure and had a history of urinary tract problems. You know how painful that procedure is.

Mom: I certainly do. It's very painful.

Christie: Well, as soon as the physician completed the procedure he said to her, "That didn't need to be done." The patient was visibly upset. She asked, "What do you mean that didn't need to be done?" He said, "The only way to know whether a dilatation is required or not is to do one." Now what made this really bad was that he told her this while standing with his hand on the door—ready to walk out of the room without giving her any alternative explanations for what might be causing her problem.

Mom: What did you do?

Christie: I stayed in the room with her after the other physician left and talked to her about other possibilities. In the end I recommended she see her GYN since the patient could track the symptoms to her menstrual cycle.

Mom: I'm sure she was happy you were there to help her.

Christie: I think the physician was too detached and not attentive to what the patient was really asking for, which was not a definite answer but at least some form of validation that her symptoms weren't a figment of her imagination.

During Christie's ER rotation, a young man, 25, was brought in because of injuries he suffered during an automobile accident. Despite the staff's attempts to save his life, Jason was declared brain dead. They kept his body alive through life support while they attempted to secure consent for organ donation from the family. The attending physician on that shift took it upon himself to ask Jason's parents for permission for organ donation. Jason had signed his driver's license, but family consent also is required. Jason's parents were confused when the physician said, "I'm sorry to tell you that your son is brain dead, and by law I'm required to ask your permission to donate Jason's organs." The Organ Procurement Officer, Anne Bennett, had a thing or two to say to this physician later. She reminded him that it is not the physician's legal responsibility to ask for the permission for the donation—it is the responsibility of the Organ Procurement Officer. Christie was able to witness the procurement process from start to finish on this case, and gained a new alliance and friendship with Anne Bennett. One day, Anne and Christie went to lunch together in the hospital cafeteria.

Christie: What is the worst delivery of brain death news you have witnessed Anne?

Anne: Actually it was that ER case you worked on a month ago—you know Jason, the young man who died in the automobile accident.

Christie: Why was that the worst example?

Anne: First because the physician violated his role in the procedure. He is supposed to deliver the news, but not request the organs. Second because he didn't allow for the decoupling process to occur.

Christie: What's decoupling?

Anne: Decoupling is the separation of the delivery of the news—death—from donation. Our philosophy is that there needs to be a distinction in time between telling the family that their loved one is dead and seeking procurement of the organs. Additionally, it's a conflict of interest for him to make the donation request. It's really our legal responsibility to seek consent.

Christie: How would you rate the physicians at this hospital in delivering the death news?

Anne: I would say they're about average. You would be shocked at the number of families who misunderstand what brain death means.

Christie: Misunderstand in what way?

Anne: They often confuse brain death with coma. I would estimate that five out of ten families are confused. They often don't understand that the person *is* dead and if they refuse donation, by law, the life support will be turned off.

Christie: Do you feel it's the physicians causing this confusion?

Anne: Sometimes it is because, in my opinion, it's all in the delivery of the bad news. Some physicians hide behind the medical terminology during the delivery and explanation of brain death. I mean who really wants to be the one to tell someone that we didn't save your loved one?

SOME GOOD EXAMPLES

There were some health care providers whom Christie had an opportunity to observe who inspired her, however. Dr. Chapman, she discovered, always began bad news delivery with a variation on the words, "I'm really sorry. . . . " More broadly, Dr. Chapman and other good doctors continually showed caring and compassion throughout their interactions with the patient and family, while still telling them the truth. Those physicians who communicated the bad news more neutrally or in a matter-of-fact manner tended to have patients who were more likely to deny the diagnosis and prognosis or experience severe depression and difficulty coping with the illness.

Christie had the pleasure of observing one fellow resident who worked very hard to help a young woman in her mid-twenties face her breast cancer diagnosis. The patient had just left her job, so her insurance was about to run out. She had been in denial of a possible problem—a lump underneath her arm. When Christie's colleague, Dr. Jim Franko, completed a breast exam, he not only found a lump under her arm, but also one in her left breast. Jim knew that the young woman must have been in denial because she said that she thought the lump under her arm was caused by an infected hair. He was wonderful with her. He asked her to complete a self-breast exam right then and there in front of him, so that he could get her to acknowledge both lumps. He suspected that they were malignant, so he ordered as many tests as he could for her that same day before her insurance expired. He also set up an appointment the same day with a surgeon and oncologist. He later told me that he didn't want to rush this woman through the diagnosis and treatment process without allowing her time to absorb the news, but also knew that her financial situation would be changing very quickly and he didn't want her worrying about paying for all the necessary tests.

In a later phone call home, Christie shared what she had thought was another especially interesting example concerning breast cancer with her mom.

Christie: Gosh, Mom, I have to tell you about this interaction I observed the other day. Remember that great Dr. Chapman I've mentioned to you? Well, she was treating this patient in whose breast they'd just found a lump. I just thought she handled a bad situation so well.

Mom: How so?

Christie: She started by sitting pretty close to the patient, and looking at her directly, with a concerned expression on her face. They call each other by their first names, so Dr. Chapman said, "Joan, I'm really sorry, but I'm afraid that the biopsy showed that the lump is indeed malignant. It's stage 3, which is not as bad as it could be, and we've caught it pretty early. It's not very big, but we do need to attend to it.

We can handle this. I think we should shrink it with some chemo, then take out the lump, and then follow up with some radiation. I know this isn't good news, but I think we can handle this."

Mom: How did the patient react?

Christie: Well, of course she was upset, but I think she felt better about having Dr. Chapman as an advocate and encouraged by as much hope as Dr. Chapman showed. Dr. Chapman managed to convey the news without completely devastating the patient or taking away all hope. She gave her the bad news, but then let her know that something could be done about it without giving her so much information that she couldn't process it.

Mom: It can't be easy to tell someone they have cancer. It sounds like she handled it as well as can be expected given that no one really wants to be the bearer of bad news.

Christie: Yeah, I hope I'm that good when I'm faced with being the messenger.

Christie saw that it was possible to communicate bad news while still giving hope to people, because physicians are not all-knowing and can't predict the future with any certainty. Besides that, they are trained to cure, not just treat, and sometimes telling someone they can't be helped by modern medicine feels like a failure on the part of the health care provider. There was one case that moved her in particular. On her first day in the Neonatal Intensive Care Unit, Christie witnessed one of the neonatalogists inform a father that his newborn baby was going to die. He asked the father's permission to cease the life support. Christie was impressed with the physician's demeanor and compassion. He stood very close to the father, touched his arm, and even cried with him. The only thing that Christie would have done differently herself would have been to tell the father in a quiet, private place. The physician broke the news right in front of the nurse's station by the unit's door, with the head nurse and unit clerk standing behind the desk.

It was after watching this interaction that Christie realized the many levels there are to bad-news delivery. There is initial bad-news delivery. There is bad news delivery coupled with requests for organ donations. There is bad news of sudden and unexpected death. There is bad news regarding chronic but treatable diseases, such as diabetes and high blood pressure. There is bad news regarding lifelong genetic disorders found in children. There is also some relativity to bad-news delivery in that what is bad to one person may not be perceived as bad news by someone else. Finally, there is bad news regarding going from curable to incurable states.

Through her observation and experiences, Christie found that it was best to communicate bad news slowly and in nonmedical terms, giving limited information at first but with planned follow-up. When she found herself launching into medicalese, she forced herself to think about how her grandmother would process the information she was communicating and tried to phrase things so that Grandma Bess would be able to understand them. It was a balancing act between being clear but not patronizing the patient. She found that it was better to make things too basic and let people indicate to her that they could handle more sophistication than it was to start at too high a level and have people not understand her. Even though she tried to be down-to-earth with her patients and their families, some people were intimidated enough by physicians that they felt reluctant to indicate that they didn't understand what she was saying. Christie found that it was one thing to know what to do, however, and quite another to be able to actually do it.

In another call home, Christie shared with her mom one of her early experiences of giving bad news when she was a third-year medical student.

Christie: Oh, Mom, I didn't want to do it! I had to tell this young man that he was HIV positive!

Mom: What did you say?

Christie: I was so flustered and upset that I launched right into doctor-talk. I told him that the test results were positive and that we were sure of this because we had run an ELISA test, which is the gold-standard of testing. Can you believe that I said it that way? I was actually upbeat when talking about the quality of the testing, as if he should be excited that we were certain that he is HIV positive.

Mom: I'm sure you didn't mean to sound excited about it Christie. Don't be so hard on yourself.

Christie: I can barely forgive myself for being so wrapped up in the clinical that I forgot that this man's life will never be the same.

Mom: I'm sure that he was more stunned about the news than how you said it.

Christie: Mom, that is the point, how I said it may have made a bad situation worse.

Mom: Did you ask him how he felt?

Christie: Once I took my foot out of my mouth I said, "What this means is that you're HIV positive." He said, "You mean I have AIDS?" I said, "No, it doesn't mean you have AIDS yet, but it does mean that you have been infected with the HIV virus. You could stay HIV+ for years without actually developing any of the symptoms of AIDS, and during that time research may find a cure."

Mom: What did he say next?

Christie: He still didn't know quite what I meant, and then I started babbling about treatment options and all kinds of stuff that he couldn't possibly understand. I was just terrible. I feel awful.

Mom: I still think you're being too hard on yourself. You're just learning, Christie. You'll get better in time and with more experience.

Christie: Yeah, but how many lives will I shatter in the meantime?

Christie also discovered some things about just why it was so difficult to give people bad news in an effective and appropriate manner. As a fledgling health care provider, she was being trained to cure people, not let them go. Giving bad news goes against all of the reasons that most people enter medical schoo—they want to save people, not tell them bad news. Bad-news delivery forced her to focus on her limitations and, ultimately, on her own mortality. She experienced a feeling of helplessness when giving bad news, and she quickly realized that most health care providers have pretty high control needs. That was one of the reasons they went into health care to begin with.

ADAPTATION

Christie realized that delivering bad news also requires trying to think about how this message will be received by both the patient and the family. This assessment is not always easy and requires taking into consideration both knowledge about the individual and an understanding of the culture from which the individual comes. She learned that some cultures perceive that the sharing of bad news functions to *bring about* that bad news. She told her mom about one Navajo woman she treated who wouldn't let her even finish her sentence.

Christie: So, Mom, I started saying, "I'm afraid I have some bad news. The tests show that your cancer has progressed far beyond what we had originally thought. I'm afraid that . . ." and the woman said, "No!" So I said, "I'm sorry?" and she said, "No, don't say anything more," and I kind of blubbered a bit.

Mom: Didn't she want to know the status of her health?

Christie: I found out later that most Native Americans prefer story-telling and reliance on metaphors to direct communication about illness.

Christie's subsequent experiences taught her that many other cultural groups share this aversion to direct communication about illness. Apart from cultural adaptation requirements, she also found that some people immediately want lots of information, but that most people need time to just absorb the initial diagnosis before they can process the details of the prognosis and treatment plan. Individuals differ in how much uncertainty they can tolerate and how much information they can process at once. So Christie discovered that this whole bad-news delivery job is much more complex than she had first imagined.

Although Christie knew that too much information when initially delivering bad news was counterproductive and overwhelming, she also came to see how information helped people cope with bad news, pain, and illness. Her mom agreed with her assessment.

Christie: It's fascinating, Mom. I saw these two kids undergo the same procedure this week. One of them was with Dr. Miller, who didn't tell this poor kid anything about what was going to happen to him. The little guy got hysterical when he saw this massive equipment surrounding him and felt the doctors begin poking and prodding. The other boy was a patient of Dr. Chapman's. She told him everything that was going to happen before he experienced it. The boy didn't like it—it's a very uncomfortable procedure—but he stayed calm and handled it all.

Mom: Every child is different, just like every adult. Some people want to know the most minute details and others don't want to know anything. It's a hard call sometimes. But you're right that information helps coping more often than not.

Christie: Maybe it's just the difference between these kids, but I think it takes an effort from us to find out what each patient wants.

READING THE RESEARCH

In addition to observing bad-news delivery, Christie found an opportunity to read literature on the issue. Most of this writing fell into the "how-to" category rather than being based on empirical examination or theoretical framing of the topic. The empirical research she did find typically looked at the impact of bad-news delivery training programs on satisfaction levels and perceptions of effectiveness, but didn't test to see if the programs had any real impact on how subsequent bad news was delivered and on real-world outcomes of this delivery. She found several recurring themes in the literature, however. She discovered that, according to the academic experts, her mother had been right—it should be the treating physician who delivers the bad news—not anyone else, even though the research recounts many instances when the job is deliberately or inadvertently handed off to someone else. She observed another example of this with a family who was told by a hospice worker, "Honey, she's dyin'—that's why her body's doing those things." Although the family knew that the woman was terminal, or she wouldn't have been in hospice, they were shocked to receive the news of imminent death in this way. Not having heard the news from the physician, they didn't know whether to believe it. As it happened, they didn't take her seriously, and only the hospice worker was with the woman when she died later that day.

Some writers on the topic suggested starting with a "warning shot," to let the patient know that bad news is coming. Yet others reminded care providers to give the news at a pace at which the patient or family can best process it, which might be slower for some people and faster for others. Many urged trying to pick up on cues from the patient in regard to all of these issues. Christie saw Dr. Chapman do this on repeated occasions. She would see Dr. Chapman look at the patient and the family intently, and then begin to slow her rate of speech and repeat important points. With other families, Dr. Chapman would notice that they were nodding attentively, as if they understood, and she would begin to explain things in more detail. Christie observed other doctors who seemed completely oblivious to the cues of the patient or family. They'd continue rattling on, even though it was obvious to Christie that the patient and the family were lost, or they'd plod along slowly with a family that, it seemed to Christie, was following well and could handle more information at a faster rate.

As she talked to her mom about all of the research she had been reading, she wondered aloud, "You know, there's all this writing about bad-news delivery, and all this work on it. I did this search on Medline and found over a hundred articles on it! So, with all these experts telling us what to do, how come so few people do it well?"

STORIES

As Christie moved into her rotations, internship, and residency, she found not only plenty of opportunities to practice bad-news delivery, but also heard plenty of stories from patients about ineffective bad-news delivery from other care providers. Frankly, she didn't hear a lot of stories about particularly good bad-news delivery because people didn't tend to share those stories. Those people who had been the recipients of effective delivery also didn't tend to leave their physicians as frequently and seek a second opinion as did those to whom the information had been ineffectively communicated. Nor, the literature told her, did they file malpractice suites as frequently. She was quite interested to discover that it was rare for malpractice suits to be filed based solely on medical malpractice. Most of the suits were characterized by some kind of perceived medical malpractice coupled with a lack of information or a lack of caring communication from the health care provider. She told her mother:

> *Christie:* Mom, I had a patient come right out and tell me, "I wouldn't have sued him if he'd even acted like he cared about his mistakes or about me. But he was just so darn cold about the whole thing. People like that shouldn't even become doctors."

As she progressed through medical school, Christie also noticed something interesting occurring among her cohorts.

> *Christie:* You know, Mom, it's like they're all cookies from the same cutter. We had that one lecture in that doctor–patient relations class about bad-news delivery. First of all, the professor, a medical doctor, was basing his recommendations on one source of information, and then he likened communicating with patients to moving a barge.
> *Mom:* He what?
> *Christie:* He basically acted like patients need to be led by the hand in the interaction.
> *Mom:* Obviously, he has a very high opinion of himself and not much faith in his patients.
> *Christie:* What I found to be problematic was the advice we were given. He gave us a series of rudimentary steps on carrying on a conversation as if we have never done that before.
> *Mom:* Well, there are some things you have to say by law, aren't there?
> *Christie:* Yes, like we need to identify ourselves and state what our level of training is, and verify that we have the right patient, etc. But the thing that was off-putting was

that he acted like all our patients were going to need the same steps to be followed in the same order. No matter what the situation is, what the problem is, and how the patient is reacting, they just do 1-2-3-4.

Mom: It seems very contrived. The doctors at my office sort of have their own style for breaking bad news with their patients, but it isn't always the same words in the same order.

Christie: Exactly, I know that if it were me, I would want to be treated as an individual. Otherwise it's just disingenuous. I guess the thing that surprised me the most, though, was when we finally got to talking about being empathic—something of real value—I overheard my classmates mocking the professor.

Mom: What did they say? Did the professor hear them?

Christie: They said facetiously, "I understand your feelings . . . I empathize with you."

Mom: Did you call them out on it?

Christie: No, because the class was still in session. I think they were so bored and so annoyed by the earlier cookie-cutter approach that they didn't take anything of value from the class.

With her strong interest in the topic, Christie was particularly delighted one day to find a notice of an upcoming seminar for continuing education credits titled, appropriately enough, "Bad-News Delivery." She signed up and attended the seminar with great enthusiasm. It was conducted by a graduate student working on his doctorate in Health Communication, and he provided a more sophisticated overview of the topic than she had heard so far. He shared with the seminar attendees both empirical research on the topic and a theoretical framework for providing some understanding of the complexities of the process. One of the things he addressed was the whole "recipe" approach to bad-news delivery that Christie had spoken to her mom about in the past, except he referred to it as a script.

After the seminar, Christie sought out the presenter, Terry McMillan, to talk with him about the topic in more detail and share with him her experiences. Terry was studying the individual differences among third-year medical students in their abilities to deliver bad news effectively and appropriately to a simulated patient. Although this was a role-play interaction, it was part of the students' clinical performance examination during their internal medicine/surgical clerkship, so the students treated the interaction quite seriously.

Terry: Christie, thank you so much for taking an interest in my study.

Christie: You're quite welcome. I've been intrigued by bad-news delivery for some time.

Terry: Oh yeah. Is that because of your medical training?

Christie: Well, yes partially. It really all began when I was back in high school and my older brother Matt was given some bad news in a rather inappropriate manner. . . . But that is a really long story that I'll save for another time. I'm really interested in hearing more about your study.

Terry: Well, it really boils down to being person-centered or in this case patient-centered. Being patient-centered means meeting the instrumental goals of the interaction—delivering the bad news—while still validating the perspective and feelings of the patient.

Christie: It seems reasonable to do that. Why do you think that it doesn't happen every time?

Terry: Well, from a theoretical perspective, we would explain a physician's inability, or anyone for that matter, to be person-centered to be linked back to the level of their interpersonal cognitive complexity, which is a measure of how large a repertoire of skills and experiences a person has regarding interpersonal interactions.

Christie: I'm confused. It has been a while since I studied cognitive psychology. Are you talking about IQ?

Terry: Actually, Interpersonal Cognitive Complexity is *not* IQ. The higher a person's Interpersonal Cognitive Complexity, the more person-centered they are capable of being in an interaction.

Christie: I see. So you're linking cognitive development with actual behavior?

Terry: Yes, and not just verbal behavior but nonverbal behavior as well. Going back to what I was saying earlier about goals, delivering bad news and validating the patient do not have to be mutually exclusive. Most of the students in my study effectively delivered the bad news to the "patient" and most of their discourse was characterized as a script. In particular, in over 10 hours of videotaped interaction, you can hear the medical interview repeated over and over again.

Christie: I call the "script" the cookie-cutter approach. The patients are treated like the cookies, no variation.

Terry: Your analogy is a good one. My argument is that we are all individuals and wish to be treated as individuals. I gave this presentation at a hospital in the city recently, and I had an attending physician say to me, "Well, I know patients who don't want to be validated. They just want me to bottom line it and be blunt."

Christie: What did you say to him?

Terry: I told him that technically, if he knew that that is truly how the patient wanted to be told the news then he was being person-centered by adapting to the patient's wishes for how the interaction should go.

Christie: What did he say to that?

Terry: He just smiled. I think he just disregarded everything I said, which is okay because I think other physicians at the seminar understood my point. Getting back to that cookie-cutter analogy. I call it Cooking Up Communication, and, trust me, all too often I think that we are guilty of handing out recipes instead of teaching people skills that allow them to adapt to the interaction at hand.

Christie: So you don't believe in the scripts?

Terry: Actually, following a script is not necessarily a bad thing. It isn't a conversational felony to use a script. However, it can impede providers from being appropriate and person-centered if they don't deviate from the script when it's necessary to do so.

Christie and Terry continued their conversation for several more hours. Terry was able to steer Christie in the direction of more research that went beyond the many how-to articles she had found to date. Christie found these articles much more grounded and insightful. She was especially interested in work like that of Doug Maynard, who did discourse analytic studies of bad-news delivery. He described bad news as bringing about a rupture in the reality of the receiver and looked at how the communication of this information was foreshadowed. Some of Maynard's earlier work on the subject brought this point into clear view. Christie read that Maynard studied bad-news delivery to parents whose children had been diagnosed with mental disabilities. He found that if physicians start these bad-news delivery interactions by having the parents describe their child's behavior and reiterate their concerns for why they initiated medical treatment and diagnosis, the parents were more likely to accept the news. In other words, it was a way to confirm what the parents suspected and to help them in their process of acceptance. Christie thought of Terry's person-centered approach when she read about these studies.

FAMILY ISSUES

As Terry and Christie talked more about bad-news delivery, she began to think about differences in bad-news delivery to the patient and bad-news delivery to the patient's family. There were different constraints in the two situations. Terry had told her about a study that traced the history of medical disclosure in this country. He said that it was in the 1950s that a shift occurred where patients began to demand the truth about their conditions. This still left the issue of telling family members. For instance, it's the family who has to be told that a patient has died, and Christie soon came to realize that the family should not be asked for permission to do an autopsy at the same time they are being given the news of the death. It is similar to what Anne always talked about with decoupling the news from asking for organ donation. Also, the family should be warned about how the deceased will look before they see the body.

REACTIONS TO BAD NEWS

Christie discovered some pretty consistent reactions to bad news from patients and their families, too, both in her own experiences and in the literature. As she thought and read about it, she found that the reactions tended to fall into one of six categories: acceptance, overwhelming distress, denial, ambivalence, unrealistic expectations, or collusion. She found the ideas of acceptance, distress, and denial pretty straightforward, but had to do some additional reading about the others. Ambivalence, as described in the literature, involves going back and forth from acceptance to denial. Similarly, people with unrealistic expectations appear to understand and accept the bad news, but then request or expect things that are completely inappropriate for their state or that of their family members. Collusion involves a family member, and occurs when either the patient or someone from the family tries to convince the care provider that someone else not be told the bad news. It's all right for a patient to request this, but it's problematic when a family member requests that the patient not be told, as this violates the patient's legal rights.

Christie observed denial in the daughter of a terminally ill patient. She spent a long time talking to Cathy about her father's cancer treatment and prognosis. They then talked a bit about coping, and Cathy, who was enrolled in the same doctoral program in Communication as Terry, expressed interest in writing something about her experiences and those of her father. She talked about the language that she heard being used to describe him and his situation, and described an interesting piece of rhetorical analysis that she saw coming out of that.

Christie: Yes, I can see it, too. "The Rhetoric of Terminality."
Cathy: Yeah, "The Rhetoric of Survival."

"Wow," Christie thought, but didn't say. "The rhetoric of 'terminality' vs. the rhetoric of 'survival.' That's a big difference. She still hasn't accepted the fact that he's going to die."

EPILOGUE

Terry, whom Christie later married, and all of her family were very proud of the fine doctor she became. Although, like many doctors, she was a very good provider of medical care, they were even more pleased with the interpersonal skills she developed and with her ability to sensitively adapt to individual patients and their families during those times that she had to deliver bad news to them. Importantly, Christie felt better about herself as a doctor when she saw patients suffering a bit less because of how she told them bad news that had to be shared. Even her brother George came to appreciate the importance of this issue, as he "came to" after prostate surgery to find that his prostate had been completely removed during surgery, which was not the outcome he had expected. When the doctor bluntly told him this, followed by the news that he would no longer be able to obtain an erection unaided, George realized the difference a little sensitivity from the doctor might have made.

"It would have been bad news, anyway," George told Christie, "but I see what you mean now—it would have cushioned the blow a bit if he had told me ahead of time that this might be a possibility and that there are some options available if it does happen. I would have felt better if he had acted like he even cared a little. I felt like I'd been blind-sided!"

All that Christie could do was hug her brother—yet another victim of poor bad news delivery. As Christie moved through her career as a doctor, she let the words of authors Rabow and McPhee (1999) ring in her mind every time she delivered bad news: "Clinicians are not responsible for knowing the answers to patients' deeply personal and existential questions; they are called on to be present as witnesses to their patients' suffering and to respect the vulnerability created by the news they bear" (p. 263).

RELEVANT CONCEPTS

Bad-news delivery: The verbal and nonverbal communication of medical information that will be perceived by the patient and/or the patient's family as negative.

Decoupling: The separation of the delivery of the news that the patient has died from the request for the donation of the patient's organs.

Disconfirmation: A verbal and/or nonverbal message that invalidates the perspective or feelings of the other interactant.

High-context cultures: Cultures that place a higher emphasis on nonverbal communication and look to the environment (i.e., physical setting, social norms) for cues in interpretation of messages.

Interpersonal cognitive complexity: A measure of the social-cognitive development of the individuals in terms of the integration of their psychological construct system.

Medical disclosure: The communication of medical information from a care provider to a patient.

Person-centeredness: The ability to value and legitimize the perspective and emotions of the other person(s) in the interaction, such that you help them achieve their interactional goals without sacrificing your own.

DISCUSSION QUESTIONS

1. Why is it difficult for care providers to communicate bad news to patients and their families?
2. What are some different constraints that affect the communication of bad news to patients vs. their families?
3. What individual and cultural characteristics are important to adapt to in the process of delivering bad news?
4. How can reassurance be disconfirming? How can it be communicated in a more confirming way? How can bad news be delivered in a disconfirming way?
5. What is person-centeredness? What is its relevance to bad-news delivery?

REFERENCES/SUGGESTED READINGS

Gillotti, C. M., & Applegate, J. L. (2000). Explaining illness as bad news: Individual differences in explaining illness-related information. In B. Whaley (Ed.), *Explaining illness: Research, theory, and strategies* (pp. 101–122). Mahwah, NJ: Lawrence Erlbaum Associates.

Gillotti, C. M. (2003). Medical disclosure and decision-making: Excavating the complexities of physician-patient information exchange. In T. Thompson, A. Dorsey, K. Miller, & R. Parrott (Eds.), *Handbook of health communication* (pp. 163–181). Mahwah, NJ: Lawrence Erlbaum Associates.

Gillotti, C. M., Thompson, T. L., & McNeilis, K. (2002). Communicative competence in the delivery of bad news. *Social Science and Medicine, 54*, 1011–1023.

Hafferty, F. W. (1989). *Into the valley: Death and the socialization of medical students.* New Haven, CT: Yale University Press.

Maynard, D. W. (1989). Notes on the delivery and reception of diagnostic news regarding mental disabilities. In D. T. Helm, W. T. Anders, A. J. Meehan, & A. W. Rawls (Eds.), *The interactional order: New directions in the study of social order* (pp. 54–67). New York: Irvington.

Rabow, M. W., & McPhee, S. J. (1999). Beyond breaking bad news: How to help patients who suffer. *Western Journal of Medicine, 171*, 260–263.

Additional Resources

Web sites:
www.hematology.org/meeting/2002/newsdaily/BadNews.cfm
www.acponline.org/journals/news/jan03/communication.htm
www.uiowa.edu/~ournews/2002/october/1030bad-news.html
www.biomed.lib.umn.edu/hmcd/990901_bad.html
www.articles911.com/Communication/Delivering_Bad_News

Suggested Movies:
The Doctor
Patch Adams
Terms of Endearment
Marvin's Room
Lorenzo's Oil
Forest Gump

3

Problematic Discharge From Physical Therapy: Communicating About Uncertainty and Profound Values

Austin S. Babrow
David O'Connor Dinn
Purdue University

Charlie muttered an oath. The simple knot in his shoelace was defeating him. He knew the knot was not very tight and could see exactly how to disentangle it. It was just that his right arm felt leaden, his hand a numb claw. Try as he might, and he had been trying to put on his second shoe for a couple of minutes, he was unable to pull apart the knot. On top of the frustration of being unable to accomplish a simple task that he'd mastered 60 years ago, Charlie was vexed by the choice that remained: either ask his wife for help when he'd assured her minutes ago that he needed none, or wear the ridiculous pair of loafers his daughter had bought for him at that ritzy fashion mall in Indianapolis. Growing up on the farm as a child, and then working on it until he was forced to sell just after his 66th birthday 2 years before, he had never owned a pair of these useless shoes. On the farm, he wore sturdy work boots, except when the ground was so rain-sodden that he had to put on a pair of rubber boots. He had always worn a respectable pair of black lace shoes to church. These had been his standard footwear since selling the farm. So Charlie had no use for loafers. Even the name irritated him.

Looking up at the clock, Charlie saw that it was nearly time to leave for a physical therapy (PT) appointment. This frustrated him even more; he had wanted to report to Connor Morrison, the young therapist, that he had tied both of his own shoes today.[1] It would be embarrassing to admit that a simple knot had defeated him. Still, it was better than wearing loafers. And, he had managed to tie one shoe. With these reassuring thoughts in mind, he called his wife for help.

In this, the most difficult time in his life, Charlie kept hearing that it was important to think about small successes. His doctors told him that setting too high a goal would set him up for failure and disappointment. Charlie felt uncomfortable with this advice. He had always considered himself to be a man unafraid of aiming high. Hadn't he bought the neighboring farm when old man Deutsch passed away? Hadn't he been able to keep the new land until the burden of farming it without good help had forced him to sell off the excess acreage? He had taken it in stride when neither his daughters nor their husbands wanted to take over the family farm. Not everyone had the grit to keep farming these days. And many farmers were not shrewd enough to sell their farms; even though the price he got was pretty low, at least he had not gone completely bust and had the place sold out from under him by the bank.

Charlie also disliked the advice to "think small" (as the advice seemed to him) because it meant having to watch his thoughts like a mother hen. It seemed false and unnatural, sort of like he'd be lying to himself. What he honestly wanted was hope. So he also disliked the advice to think small because he thought it implied that things would never return to normal. And he wanted desperately to be his old self. He had lost so much. Although it was true that he had regained his voice and some function in his arm and leg, how much more would return? How long would it take? What could he do to improve his situation? It hurt to think about all of this.

Charlie could actually see some value in small successes. They brought a brief rush of hope and distracted him for a time from thinking about how much the stroke had changed him. Still, this didn't mean that he should think small. When little improvements were few and far between, hoping for small gains felt like giving up on a fuller recovery. And all this thought-management was both unnatural and hard work. So, in addition to the knot in his shoelaces, a mental knot bedeviled Charlie. Still, his condition had improved.

In the days immediately after his stroke, Charlie had ridden a nightmarish roller coaster ride. Unsuccessful efforts to speak coherently or move his right arm and leg brought him close to panic. Would he never regain his speech?[2] Was he paralyzed on one side for the rest of his life? The doctors' brusque confidence and the nurses' cheerful encouragement calmed him somewhat, but these periods of relief gave way to fear when he saw the worry in the faces of his family members.

The roller coaster of panic and relief gradually gave way to new thoughts and emotions in the following weeks. Although he was still afraid from time to time, more often Charlie felt anger, sorrow, frustration, hope, satisfaction, and joy. These feelings seemed to change, depending on his body, his ruminations, and interactions with health care providers, family, and friends.

When he regained speech and limited mobility on his right side, Charlie was emboldened. He told himself that he would return soon to the body and life of a vigorous, independent, 68-year-old. However, when he had trouble doing something that seemed simple, such as cutting a piece of food or tucking in his shirt, or when he lost balance maneuvering around the old farmhouse, he'd feel a flash of fear and become angry. Why had this happened to him? Why was his wife always pestering him to do things for himself? Why wouldn't she help more? She had always been so helpful around the farm before he got sick. Why was his house such a cluttered mess? Surely it had not always been this way. Did she need help? Why were his daughters working full time instead of staying home to raise their kids and help out their mother and father? Could Charlie and his wife Meg afford paid help at home? Why weren't his doctors and therapists giving him better care? Why weren't they more understanding and encouraging?

Interactions with his family doctor and the hotshot, overpriced neurologist were not always what he wanted them to be like. He expected his doctors to "shoot straight," to tell him what was going on. Although they had been willing to tell him what had happened to his body, the doctors seemed reluctant to talk about his prognosis. He wanted them to be clearer about what to expect in terms of his recovery. When would he be able to do more things for himself? When would he be able to drive? Why were his arm and leg recovering so slowly? When would his sense of balance return to normal?

When he asked about these things, his doctors seemed evasive; they became downright slippery when he tried to pin them down. A couple of times, the doctors had told him that he might not recover much at all. That really got him mad. He had known folks who had never recovered from devastating strokes, but they were older and really sick. By contrast, Ned Miller, a farmer out in the western end of the county who had a stroke a few years back, eventually got back to farming as if nothing had ever happened to him. When Charlie insisted that his stroke was no worse than Ned's, his family doc seemed to back off and admit that he might eventually regain much more use of his arm and leg, although "that worthless neurologist" said that no two strokes were the same. Still, both docs told him that it was important to remain hopeful. So, why did they disagree about his prospects? Generally, why weren't they more encouraging and optimistic?

Why weren't his doctors willing to shoot straight about his prognosis? Were they hiding something from him? Were they treating him like a child just because he was old and had been sick? Were they competent? His family doc was nearly as old as himself, so maybe he didn't know all the latest treatments. And Charlie had heard from a few of his cronies at the Downtowner restaurant that the docs at the county hospital were not that great. Did all the really good docs work at one of the big-city hospitals in Indianapolis? Some of the guys at the Downtowner thought there were excellent docs right in town. Who was right? If he drove up to Indy, would he receive better care?

Interactions with his family were only somewhat more helpful. Charlie was happiest talking with his daughters, Sarah and Grace, because they were so optimistic compared with his doctors and his wife. However, even conversations with his daughters at times made the situation harder to bear. Both talked like Charlie's condition was improving rapidly and substantially, and encouraged him to believe he would soon be back to his old self. They also brought him printouts of articles from the Internet. At first, he found this useful, but he soon became overloaded by all the information. It was just more than he could manage, so he stopped reading the printouts.

Although Charlie wanted very much to hear his daughters' encouragement, these conversations had come to upset him. He knew Sarah and Grace loved him, but they were unwilling to hear about what a hard time he was having, how much he needed help from their mom, and how tough he was finding the PT with Connor. Why did they brush off his concerns? Why did they insist that everything was going so well and keep pushing those Internet clippings on him? And why did there seem to be so much anxiety behind their smiles and encouraging words? Were they hiding something from him? Were they really feeling pessimistic but afraid to admit it?

Meg, Charlie's wife of more than 40 years, was mostly the blessing she had always been, but she had also started to become a source of frustration. She was her old cheerful self, full of energy and generosity when he returned from the hospital, and she continued to be a great help to him months later. However, she had also become more irritable than she had been before the stroke, and she had even become somewhat less accepting of his limits. At times, she seemed downright angry with Charlie for not trying harder to get around or do things for himself. She was especially unforgiving when it came to his diet and therapy exercises. Did she expect him to eat that bland pap the dietician had prescribed for the rest of his life? To eat without any salt whatsoever? To become a vegetarian? To exercise from sun-up to sundown?

Meg was indeed trying to be cheerful and upbeat, but she was worried. She had grown tired in the months since Charlie came home from the nursing home. As a healthy 63-year-old farm wife, she was able to manage Charlie's needs for physical help. Still, his needs were quite demanding. Would they remain so forever, or would they decrease significantly? And if he were to improve much, when would this progress happen? How much would he be able to do for himself? How much would she have to do? These and many other questions came to mind whenever she thought about his very slow and limited recovery to date.

As time passed, Meg found herself no less willing to help Charlie, but she was beginning to feel resentful. She became frustrated with him at times. Rather than appreciating her efforts to learn a new way to cook, he grumbled. He always asked to be dropped off so he could have a cup of coffee at the Downtowner when she went to town on errands. She suspected that he cheated on his diet when out of her sight. It also bothered Meg when Charlie did not complete the exercises Connor had assigned in PT. Were they too hard, as Charlie said? Could he not try harder? Had the stroke affected his personality in some way, perhaps damaging his pride or self-confidence, perhaps making him take advantage of his situation, doing less and demanding more? As these thoughts crossed her mind, Meg found herself in a swirl of anger, sorrow, anxiety, and guilt.

Making matters worse, Meg wanted very much to talk about these uncertainties and worries, but she found few satisfying opportunities to do so. How could she talk to Charlie about her thoughts and feelings? Would he understand and respond well, or would he be hurt? Would he feel that she distrusted him? That she thought he was irresponsible? That she was disappointed in him? She also hated that, despite her best efforts to be supportive, she leaked her frustration and worry. Talking about her feelings with Sarah and Grace was impossible. Meg could see that they needed to think of their father as the vigorous and self-assured man he had been before the stroke. They were guided more by their hearts than their heads and seemed incapable of accepting the possibility that their father had been changed forever. Meg hoped her daughters would soon come to see and begin to accept the changes, but she was afraid to confront the girls by telling them how little their father had regained since his speech had returned.

Even though she could see the situation more clearly than her daughters, and perhaps more clearly than the doctors or physical therapist, Meg was unwilling to express out loud to anyone just how frightened she was that Charlie would recover little more. Would giving voice to her innermost worries somehow make them come true? Would she cross an invisible line and anger God by expressing such faithlessness? Indeed, she was not even sure what to hope for. What should she ask of God?

Talking to her minister and friends was a mixed blessing. One friend simply dismissed any expression of uncertainty; all would be well, she insisted. Another friend encouraged her to look into getting a visiting nurse or housekeeper. Still another friend encouraged her and Charlie to move in with her oldest daughter. Were things that bleak?

Everyone, friends and minister alike, assured her that God would help her family in its hour of need. But what did this mean? What was she to pray for? At the end of the day, when she lay in bed next to her frail husband, exhausted and beset by worry, she wanted to ask God to return Charlie to his old self. At the same time, she knew better than anyone, except God, how much Charlie had lost and therefore how much it was to ask for Him to return Charlie to his healthy pre-stroke self.

In sum, as Charlie's main care provider, Meg saw clearly that she needed to understand just where things stood. She also intuited the vital importance of hopefulness—for her husband, herself, and their children. Her minister reminded her of a prayer that had given her comfort in the past when confronted by smaller trials: "God give me the strength to change those things I can, the serenity to accept those things that I cannot change, and the wisdom to know the difference." Unfortunately, since Charlie's stroke, although she prayed for strength, serenity, and wisdom, she was confronted daily by her limits. So she ended each day simply asking for God's mercy, whatever it might be in His infinite wisdom and compassion. She took what solace she could from this vague, open-ended entreaty.

In short, Charlie, Meg, and the girls were trying to keep an optimistic outlook, but it was getting tougher to do so. Charlie was improving so slowly that at times it was hard to see change. Moreover, he was getting little definitive information about his prognosis from doctors that he saw less and less frequently as time passed. Even though he had found them mostly frustrating this last month, Charlie believed that the weekly PT sessions were his best hope for information and help at this point. So, it was with mixed feelings that Charlie sat by Meg as she drove him to yet another PT session.

Charlie liked his therapist and the friends he had made at the PT clinic, and it was a pleasure to see them most days. Still, therapy itself was no great pleasure. It was a lot of hard work, and lately there had been little reward. After a lifetime in the fields, Charlie had adapted rather well to the easy life he had found in the first two years of his retirement. So, each week he told himself to have a positive attitude and to try hard to do what Connor asked. He thought he did pretty well, too, even if the boy sometimes asked him to do what seemed impossible. At times, he was even happy to try because Connor was so encouraging. However, lately, the therapy sessions had been getting more frustrating, and Charlie could tell that he was not alone in this feeling.

When he thought that Connor was frustrated with him, Charlie would get mad, although he would never show it. Why did the young "whipper-snapper" give him exercises he could not do? Why did the home exercise assignments take so long? Did he think Charlie would spend his entire life doing nothing but working his afflicted arm and leg? Was there no more efficient therapy available? Was this youngster, who barely had a beard to shave, really an expert at PT? Was he as good as the therapists in the city? These troublesome thoughts dogged Charlie whenever he felt frustrated, and particularly when he sensed frustration in Connor's manner. The thoughts and unpleasant feelings would linger until Charlie had one of those small successes that everyone told him to aim for. He would then feel hope return, and he would congratulate himself and whoever else was around. But when there were so few successes, there was little to say.

Lately, conversations with Connor also had become less satisfying. Charlie wanted to reveal his worries, but he felt uncomfortable talking with a stranger, especially a "kid," about his feelings. He was also unwilling to tell Connor how hard it was to do the strengthening and flexibility exercises at home. He felt embarrassed about admitting that he was not sure he was doing them right, even though they had been going over his home program for many weeks. How would Connor react if Charlie suggested that there might be better exercises? That better PT might be available in Indianapolis? He did not want to hurt Connor's feelings. He liked the young man. So when the sessions turned frustrating, Charlie generally tried to get Connor to tell him what to expect in the coming weeks. This dialogue was unsatisfying because Connor was never definite about the timetable for recovery. Instead of talking directly about his client's prognosis, Connor encouraged Charlie to work harder than ever to get over the "plateau" in his recovery. Maybe today would be different. Perhaps Connor would give him new exercises. Maybe today Charlie would show everyone, including himself, that he had gained more than they thought. After all, he had tied a shoelace for the first time today!

THE PHYSICAL THERAPIST

Despite the constant demands of his very busy practice, Connor Morrison found himself thinking of the coming afternoon appointment with Charlie whenever he was involved in a routine task. He knew it was important to give each patient undivided attention, and he had a steady, uninterrupted stream of patients these days, but Charlie's case was troubling. It intruded again and again into his thoughts.

As a licensed physical therapist in practice since earning his master's degree 3 years earlier, Connor felt comfortable dealing with involved neurological cases. He knew that he was quite competent; clients, coworkers, and supervisors often attested to this fact. However, Connor was uncomfortable with some important and recurring communication situations. Today, he was facing just such a challenge.

Connor had started his work with Charlie Van Sleet under fairly typical circumstances. Several months ago, and shortly after his 68th birthday, Charlie suffered a left-sided cerebral vascular accident with consequent right-sided hemiparesis, a stroke that left him partially paralyzed on his right side. Connor had taken the outpatient case a short time after the elderly man's discharge from the hospital.

Although Charlie presented with some important physical limitations, his stroke appeared to have had little impact on his cognitive abilities. He was generally able to follow one- and two-step commands; was oriented to time, person, and place; and had good safety awareness. He did have some difficulty with solving problems in new or complex situations,[3] but his major limitations were in the area of functional mobility.

In his first weeks back at home, Charlie had considerable difficulty with transferring (i.e., moving from one position to another, such as moving from a seated position in a chair to a standing posture), balance, and ambulation. These limits severely restricted his independence, a loss that is common for the growing number of older individuals who suffer strokes. Indeed, Charlie was completely reliant on Meg for instrumental activities of daily living when he was first released from the hospital.

After nearly 4 months of therapy, Charlie was now able to get around the first floor of his home using a quad-cane, or "walker." He also could sit and get up from chairs with reasonably high seats, but he still needed his wife's help with transfers to his favorite lounge chair or to the commode and getting up and down the stairs on their front porch. (Charlie's family had apparently rearranged his home so that his bedroom was now on the first floor.) Although these improvements seemed to bring Charlie some happiness, Connor could tell that Charlie was having trouble adjusting to the remaining limitations. Indeed, since they started working together, Charlie seemed to want to improve physical function faster and more substantially than it was reasonable to expect. Connor had tried to encourage him to be realistic, but his words seemed to have had little impact on his client's expectations.

Connor was also troubled by Charlie's apparent unwillingness to admit that he had not been making much progress for the last several weeks. In fact, by the standards of care dictated by Medicare, Charlie's therapy might have been discontinued a few weeks earlier; he had hit a plateau between weeks 7 through 11, and Connor had very seriously considered calling an end to therapy. The Medicare rules were pretty clear on this: if, in Connor's clinical judgment, his client would make no further significant progress with skilled therapy, Medicare would no longer pay for PT. At that time, it would be up to the client to pay in full for the costs of regular visits or to discontinue PT and shift instead to self-care. Few elderly stroke patients in Connor's practice had been able to pay for therapy by themselves. Most typically had debts from the stroke as well as other expenses from chronic illnesses, and many, including Charlie, had essentially no coverage outside of that provided by the Medicare program.

At the time of his first plateau in improvement, Charlie seemed both unaware of the stall in his progress and not yet adjusted emotionally to his limitations. Connor had continued skilled PT, writing up progress reports that, if not strictly a reflection of his innermost thoughts, were not outright distortions of Charlie's prognosis. In this way, Connor had been able to ensure continued Medicare reimbursement, and PT had continued. Fortunately, if somewhat unexpectedly, Charlie had actually improved a bit more during weeks 12 through 14, but he had now passed another 4 weeks at a plateau. In spite of this, Charlie continued to hope for more changes in his physical functioning, and he pressed Connor for an optimistic prognosis. But Connor knew that, following Medicare treatment and compensation guidelines, he could not justify continuing Charlie's plan of care for another 30 days. His treatment would no longer be covered. Although it was time for his discharge, Connor dreaded the interaction that lay ahead.

It was unusual for Connor to greet Charlie in the reception area when the generally affable old man arrived, but Connor finished quickly with his 1 o'clock appointment and waited anxiously as he watched Charlie move slowly through the door held open by his wife. Charlie was surprised to see the young man waiting and gave him a big smile. Connor knew that Charlie was looking forward to talking with him. He knew Charlie had been feeling housebound since the stroke and enjoyed the sessions with his physical therapist. He also felt that Charlie admired him for his expertise and dedication.

For his part, Connor liked Charlie, although his client was also frustrating. The old man was affable and cooperative in the clinic; he generally tried hard to do the exercises while Connor supervised in the clinic, although he was at times more balky than Connor wished. Connor also suspected that Charlie was not always responsible when it came to the home exercise assignments he had been given. It wasn't that Charlie seemed unwilling to work. Rather, it seemed like he wanted to improve faster and more substantially than it was reasonable to expect, and he also didn't seem to understand just how hard it would be to recover much more than he had already.

THE INTERACTION

After Connor's initial greeting, Charlie managed a partial smile but strained a bit to give a genuine handshake with his affected right hand. He noticed that Connor was more restrained than usual, but he was too preoccupied with thoughts about the difficult communication task that lay ahead: getting Connor to tell him clearly when he'd start to improve again or give him better exercises.

Connor followed Charlie's slow, quad-cane–assisted walk from the waiting room to the rehab area. The area was a large open room with various forms of equipment, including treadmills, stationary bicycles, and parallel bars. It was bordered on two sides by a few smaller examination cubicles with curtains for privacy (along the side facing the rehab area). On this day, all of the semiprivate curtained examining cubicles were taken, so Connor asked Charlie to sit on a folding chair by a table in the open rehab room.

The therapist observed his client's difficulty seating himself in the chair, but Charlie felt good about the fact that he was able to sit without help. Feeling smug, Charlie turned to his therapist and asked his standard opening question, "So how are you going to torture me today, Doc?" Connor and Charlie both smiled and laughed, but Connor felt the knot in his stomach tighten at the thought of what lay ahead.

Reluctant to jump right into the discharge, Connor asked his client to stand so that they could work on his balance. Connor positioned himself by Charlie's side as he had him stand on a balance pad that they had been using the last several weeks to improve his ability to maintain his balance, especially while ambulating over uneven surfaces. Before long, Charlie asked to move on to something more difficult. Connor asked him to close his eyes while his feet were together. When he did, it was soon apparent that Charlie had made no gains during the past week, so before Charlie was done trying to stand with eyes closed, Connor said, "Alright, Charlie. You can stop now. That's enough for today. Why don't you sit down so we can talk about some important issues?"

Charlie smiled as he sat, thinking that the therapist stopped him because he had done well. He hoped to press this good news by insisting on a clearer and more hopeful prognosis. Why, he might even insist on new, more efficient exercises instead of hinting about it as he had in the past.

"I oughta give that neurologist a call and let him know how wrong he was to tell me I'd never come all the way back. Maybe I've got some ways to go, but he sure didn't think I'd come this far. So what's next, Doc?"

Still reluctant to jump into the unpleasantness, Connor said, "Well, Charlie, we'll get to that in a sec, but let's first review how often and how long you've been exercising each day at home this last week."

"You know, Doc, I do as much as I can, near every day. Them exercises are hard, but I stick with 'em. Near ever' day. So what's next? Anything new?" Charlie thought with some anxiety about what Connor would say if he knew how much trouble Charlie had with the exercises and how often he skipped them. If only Charlie could get something new to try, something more efficient.

Hearing Charlie evading his question again, Connor considered pressing for more information, but he did not know where to begin. Charlie just seemed unwilling to take more responsibility for his PT. It was time to prepare his client for the bad news (what his PT professors had called "firing the warning shot").

"We have to talk now about something that you might not like," Connor said.

"What's that? Do you want me to do even more of them same old exercises?"

Seeing the frustration in the elderly man's eyes and hearing it in his voice, Connor asked, "Do you want to get better, Charlie?"

"Of course I do! Why would you ask that?" Charlie snapped.

Unnerved by his client's indignation, Connor felt himself become defensive, and his aim to move to the bad news was momentarily forgotten.

"Well then, why aren't you pulling your weight at home?"

"I'm pullin'. I'm pullin'. It's just these exercises ain't right," Charlie blurted out in his anger. The conversation was not going like he had expected. What was Connor trying to accuse him of? What could he say to learn what he wanted to know? What did he want to know? His thoughts were blurred by anxiety.

For Connor, too, the interaction had gone off on a very unfortunate tangent. He had meant well. Indeed, he hated to offend the frail but usually genial old man and was doing his best to avoid that end. Moreover, the termination of therapy felt a bit like a failure despite his best efforts to see Charlie's stall in progress as something that just happens sometimes. So, not knowing what else to do, Connor decided it was time to tell Charlie that their work together was at an end.

"Well, I sure wish you could have gotten more out of them, Charlie. The problem is, you've reached a plateau in your function, and this has to be our last meeting."

Charlie sat in stunned silence. After an uncomfortably long interval, Connor went on, thinking that perhaps Charlie was feeling offended or sad.

"It's nothing personal. Medicare requires that we make consistent functional progress, but for the last several weeks, I haven't seen any improvement in your status."

"I'd be willing to work harder at home," said Charlie.

"If it were up to me, I'd continue with you indefinitely, Charlie. It's just that 600-pound gorilla, Medicare. They just won't pay for visits unless there is progress to report," Connor stated.

"Ain't I been progressing?"

"Well yes, but not lately."

"What's that mean?"

"As I said, it means that we have to terminate therapy sessions."

"So I ain't gonna get any better'n this? I gotta live like this forever?"

"Charlie, it's hard to say just what might happen in 3 or 6 months' time, what'll happen in a year. I'll give you some exercises to work on yourself. If you do them, there's no telling what you'll accomplish."

"You mean you'll give me new exercises, but you won't see me no more?" Charlie replied. "What'll I tell Meg and the kids?"

"Oh, you can keep in touch with me, give a call now and again. I'd like to hear how you're doing. And of course we can continue therapy if your physicians order it and you can afford to pay for it out of your own pocket."

"Is this decision final? I can't afford to pay you without Medicare. Could I get coverage to start therapy with another doc?"

"No, Charlie. Medicare will know that your PT sessions have run their course. Let's talk some about what you can do at home from now on, and then I'll walk you up front and say goodbye to Meg."

And just like that, with Charlie's questions hanging in the air, and many more questions in mind, Charlie and Connor brought their therapeutic relationship to an end.

IMPROVING HEALTH COMMUNICATION BY UNDERSTANDING UNCERTAINTY

Many uncertainties characterize illness. Communication about illness is often about these uncertainties. A fundamental premise in a growing body of health communication literature is that competent communication requires a clear understanding of the uncertainties patients, care providers, and families might be experiencing. One of us (A.B.) has developed a framework called Problematic Integration Theory, which we believe to be useful for developing this sort of sensitivity or awareness. It involves several important distinctions and their implications.

A simple but useful way to distinguish and identify illness-related uncertainties is to notice that illness makes us uncertain about lots of different issues. Think, for example, about Charlie. Obviously, he is uncertain about (a) how much his arm and leg will improve, and (b) when to expect these improvements. What are Charlie's other uncertainties in relation to his present physical condition, prognosis, and treatment; his personal identity; his relationships with Meg, their daughters, his doctors, and Connor; and family finances?

Answering these questions identifies the *content* of Charlie's uncertainties. Effective health communication depends in part on sensitivity to the range of this content, the many issues about which participants may be uncertain. For example, Connor's efforts to terminate therapy well (that is, effectively and in a socially appropriate manner) depend on the extent to which he accurately understands the specific contents of Charlie's uncertainty.

Another, more subtle, but equally important way to distinguish uncertainties, aside from their different content, is in terms of their *forms*. What we mean by this is that a person can experience various senses of uncertainty for any single specific issue or content. Indeed, uncertainty takes many different forms. For example, it can reflect perceived (personal or universal) ignorance, ambiguous information, concerns about the reliability or validity of available information (e.g., the process that produced it or the sources that relayed it), a superabundance of information ("overload"), or the realization that something we wish to predict is essentially a random outcome.

Again, we can experience these many *forms* of uncertainty in relation to any particular content. For example, Charlie is clearly uncertain about when his "arm and leg will be back to normal." He might experience uncertainty about this because he feels his doctors are with-holding information (only he is ignorant), because nobody knows this information (universal ignorance), because he has been given ambiguous information, because various sources of this information are inconsistent, because the sources are incompetent or otherwise untrustworthy, and so on. The important point here is that, for Connor to terminate therapy competently, he must understand not only the *content* of Charlie's uncertainties, but also the *form* (or forms) of each important uncertainty. For example, if he recognizes that Charlie wants to know when his body will return to "normal," he needs to ascertain just why he is uncertain about this issue. In what sense(s) is he uncertain about this issue?

A third distinction essential to effective health communication is among the many ways of living with and communicating about uncertainty. We can see this in part by rephrasing the point of the previous paragraph; effective communication requires varied types of messages, or messages adapted to fit specific forms (as well as contents) of uncertainty that concern the patient (or care providers, family members, and friends). If, for example, Charlie is uncertain about whether he is getting the right sort of therapy, Connor must ascertain whether his client has received inconsistent messages about his treatment, whether the messages were ambiguous, whether he is suspicious of Connor's competence, etc. There is no simple way to know which is the case. Effective health communication requires not merely good technical interviewing and listening skills; it also requires knowledge of the forms of uncertainty so that questioning and listening can be focused in the most profitable directions. In other words, the competent health communicator must listen for and explore the form of expressed uncertainties (e.g., probe when Charlie asks, "So what's next? Anything new?" or "Do you want me to do even more of them same old exercises?").

We said previously that one way to differentiate approaches to communicating about uncertainty is to recognize that messages must be adapted to the form of uncertainty that is challenging the intended message receiver. There is another way to distinguish among different approaches to communicating about and experiencing uncertainty. To understand this, we introduce one other distinction that is essential to effective health communication: *the difference between uncertainty and evaluation*. What we mean here is that uncertainties are only worth noting and grappling with communicatively when they involve issues that are judged to be very valuable (either positively or negatively) by those involved in the interaction.

Indeed, uncertainties become both more crucial and more difficult to deal with as they relate to more positive or negative issues or events. For example, it is more important and difficult to talk about a life-threatening illness than about an unpleasant but not particularly dangerous one. As another example, for most people, it is probably more important and more difficult to talk about the prospects for regaining full use of one's body after stroke-induced paralysis than about having to live with the typical dietary restrictions prescribed for stroke survivors. Although this may seem obvious, its implications are sometimes unnoticed by people who are ill and their care providers.

It is important to know that people generally have a tendency to be somewhat optimistic about their own health and happiness. Although this *optimistic bias* appears to be the norm, there are wide variations in personal styles, ranging from the "cock-eyed optimist" to the prophet of "doom-and-gloom." Another important implication of the distinction between uncertainty and evaluation is that, although distinct, they are interrelated. For example, desires shape expectations about the future. Think not only of the habitual optimists and pessimists noted above, but also of the effect of desire on our motivation and actual achievement. That is, our desire and motivation can prompt action that itself shapes our chances of achieving our dreams. Similarly, expectation or uncertainty shapes desires, for example, either sustaining or killing hope. In addition, any given uncertainty and evaluation are interwoven within surrounding complexes of related beliefs, opinions, values, and intentions. For this reason, when we address a particular uncertainty in our talk or actions, we often uncover other uncertainties. For example, new information may reduce our ignorance (uncertainty) about one issue and in turn give rise to a cascading sequence of new uncertainties. As a more concrete example, Charlie might ask Meg why she is pestering him, and her answer might reduce his uncertainty about her motives (e.g., she reveals that she thinks he hasn't tried hard enough to get better), but he may then experience various new uncertainties (e.g., is she right? How much harder could he try? Has she lost some respect for him? Has she said this to their children or friends?).

Recognizing these implications of the distinction between uncertainties and values is crucial to health communication. The implications reveal that, although we should generally expect optimism, this response will not be universal. They reveal that effective health communication will often require us to grapple with more than a single isolated uncertainty. They reveal that, when we try to deal with any single or very closely interrelated uncertainty, we should be attentive to the many ripples of uncertainty in surrounding beliefs about the person's condition, identity, relationships with others, and so on. There is a good chance that, even as we speak *in a single turn at talk* about a very specific form of uncertainty raised in another person's previous turn, that other person's thoughts will have turned to another issue or form of uncertainty *before our turn is through*.

A fifth and final distinction that is essential to health communication has to do with how we think about ways of living with uncertainty. For many years, and for many good reasons, communication researchers believed that uncertainty itself is bad and that it is best managed by its reduction or complete eradication. Many scholars have come to realize that uncertainty also can be good (e.g., Rintamaki & Brashers, Chapter 12, this volume), in that it can sustain hope when prospects for recovery from an illness are quite bleak. Hence, sometimes it is good to seek or to maintain existing uncertainty. Together, these ideas constitute the idea that uncertainty must be "managed."

Yet another way to think about uncertainty is to conceive of it simply as a natural, and perhaps the most fundamental, truth in life. In this view, we surrender the illusion of being able to manage uncertainty and seek simply to live with it. At times, we may be able to reduce or otherwise manage uncertainty (i.e., willfully shape it in adaptive or comforting ways). At others times, we are simply powerless to shape uncertainty and must learn to live with it. Most notably, we can seek to free ourselves from compulsive attachments, such as yearning to be in control. This sort of thinking is characteristic of some interpretations of western religions (i.e., trusting completely in a higher power) and eastern cultures and religions (i.e., accepting uncertainty as the essence of existence, see Levine, 2000). It is, however, uncommon in the United States. We believe that it represents a powerful alternative, another path for living with uncertainty. In short, we offer this last set of distinctions to further enrich the health communication resources of patients and care providers, of the ill and the well.

RELEVANT CONCEPTS

Adapting the message to forms of uncertainty: One must know the specific form of uncertainty another person is experiencing to formulate an appropriate message (e.g., give more information if the person lacks it, or provide strategies for coping with too much information if that is the problem).

Content of uncertainty: The specific issue or issues about which a person might be uncertain (e.g., diagnosis, prognosis, treatment, cause of illness, costs of treatment, and so on).

Distinguishing uncertainty from evaluation: Recognizing that uncertainty and evaluation are two different, though interdependent, issues. To communicate effectively, we must determine if a person is uncertain or uncertain about a given issue *as well as* whether they appraise that issue and attendant uncertainty (if there is any) as something good or bad.

Forms of uncertainty: The ways that we may be uncertain about any specific issue (e.g., seeing something as fundamentally unpredictable; having too much, too little, or contradictory information; suspecting that the information is irrelevant to one's case, unreliable, or invalid).

Interdependence of uncertainty and evaluation: Uncertainty can make some issues seem better or worse than they might otherwise have seemed. In addition, our likes and dislikes can influence what we believe to be so (e.g., making us more or less hopeful, rationalizing the way things are, etc.).

Living with uncertainty: Accepting limits on our control of uncertainty.

Managing uncertainty: Being in control of uncertainty in some fashion.

DISCUSSION QUESTIONS

1. What were Charlie's uncertainties when he went into therapy on the final day? (You might also think about what other uncertainties he had been experiencing. Also, what were Meg's uncertainties?) What did Charlie do to communicate these uncertainties?
2. What were Connor's uncertainties going into the PT session? What did Connor do to ascertain what was troubling Charlie, particularly to learn what his uncertainties were and what he wanted?
3. What would have been some communicative strategies for dealing effectively with Charlie's uncertainties? From the uncertainty reduction standpoint? From the uncertainty management standpoint? From the perspective that uncertainty is the inescapable and fundamentally unmanageable truth of human experience?
4. What issues or forms of uncertainty were Charlie and Meg concerned about? In relation to Charlie's condition, their future together, and communication about these concerns?

ENDNOTES

[1] Generally speaking, occupational therapists (OT) are responsible for helping an individual restore upper limb function (among other things). For clarity of the exposition, we have collapsed this important distinction between physical and occupational therapy.

[2] Charlie would have seen a speech therapist for difficulties related to speech and some cognitive deficits, such as difficulty problem solving (see below).

[3] As noted previously, these sorts of cognitive issues would likely be dealt with in speech therapy rather than PT, although Connor would have been aware of them and the uncertainties they introduce into PT.

REFERENCES/SUGGESTED READINGS

Babrow, A. S. (1992). Communication and problematic integration: Understanding diverging probability and value, ambiguity, ambivalence, and impossibility. *Communication Theory, 2*, 95–130.

Babrow, A. S. (in press). Problematic integration theory. In B. B. Whaley & W. Samter (Eds.), *Explaining communication: Contemporary theories and exemplars.* Hillsdale, NJ: Lawrence Erlbaum Associates.

Babrow, A. S., Hines, S. C., & Kasch, C. R. (2000). Illness and uncertainty: Problematic integration and strategies for communicating about medical uncertainty and ambiguity. In B. Whaley (Ed.), *Explaining illness: Messages, strategies and contexts* (pp. 41–67). Hillsdale, NJ: Lawrence Erlbaum Associates.

Babrow, A. S., Kasch, C. R., & Ford, L. A. (1998). The many meanings of "uncertainty" in illness: Toward a systematic accounting. *Health Communication, 10*, 1–24.

Ford, L. A., Babrow, A. S., & Stohl, C. (1996). Social support messages and the management of uncertainty in the experience of breast cancer: An application of problematic integration theory. *Communication Monographs, 63*, 189–207.

Levine, M. (2000). *The positive psychology of Buddhism and Yoga: Paths to a mature happiness.* Hillsdale, NJ: Lawrence Erlbaum Associates.

4

"I Want You to Put Me in the Grave With All My Limbs": The Meaning of Active Health Participation

Barbara F. Sharf
Texas A&M University

Paul Haidet
*Baylor College of Medicine and
Houston Center for Quality of Care and Utilization Studies*

Tony L. Kroll
*Texas A&M University and
Houston Center for Quality of Care and Utilization Studies*

. . . we'll work back and forth. I still come in, I still ask questions. He still gives me information that he thinks is useful for me and that will help me. But right now, he does have more control of it because he has to prod me and he has to give me the stronger medications, because I don't have control on the other end.

These are the words of Joanne, a 34-year-old woman with diabetes, during a research interview in which she talks about her struggle to feel "in control" of managing her illness. The "he" referred to is her endocrinologist, Dr. Winner. Though she has seen several physicians for various health problems, Joanne has chosen him as her primary doctor, the one she turns to regularly to discuss health issues, the one in whom she has the most confidence and trust. Like many contemporary patients, especially those with chronic conditions like diabetes that require a reorientation of lifestyle, Joanne is striving to be an active participant in her own health care. Unlike health professionals, who receive training in communication skills, there is no formal education and few informal guidelines for "activating" patients. For each person, being an active health care participant may mean something different. Furthermore, this meaning may transition and evolve over time, as an individual gains experience, the conditions of illness change, and social expectations of the patient–physician relation undergo modifications. As Joanne tells the interviewer the story of her diabetes, she expresses her efforts—and sometimes tensions—in striking a balance between accepting advice and guidance from Dr. Winner while aspiring to have more control. She concurs with the interviewer that, in the future, she'd like Dr. Winner to be "more of a consultant than a controller."

The purpose of this chapter is to examine Joanne's case to better understand how a patient makes sense of the idea of being and becoming an active health care participant. In the process, we examine two important related concepts. Several scholars in health communication have promoted the notion of partnerships between patients and doctors. What constitutes such a partnership and how does this working interaction relate to the meaning of active patient participation? Second, our investigation is based on Joanne's narration of her health-related experiences, including how she views diabetes as part of a larger family saga. We seek to illuminate the connection between the creation (or in Joanne's case, the re-creation) of a health narrative and the meaning of active participation in health care.

Before delving further into Joanne's story, we provide a brief overview of the scholarship concerning the ways in which patients play a crucial and unique part in affecting the process of the medical consultation and subsequent health outcomes. After presenting this background material, we resume Joanne's story. Because this case revolves around Joanne's telling her tale of living with diabetes in her own words, throughout the chapter, we give particular emphasis to the concept of narrative and its importance in shaping how patients respond to both the experience of serious illness and the quality of the patient–physician relationship.[1]

SETTING THE STAGE: ACTIVE PARTICIPATION
IN HEALTH CARE

> When the doctor tells my family something, they accept it for gold. It's as good as gold. You know, there's no questioning it. *I* will question it.

To begin thinking about what it means to participate actively while communicating with a physician, you might want to reflect on the last interaction you had with a doctor or other health provider. Did you feel free to talk about anything that was on your mind? Were you free to talk about your condition or concerns in the way you wanted? Who spoke first, you or your physician? Who spoke more often during the conversation? Had you planned in advance what should be discussed or did you write specific questions that you wanted answered during the visit? If so, was that plan followed and were those questions answered? Did both you and your physician ask questions? Did you feel that the doctor really listened to what you had to say? When you left, were there issues you had hoped to discuss that never were voiced? As you mentally respond to these questions, consider also who or what has influenced your notion of how a patient is "supposed" to behave.

The tradition of medical paternalism has existed for centuries across many cultures. It emphasizes the dominant role of the physician in providing authoritative advice. From a communication perspective, physicians have tended to be socialized into a "high control" style of interaction in which they talk a greater amount of time, ask more questions, give more directives, and interrupt more frequently than do patients (Waitzkin, 1984). Correspondingly, within this model, patients assume a reactive role in which they voice their health complaints and comply with medical recommendations. However, the past 25 years of scholarship in patient–physician communication in the United States reflects an alternate representation of how patients and physicians may interact, differentiated by elements of more active patient participation. The movement toward patient activation has had an impact on changing the way that physicians are educated, with a shift toward "patient-centered medicine" (Stewart et al., 1995).

Several conceptual models have envisioned what the role of a more active patient might be. Physician Timothy Quill (1983) was the first to introduce the notion of the doctor–patient relationship as a partnership, which he described as a contract developed through interaction in which both parties consent to the relationship, have unique responsibilities, are willing to negotiate, and benefit through the interchange. The importance of mutually exchanged information has been recognized as an essential component of health care partnerships. Patients' expertise regarding their own personal capabilities, constraints, resources, and values, as well as self-knowledge of their own bodies and emotions, can be seen as an essential counterpart to health professionals' clinical judgment. Both forms of knowledge—the physician's expertise with medical science and the patient's expertise with the subjective experience of health problems—need to be combined through interpersonal communication to effectively reach a diagnosis and to develop a plan of care (Sharf, 1984).

Other ways of examining the patient–physician relationship emphasize the concepts of power and control. Whereas medical paternalism accords power to the physician, the market-based model of health care consumerism and the ethical model of patient autonomy position the patient as the more powerful, and possibly sole, decision-making agent. Public health researcher Debra Roter and her colleagues (Roter & Hall, 1993; Roter & McNeilis, 2003) have developed a four-point matrix that plots a comparative level of control, high and low, in the context of physician–patient interaction. As a dynamic interpersonal exchange, the behaviors and activities of either participant have the potential to change the nature of the relationship. The matrix describes different types of physician–patient relationships (three of which have been mentioned previously): default, in which there is low control for both patient and physician; consumerism, in which the patient exhibits high control and the physician low control; paternalism, in which the physician exhibits high control and the patient low control; and, mutuality, in which power is balanced between the patient and physician so that goals, agendas, and decisions related to patient care are negotiated. Mutuality, then, is another way of describing partnership.

Focusing on communicative behaviors, health communication scholar Richard L. Street, Jr. (2001) identified four verbal features of active patient participation during medical consultations. These include asking questions to obtain and clarify information; expressing concerns such as worry, fear, or anger; being assertive in stating opinions and preferences, making suggestions, disagreeing with the clinician, and interrupting to be able to speak; and sharing one's health narrative, which will be explained in detail as we present Joanne's case.

Numerous studies provide evidence of the beneficial outcomes of patient activity. Several investigations have documented that simply coaching patients to ask questions of their health providers can result in increased satisfaction and adherence by the patient to providers' recommendations. A major breakthrough came with studies (e.g., Greenfield, Kaplan & Ware, 1985) that demonstrated a correlation between increased patient question-asking and other forms of involvement during encounters with physicians and improved health outcomes, such as briefer recoveries, decreased discomfort and need for medication, and improvement in chronic symptoms. Patients enacting participative behaviors also receive more information, elicit more support, and may influence the quality of care received from health providers. These results contrast strikingly with documentation of negative outcomes when patients, especially those hampered by the effects of illness, don't have the skills, motivation, or strength to press for clearer explanations from physicians, especially on such important topics as unexpected treatment outcomes and medication side effects, as well as confusion about whom to approach for help (Heymann, 1995).

This brief review of active patient participation sets the stage for examining Joanne's story in detail. For her, active patient participation, enacted through her questions and open communication with her endocrinologist, has the objective of eventually achieving physician–patient mutuality and partnership, as well as improved health outcomes. With this background in mind, we re-enter Joanne's situation based on the health narrative she told to an interviewer. What the research literature does not adequately describe is the process through which a patient works toward a self-perception of being active and in control of her health care. Being an active patient and a partner with one's health provider is not an all-or-nothing nor a once-and-for-all state of affairs. In exploring Joanne's experience in some depth, we are able to glimpse personal development in progress.

JOANNE'S STORY[2]

> At my first visit with Dr. Winner, I wanted to see if he was going to be my doctor, and so I made my usual statements: "My goal here is to be in the best health possible. Diabetes affects everything that I do; it's become a major part of my life. I want you to put me in the grave with all my limbs. In other words, when I go, I want to go with all my limbs if possible, and if that means dying early by age 60, that's fine, just so that I can have all my limbs." He was kind of shocked. In my mind, I was being an optimist and I was pushing it, going for [age] 60, but he just sat back in his chair. I started to go into details, and then he said, "Okay, I understand . . . but I don't think it has to be that way. I'm going to treat you and do these tests and then I'm going to call you back in," and that next visit was when we started to have the open dialogue. . . . The second time that I saw Dr. Winner, I made up in my mind that he was my doctor.

Being able to tell the story of one's sickness to physicians, as well as to family, friends, and coworkers, is another way patients communicate active participation in their health care (Street, 2001). Individuals use story formats to make a disorderly world coherent and to justify their chosen ideas and actions (Bruner, 1990; Fisher, 1987). In addition to sense-making and warranting decisions, illness narratives also serve the functions of asserting control (especially in the case of diseases that seem to defy control), transforming the identity of the storyteller, and building community with fellow sufferers (Arntson & Droge, 1987; Sharf & Vanderford, 2003). During the process of telling the story, the distinct voice and style of the narrator becomes apparent.

In response to the patient's narrating her illness during a medical consultation, the doctor may not listen well or give credit to the patient's rendition. On the other hand, the physician may provide a very understanding hearing of that account and take part in its further development. Thus, a patient's illness narrative may sometimes serve an additional purpose. The patient–physician relationship may be transformed and strengthened as a partnership when both contribute to a mutually understood story of the patient's sickness.

The overarching plotline that Joanne emphasizes within her story is her struggle against diabetes by seeking ways to change her primary health narrative of how she lives and deals with this disease. Diabetes has existed in her family for a long time, and Joanne has witnessed many of its ravages. She speaks of these consequences in a rather matter-of-fact tone, as they are a regular occurrence and a natural part of her existence, even though the topics she talks about are of grave significance to her family and her own health:

> *Joanne:* I found out that I had diabetes at 25. You see, I come from a family of
> diabetics and we call it "the curse." On my mom's side of the family, her
> mother and her father had it. My grandmother was blind all my life, and
> she died of kidney failure as a result of diabetes. Half of my mom's
> brothers and sisters—there are nine of them—have diabetes and related
> illnesses that suggest heart problems and so forth. And on my dad's side of
> the family, it's worse, it's bad. Everybody on my dad's side of the family
> takes insulin and have had parts missing because—
> *Interviewer:* By "parts missing," you mean amputation?

Joanne: Yes. My grandfather had no legs; my dad has no legs, and part of his chest is missing, and part of one hand missing, and he can only see out of one eye, but not very good. Also, my dad's brother has one hand missing, and one leg missing and so forth. And so it goes in the family. There are seven kids on my dad's side of the family; all of them have diabetes.

Stories are not an exact recounting of real-time events, but instead are a re-creation of what happened in a way intended to advance a particular purpose for certain listeners. Narrative construction includes emphasizing certain scenes and sub-plots, while focusing on selected time sequences, motives, and values. Stories are told in the present time about past events, providing opportunities for the narrator to create a certain point of view or perspective. As Joanne adds to the background information about the disease that is central to her life, she describes her family's patterns of behavior with respect to diabetic management as extremely passive. In the process of characterizing her family, their symptoms, and the physicians who have treated them, Joanne identifies a hero (her current physician), villains (other doctors), and by-standers who are both innocent and complicit (her extended family). Most of her family has received care from local doctors, who she perceives as not aggressive enough in their care of diabetes. Joanne prefers a doctor who will take a more vigorous approach to dealing with diabetes, and this has set up a tension between her and the rest of her family members:

And so when I told everybody at the family reunions that I was seeing an endocrinologist on a regular basis and that he demanded that I have lab tests and so forth, they were all shocked. And I told them it's the best thing that's happened because I actually feel good sometimes instead of feeling bad and tired and weak. I feel good, and when I start to feel bad, I know to call him and say, "Okay, something's not right, my sugar levels are out of whack, what's going on here? I need to come in and have this checked." And I said [to the family], "It's good to have an endocrinologist." No one had one, no one had heard of one, and by this time my dad already had one leg amputated, and he had never seen one. Most of us have the same family doctor, and nobody wanted to switch. So, when I started seeing another endocrinologist, it took my dad another year or two to see one.

Human beings are not only storytelling beings (Fisher, 1987), but also "storyliving" creatures (Allison, 1994). Any story about current life experiences shared with others is one in which the narrator is both in the midst of telling and in the midst of living or experiencing. Joanne's account highlights two critical conflicts ongoing in her life. The first is the tension between Joanne and her family regarding the treatment they have received, including her strong feelings toward doctors that she feels are not aggressive enough in their approach to diabetes. Her stance is evident in her discussions regarding actions taken about high cholesterol levels:

And so Dr. Winner showed me what a good cholesterol level was and I was upset, because I didn't find that out until I was 34 years old and, apparently, I've had high cholesterol for the longest time. No one else in the family knew anything about cholesterol being an issue. So when I went home for Christmas I said, "I'm taking Zocor now. Anybody else taking anything for high cholesterol?" And they said, "Oh, no, no, no." I had an aunt that asked, "Is your cholesterol level still running over 400?" And she said, "Well, the last time I went, it was 600 and something. In fact, they're thinking about doing something because of stroke or whatever else." I said, "Thinking about doing something? My doctor is having a cow because I'm at 325 and you're at 600 and something, and they're thinking about doing something?" I said, "I think they're suppose to be doing something."

Joanne wants a relationship with a doctor that is based on sharing of information. As such, she is well prepared when she goes to the doctor, and she expects that the doctor will respond in kind. This active stance that Joanne takes has not always led to good results:

I have questioned doctors in the past and they have gotten upset about it. When I take lists of questions with me to doctors, they say, "What are you doing, auditing me?" I used to be an auditor by trade, and so they say, "Every time you come in, I feel like you're auditing me," and I have to say, "No, I'm not auditing you. I just need to know these things, so I can help you treat me."

With Dr. Winner, Joanne finds someone who is willing to listen, who understands, and who will give her the information that she wants. However, even though Joanne describes herself as a very active patient, there are limits to her participation. The second major conflict evident in Joanne's narrative is her fight with lifestyle choices that contribute to ill health. Throughout her story, she describes herself as being engaged in a struggle to gain control over her diet. She describes food and wine as being her "major vices"; she sees these indulgences as worsening her diabetes, keeping her from reaching her goal of making it through life without amputation, and being a force with which she has to contend. She looks to Dr. Winner as a powerful ally, but also as an authority. Even though she comes to the relationship as a very active communicator, she concedes much power to Dr. Winner in the struggle to contain the food and wine:

> *Interviewer:* Of anybody or anything, where does the control lie with your diabetes?
> *Joanne:* Right now, for the first time in a long time, it's Dr. Winner. Usually, I would say that I am controlled by food and wine because I don't have will power, but now the control is with Dr. Winner because he has information on his side and has been giving me better medications to not only where I feel better; there are medications that are treating both this bad habit that Joanne has and this bad illness that she has. I have the sugar level that he wants me to have and I have the cholesterol level that he wants me to have, which all are major players in diabetes.... Before, other doctors didn't have control over what medication they were giving me, and I didn't have control over my habit or my need or what I thought were my needs. The food and wine had control of the diabetes, and it was going downhill.

Interestingly, even though Joanne credits Dr. Winner as having taken control of her diabetes, at another level, she is the one in charge of choosing who is acknowledged as an expert and with whom she aspires to partner. The power *she* yields is conveyed in an incident she describes in which her doctors give conflicting advice on medications:

> ...we had a battle going between my gynecologist and Dr. Winner.... they have been trying to switch medications for each other and of course, naturally I'm going to go with Dr. Winner's recommendations because I feel best under him.... Well, Dr. Winner said, "The gynecologist didn't think about your kidneys, did he? The medication I started you on is what you need. Which one would you rather have: good kidneys or hair growth?" I said, "Well, you know, I think the good kidneys are a good thing." So, I called the gynecologist and said: "Well no, I'm going with Dr. Winner."

Despite not yet feeling that she can manage diet issues on her own, Joanne visualizes a future in which she will be able to take a more active role in terms of managing her illness:

> Because Dr. Winner and I work so closely together now, that in the future I think I will have more control over the diabetes, which is very important to me. You probably can tell that I'm kind of a control freak. I think in the future I will be able to be a major player in fighting the diabetes.

Thus far, we have highlighted the main issues that constitute Joanne's illness narrative: having diabetes as a consequence of family history, repudiating her family's passivity in dealing with this life-altering and life-threatening disease, setting her own objectives for survivorship, and affirming Dr. Winner, her endocrinologist, as the major authoritative force in coping with diabetes. In our continuing analysis of Joanne's story, we examine the complexities of her ongoing process of changing the plot of her life story and her striving to be a "major player" on her own terms.

THE PLOT THICKENS: INTERLOCKING STORIES

Dr. Winner recognized something in me and he told me, "You're extremely competitive, so, what I want you to do when you go to walking" . . . . I have to walk from the parking garage all the way down to the building that I work in. He was saying, "And how often do you do that?" I told him at least twice a day going and coming. He said, "Well, try to make an exercise out of it." Now I find in the morning that when I get out, you know, I'm looking for that person who's walking fast and [I] say, "I'm going to try and beat this person, see if I can get there before that person does."

In this interview, Joanne portrays what she has been living, a multi-layered story of diabetes. Her family's experience with this disease, strengthened genetically through marriages, constitutes an ongoing epic, affecting successive generations and taking a gruesome toll in quality and length of human life. Given its prevalence, even with the consequences of impairment and premature death, living with severe diabetes has become routinized within Joanne's extended family. Patients' ways of explaining symptoms, causes of disease, and possible remedies are known as explanatory models. An understanding of a patient's explanatory model helps a physician to decide how to approach clinical care with that individual (Kleinman, 1988). The dominant explanatory model within Joanne's family is one of diabetes as hereditary, an unavoidable fate. Driven by this explanation, the family has taken what Joanne considers a comparatively passive and reactive stance in terms of health-seeking behaviors. They see the same family doctor that they have seen for years. That practitioner provides them little information, and what information they have received has sometimes been inaccurate. Even when the family receives updated information from an endocrinologist or from Joanne herself, they usually choose to prioritize the authority of the family doctor. As Joanne's testimony reveals, the results of this routine have been disastrous for her family's well-being. For their part, Joanne and her brother (who also has the disease) cynically refer to diabetes as "the curse":

. . . it's that family curse that we have. . . . And so, yeah, we blame our parents, at least I do. "Couldn't marry a non-diabetic could you? You just had to double—or triple–our chances of getting it [by marrying each other]."

Joanne also describes a transformation of identity triggered by her diagnosis. Although she grew up in the extended family saga of diabetes that included not only the litany of missing limbs but other life-threatening problems ("Who had a stroke or a heart attack since the last family reunion? . . . and we all assume that it is related to the diabetes, and it is"), she considered herself "blessed," thinking she had been spared. However, at age 25, she discovered that she, too, shared the family's fate:

By the time I found out that I had it, it was full blown. I had the same family doctor my dad and everybody else had, who never checked me for it. The doctor that finally told me I had it said, "You probably had it all along because when you walked in the door I could tell, I knew that you were a diabetic."

Not only was Joanne faced with adapting to her illness, she also struggled with a sense of betrayal, having been denied crucial information:

All I wanted to do was try and correct it, and see if there was anything that we could reverse, if I could go back to not being a diabetic. I thought, "I don't want to be like everyone else."

At this point, emplotment, meaning a focus on "what story am I in" (Mattingly, 1998, p. 72) becomes a predominant element in Joanne's narrative. As onset and adaptation to serious illness inevitably cause patients' life stories to change in many ways, how Joanne answers this question mediates between the multiple forces that created who she was and who she has become through the illness and is critical to her ongoing well-being. Joanne made the decision to do all that she could to construct a different plotline for herself than the one enacted by the rest of her family. Her effort was facilitated by changing both the scene and the physician character within her narrative. By moving to another city and searching for an endocrinologist, in lieu of the family doctor, to advise her health care, she very purposely broke with the family epic. Although she was not able to change her diagnosis, she realized that she could change the way in which she lived the experience of illness.

By her own account, Dr. Winner played a key role in helping Joanne find an alternative, more satisfying story. Through the process of narrative collaboration, patient and physician engage in history building versus the more commonly used metaphor of the doctor taking a medical history or gathering data from the patient (Haidet & Paternini, 2003). Together, they developed a plot to "locate desire" (Mattingly, p. 107), that is, to find the motivating factors for Joanne to cope with or overcome the problems engendered by diabetes. For instance, in the excerpt at the beginning of this section, Dr. Winner uses recognition of Joanne's competitive nature to turn a daily walk to and from the parking garage into a race, so that the walk becomes good exercise for her.

At the time that Joanne gave this interview, she had transitioned from a narrative of acceptance to a narrative of struggling for control. At one level, that struggle focused on gaining control of dietary habits. This is a problem facing every individual diagnosed with diabetes. In Joanne's case, as she clearly explains, it is an issue deeply rooted in family traditions and regional culture:

We're from Louisiana. In that area of the country, food and wine will probably be the top two vices for anybody. So, getting diagnosed with diabetes was a big let down for me because I love to cook, and I also collect wines. I love wines. I look at a list of things that they recommend that people should not eat in general and things that diabetics should not eat. I mean everything, if you put those two lists together, everything on them is what we eat on a regular basis in our family.

With this background, it is not surprising that Joanne finds herself in a continuous and difficult effort to make the necessary changes in her dietary lifestyle. She credits Dr. Winner for helping her to find the motivation for coming to grips with her vices. Through her discussions with him, she comes to realize that although she cannot change the genetic script underlying her disease, it is possible for her to change her diet and exercise patterns. Taking charge of these issues can potentially change the outcomes of the diabetes saga for Joanne and allow her to achieve her objectives of living longer and with all her body parts intact.

There is a second angle to be considered in Joanne's narration of struggling for control, namely, the relational perspective. In response to the interviewer's question about where the control for her illness lies, she unhesitatingly states that it is with her physician. Her reasons for acknowledging Dr. Winner in this way are multiple; he provides information that other clinicians have not and he has prescribed medication that helps Joanne to maintain sugar and cholesterol levels in a desirable range. Repeatedly, she confirms her confidence in her endocrinologist:

Dr. Winner is my primary doctor, because sooner or later, everything gets back to him. Whatever doctor I go see is going to talk to him.

Not only does Dr. Winner's advice trump the recommendations of other physicians, to Joanne, he is the counter-balance to her own intrinsic weaknesses:

> He has the most control because he still has to do the prodding. He still has to come in with more and stronger medications because I don't have control of the food and the wine. So, to me, he has the most control over the diabetes, because if he stopped giving me the information and everything I need, then it would be out of hand completely, because I wouldn't have the will power to try to get it under control myself.

The struggle for control as depicted in Joanne's narrative is complex. In the course of telling her story, she makes very clear that she has redefined her life goals in relation to her illness; she has chosen to prioritize Dr. Winner's advice over recommendations from other physicians; she questions and monitors medical information presented to her; and she has made some progress in making lifestyle changes, such as exercising more regularly. In other words, Joanne has exerted a great deal of self-management, using her own resources in coming to grips with her illness, even though she identifies her physician as the person who is in charge.

BRINGING THE STORY TO CONCLUSION: DIFFERENTIATING PARTICIPATION AND PARTNERSHIP

> I want to be happy and have a good life, the best possible life, and that means having good health, if it's possible. I will do what I can and, Dr. Winner, he will do what he can to make sure that happens. His job is to monitor and tell me when I'm getting out of whack, or it will cause potential health problems, or I'm going down the wrong path. . . . His role is to make sure that I can maintain and have good health.

This review of Joanne's health narrative immerses us in details that are, of course, unique to this young woman's disease, family history, and cultural upbringing. Yet, in some important ways, Joanne is emblematic of many people; she longs for a story that ends "happily ever after." Though she is not pleased with herself for lacking sufficient willpower, she sees herself working toward being more in charge of her own health situation, a move that will shift the terms of her relationship with her doctor:

> *Joanne:* . . . he will probably be taking more of the role that he should have; that is, one that comes in only when there's an issue instead of having to monitor all the time. Because it's my disease; I have it. I should be the one because I have the capabilities with the testing machines and whatever that monitor my disease.
> *Interviewer:* So, when that day when you have more control arrives, Dr. Winner will be more of a consultant than a controller?
> *Joanne:* Yeah, and absolutely.

Geist-Martin, Ray, and Sharf (2003) identify communicative competencies that characterize proactive patients. The first of these is agenda-setting, meaning that highly activated patients plan in advance what issues they want to bring to their doctor's attention and state these concerns at the beginning of the interview. Second, this kind of patient takes an active role in sharing information, which means an ability to "tell your story succinctly yet assertively, highlighting those factors that describe your concerns, symptoms, and ideas about what is going on" (p. 334). Third, as mentioned previously, the ability of patients to raise questions with the physician has proven to be one of the most significant and influential communicative acts, including queries about technical terminology or alternative treatment options. On all three counts, Joanne has participated actively with Dr. Winner, as well as other practitioners she with whom she's consulted.

The fourth communication competency involves assuming an active role in negotiating treatment decisions; patients vary as to the extent they wish to be involved in participatory decision making, but the trend is toward increasing involvement (Deber, Kraetschmer, & Irvine, 1996). This is the point with which Joanne finds herself struggling in terms of needing to be directed by the endocrinologist. Eventually, she hopes to be a more proactive self-manager, with Dr. Winner as her consultant. Health empowerment is a state of feeling relatively powerful and in control of one's life on the basis of concentrating time, effort, and personal resources to improve health-related problems (Geist-Martin et al., 2003). Joanne is on her way, but she's not quite there yet.

In fact, Joanne represents many, and perhaps most, patients. Few of us are naturally well equipped to assertively collaborate with our physicians and assume the role of active health decision maker. The communication competencies required need to be further defined, honed, and practiced. People, especially people striving to cope with serious illness, are often not in the best place to counter the centuries-old attitude of deferring to medical experts and making their own opinions, values, and feelings known. At the same time, Joanne represents an increasing population suffering from chronic, ongoing diseases that will persist throughout their lifetimes and must be largely managed in patients' own environments rather than medical facilities. Though challenging, it is especially important for such seriously ill individuals to come to grips with what level of health-related participation and self-management is appropriate for them. Assuming increasing degrees of involvement and self-responsibility tends to occur and improve over time and experience.

Active patient participation, which Joanne is both enacting and striving toward, can be portrayed on two continua: the continuum of engagement with the illness experience, and the continuum of negotiated control with regard to illness decisions. In detailing these two spectrums, we are claiming a distinction about active patient participation that previously has been treated as a single entity.

The sequence of developments represented in each continuum is important conceptually. The first continuum describes the degree to which a person is either engaged with her own illness experience or not. Engagement from this perspective implies a sense that one can influence the course of one's own experience of illness and health-seeking. The opposite of engagement is fatalism, a sense that one's course of illness is predetermined and that no one (not patient, doctor, family, etc.) can change the outcome or the way that the experience will unfold. A state of high passivity makes a collaborative relationship with one's physician irrelevant, because in such a state, control over illness is not achievable. A patient in a state of passivity, therefore, is unlikely to partner with his physician, because health professionals, in the patient's eyes, are helpless as well. At the other end of this continuum is a state of high activity and deep engagement. Individuals at this end have an empowered sense of being able to influence the lived experience of illness, without discounting a realistic perception of what factors are and are not changeable. As her interview documents, Joanne is closer to the active end of the engagement continuum, though she is not yet in the most fully developed position.

Continuum 1: Engagement with the Illness Experience

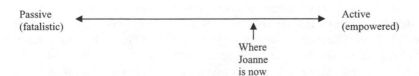

Passive
(fatalistic)   Active
                                                           (empowered)

Where
Joanne
is now

The second continuum describes the spectrum of negotiated partnership in making health care decisions and managing chronic illness. This continuum recognizes that illness presents a series of decisions that can impact the way events will unfold, as well as the meaning of such events. Both patient and practitioner can have varying levels of influence over these decisions. It is important to note that a person can be a very active participant in terms of engagement with the illness and health-seeking experiences (Continuum 1) and still cede much of the influence over health-related decisions to the doctor. In this case, the person is still an active participant by intentionally deciding to confer primary influence on the decision process to the doctor. This is Joanne's current developmental position. She aspires to eventually move nearer to the patient influence end of the continuum, though not to the extreme end; instead, she wants to modify the collaboration she has already established with Dr. Winner.

Continuum 2: Negotiated Partnership in Health Decision Making and Illness Management

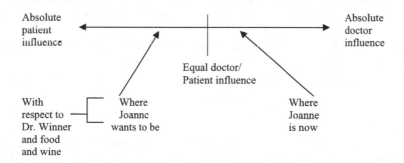

We end this chapter with an observation from a narrative point of view. Joanne ascribes power to Dr. Winner on the basis of his willingness to impart expert information, ability to prescribe helpful medications, and impact in assisting her to adopt more healthy behaviors. In addition to this list, just as important—or perhaps even more important—Dr. Winner has helped Joanne to figure out what story she is in; he has made a huge difference in serving as a coauthor in Joanne's unfolding account. More specifically, she perceives that he has been instrumental in illuminating narrative options, thus enabling her to move from the fatalistic family saga with a predictably tragic conclusion to a more optimistic plotline with feasible alternatives that she can make happen with a potential for a happier ending.

RELEVANT CONCEPTS

Active health participation: An individual's degree of participation in his or her own health care and maintenance, including how engaged one is with her or his own illness or health conditions and how one negotiates control of health care decision making with health care providers.

Emplotment: The process of an individual becoming aware of what life plot or story he or she is enacting at a particular point in time.

Engagement with illness experience: The extent to which an individual senses that he or she can influence the course of one's own experience of illness and health-seeking.

Health narrative: The story of one's illness or health conditions, typically referring to how patients relate such stories to their physicians and other health professionals, family, friends, coworkers, etc.

History building: A new metaphor to describe a physician and patient working together to construct a mutually meaningful explanatory model for understanding the patient's health conditions and how best to approach them. This metaphor contrasts with the traditional metaphors of "history taking" and "data gathering," which imply that the physician is actively eliciting selective pieces of information from the more passive patient.

Partnership between patient and physician: The spectrum of negotiated interactions and relationships enacted by a patient and a physician in making health care decisions and managing chronic illness.

DISCUSSION QUESTIONS

1. How would you describe your own narrative of health and wellness (considering heredity, culture, family events, experiences with health care, etc.; this could be a story about an episode of illness, but it doesn't have to be)? How is your narrative similar to or different from the one that other members of your family tell? In what ways have you adopted or modified that narrative over time?
2. Who are the main characters in your health narrative? How are these characters positioned within your story (heroes, villains, bystanders, victims, etc.)?
3. What functions (i.e., identity transformation, sense-making, exerting control, decision making, building community) has this health narrative served in your experience? What meaning(s) does this narrative imply in terms of your goals and desires for your health and for health care?
4. In reference to the narrative that you previously described, how would you position yourself on Continuum 1? Are you satisfied with this position or do you aspire to be elsewhere? In either case, explain why.
5. Think about the health provider you consider to be most important or influential. In relation to this practitioner, how would you position yourself on Continuum 2? Are you satisfied with this position or do you aspire to be elsewhere? In either case, explain why.
6. Identify a time when you changed a personal behavior in an effort to improve your health and wellness. What information or what person was instrumental in your choice to change the behavior? Were you able to sustain the behavior change?

ACKNOWLEDGMENTS

This project was cofunded by grant number PO1 HS10876 from the Agency for Healthcare Research and Quality and the National Center of Minority Health and Health Disparities. Dr Haidet is supported by a career development award from the Office of Research and Development, Health Services R & D Service, U.S. Department of Veterans Affairs. We are grateful to "Joanne" for contributing her story to this project.

ENDNOTES

[1] Because Joanne's story focuses on her relationship with Dr. Winner, her endocrinologist, we have limited our own review of literature and discussion to the patient–physician relationship, rather than attempting to include all types of practitioners. That said, much of what we discuss is applicable to the full range of clinical providers.

[2] Joanne's story was told in the form of a 90-minute interview, one of several conducted for research examining how patients explain how they live with chronic illness. The interviewer was one of the authors of this chapter (PH).

The interview was audiotaped and later transcribed, resulting in over 30 pages of single-spaced dialogue. In choosing excerpts to tell a brief version of Joanne's story for this chapter, we have been forced to be selective in piecing together quoted remarks, with minor editing of Joanne's original words for purposes of fluency and continuity.

REFERENCES/SUGGESTED READINGS

Allison, J. M. (1994). Narrative and time: A phenomenological reconsideration. *Text and Performance Quarterly, 14*, 108–125.

Arntson P., & Droge, D. (1987). Social support in self-help groups: The role of communication in enabling perceptions of control. In T. Albrecht & M. Adelman (Eds.), *Communicating social support* (pp. 148–171). Newbury Park, CA: Sage.

Bruner, J. (1990). *Acts of meaning.* Cambridge, MA: Harvard University Press.

Deber, R., Kraetschmer, N., & Irvine, I. (1996). What role do patients wish to play in treatment decision-making? *Archives of Internal Medicine, 156*, 1414–1420.

Fisher, W. (1987). Human communication as narration: Toward a philosophy of reason, value, and action. Columbia: University of South Carolina Press.

Geist-Martin, P., Ray, E. B., & Sharf, B. F. (2003). *Communicating health: Personal, cultural, and political complexities.* Belmont, CA: Wadsworth.

Greenfield, S., Kaplan, S. H., & Ware, J. E., Jr. (1985). Patients' participation in medical care: Effects on patient outcome. *Annals of Internal Medicine, 102*, 520–528.

Haidet, P., & Paternini, D. A. (2003). Building a history rather than taking one: A perspective on information sharing during the medical interview. *Archives of Internal Medicine, 163*, 1134–1140.

Heymann, J. (1995). *Equal partners.* Boston: Little, Brown.

Kleinman, A. (1988). The illness narratives: Suffering, healing & the human condition. New York: Basic Books.

Mattingly, C. (1998). Healing dramas and clinical plots: The narrative structure of experience. New York: Cambridge University Press.

Quill, T. E. (1983). Partnerships in patient care: A contractual approach. *Annals of Internal Medicine, 98*, 228–234.

Roter, D. L., & Hall, J. A. (1993). *Doctors talking with patients/patients talking with doctors: Improving communication in medical visits.* Westport, CT: Auburn House.

Roter, D. L., & McNeilis, K. S. (2003). The nature of the therapeutic relationship and the assessment of its discourse in routine medical visits. In T. L. Thompson, A. M. Dorsey, K. I. Miller, & R. Parrott (Eds.), *Handbook of health communication* (pp. 121–140). Mahwah, NJ: Lawrence Erlbaum Associates.

Sharf, B. F. (1984). *The physician's guide to better communication.* Glenview, IL: Scott, Foresman.

Sharf, B. F., & Vanderford, M. L. (2003). Illness narratives and the social construction of health. In T. L. Thompson, A. M. Dorsey, K. I. Miller, & R. Parrott (Eds.), *Handbook of health communication* (pp. 9–34). Mahwah, NJ: Lawrence Erlbaum Associates.

Stewart, M., Brown, J. B., Weston, W. W., McWhinney, I. R., McWilliam, C. L., & Freeman, T. R. (1995). *Patient-centered medicine: Transforming the clinical method.* Thousand Oaks, CA: Sage.

Street, R. L., Jr. (2001). Active patients as powerful communicators: The linguistic foundation of participation in health care. In W. P. Robinson & H. Giles (Eds.), *The new handbook of language and social psychology* (2nd ed., pp. 541–560). Chichester, UK: John Wiley.

Waitzkin, H. (1984). Doctor-patient communication: Clinical implications of social scientific research. *Journal of the American Medical Association, 252*, 2441–2446.

5

Direct Marketing Directs Health Care Relationships?: The Role of Direct-to-Consumer Advertising of Prescription Drugs in Physician–Patient Communication

Rebecca J. Welch Cline
*Barbara Ann Karmanos Cancer Institute/
Wayne State University*

Henry N. Young
University of California, Davis

Today, when we watch television or read our favorite magazines, we are exposed routinely to prescription drug advertising. Direct-to-consumer advertising (DTCA) of prescription drugs arguably functions to provide us with information about medical conditions and treatment options. At the same time, DTCA has sparked heated debate regarding its influence on physician–patient communication and thus on relationships with our physicians. This case explores and illustrates the issues debated among physicians regarding the value of DTCA, and variations in the nature of the advertisements, patients' communication approaches with physicians as a result of exposure to DTCA, and physicians' responses to patients' attempts to communicate with them about advertised products.

BACKGROUND

DTCA is "any promotional effort by a pharmaceutical company to present prescription drug information to the general public through the lay media" (e.g., popular magazines and television; Bradley & Zito, 1997, p. 86). Cline and Young (2004) review the history and growth of DTCA in the United States. Rapidly growing DTCA expenditures and routine exposure of consumers to DTCA suggest its potential for influence. Until the early 1980s, the pharmaceutical industry marketed drugs to physicians via advertising in medical journals and visits from company representatives. In 1981, the industry proposed marketing directly to consumers, arguing its educational benefits. Since then, the Food and Drug Administration (FDA) eased regulations on DTCA, which sparked the exponential growth of by-name advertising of prescription drugs. DTCA spending grew from $25 million in 1988 to more than $2 billion in 2002. From a consumer perspective, DTCA's magnitude lies in the number of advertisements consumers encounter. Popular magazine readers may be exposed to four or more ads in some magazines (e.g., *Better Homes and Gardens, Prevention, Reader's Digest*). Over time, this exposure continues to increase. For example, the February 2003 issue of *Reader's Digest* contained 11 prescription drug ads, several associated with serious medical conditions (e.g., preventing a second heart attack or stroke, treating diabetes and depression). In fact, 15% of the magazine's pages were devoted to DTCA.

DTCA AND THE PHYSICIAN–PATIENT RELATIONSHIP

DTCA's growth has fueled debate regarding its influence on health care. One critical issue centers on DTCA's potential to alter the health care relationship. Both proponents and opponents argue that DTCA is changing the health care relationship from a traditional paternalistic model toward a participatory and possibly consumerism model (Cline & Young, 2004). However, they disagree about the consequences of that change. Arguments vary from DTCA "builds bridges between patients and physicians" (Holmer, 1999, p. 380) to objections that DTCA undermines the relationship and promotes conflict (Hollon, 1999).

Advocates of DTCA predict positive relational and health care outcomes. They argue that DTCA empowers consumers by educating them to recognize symptoms and motivating them to initiate discussions with health care providers about conditions that otherwise may go untreated. Educated patients are better enabled to act as informed decision makers and may be more likely to comply with physicians' recommendations. Informational empowerment yields relational consequences by encouraging patients to take a more active role, thereby equalizing relational control, as they seek partnerships with physicians (e.g., Holmer, 1999). In turn, public health may be improved by enhancing safe and effective treatment of diseases that tend to be underdiagnosed and undertreated.

Opponents see growth in DTCA as driven by financial considerations, representing an alternative marketing strategy. They contend that DTCA offers "information of suspect quality and thus minimal benefit" (Hollon, 1999, p. 382). One key concern is that DTCA will lead to increased consumer demand for medications, yielding greater conflict between provider and patient, with presumed negative consequences for their relationship (Hollon, 1999). The result, opponents argue, is increased health care costs due to greater use of the health care system, prescribing of unnecessary drugs, and resulting adverse medical outcomes. Thus, both sides contend that DTCA influences the health care relationship by encouraging patients to take a more active role in their health care.

The underlying premise of DTCA's influence is that features of the advertisements encourage a more active patient role by suggesting new social norms and training consumers to interact more actively with doctors. Social cognitive theory (Bandura, 1994) helps to explain how DTCA may function in this manner. Through social modeling, individuals observe and learn to associate accompanying rewards with the behavior of others; in turn, those rewards become motivators for the observers' own behavior. Unlike most products, consumers need the cooperation of a third party to purchase prescription drugs. Thus, successful ads must motivate and train consumers to seek and interact appropriately, credibly, and persuasively with physicians. That modeling may occur visually, via text, and by way of "meta-messages" within ads that might motivate patients by associating rewards (instrumental, identity, and relational) with products and suggesting how patients might communicate with their physicians to obtain those products (Cline & Young, 2004).

DOCTORS DEBATE THE ISSUES

Five doctors, who have known each other professionally for many years, are attending a medical association meeting. They just heard a session in which representatives from pharmaceutical companies, physicians, and consumer advocates debated the impact of direct-to-consumer advertising on the physician–patient relationship. Doctors in the audience expressed strong opinions about DTCA, but were split regarding whether the impact was primarily positive or negative. Two of the five doctors had been vocal in the discussion portion of the formal session. Dr. Robert Nelson argued that DTCA ultimately hurts health care by encouraging patients to demand inappropriate medications, thereby placing undue pressure on physicians, resulting in faulty prescribing practices. In contrast, Dr. Peter Smith contended that doctors meet patients' health care needs better as a result of DTCA because the advertising gets patients interested in their health care and committed to carrying out mutually determined treatment regimens. When the meeting broke up Drs. George Capel and Joseph Callahan walked up to Drs. Nelson and Smith, who were continuing the debate. George interrupted, saying: "OK fellas, clearly we aren't all going to agree on this, but I bet we can agree to find a good steak house with some fine wine where we can do some catching up and continue this debate too." They agreed to meet for dinner.

The scene is a restaurant near the convention center. When the doctors met at the restaurant, Peter was accompanied by a fifth physician, Dr. Katherine Wallace. Peter said, "You all know Katherine." The other doctors greeted Katherine warmly, having known and respected her for years. Peter continued, "I ran into Katherine after that last meeting and she knows something about this drug advertising issue. I thought she should join us and throw in her two cents worth."

The doctors get a table, order some red wine, and spend much of the dinner catching up on events of the past year in their personal lives and professional practices. As the doctors talk, conversation returns to the DTCA debate. "You know," said George, "I feel like my practice really is changing. And I think part of it has to do with those drug ads. They put pressure on me and on how I practice medicine. I don't really see all of the benefits some of you claim." The doctors returned to the issue, debating the pros and cons of DTCA.

The group got on a roll about the down side of DTCA. Bob chimed in, "Drug advertising is causing some problems with our patients. Not only that, I think many doctors probably practice worse medicine as a result, present company excepted, of course!"

"Well, I do agree that the ads make some people think there is a 'pill for every ill,'" argued Peter. "They want a 'magic' formula, an easy solution, instead of exploring other ways of improving their health where they might actually have to make some personal effort."

"It's worse than that," said Joe. "It used to be that my patients understood that *I* had been to medical school, spent years in residency, and actually *knew* something more than *they* did about medicine. Now it seems like they all think *they* are the doctors and we just need to write the prescriptions. I get tired of patients' disrespect and distrust. I wish they would just let *me* do the doctoring. Most of them really don't know what they are talking about and just pick up on stuff from the ads. They don't understand the technical material and waste my time with questions. It's frustrating and pretty *insulting* too!"

"But you know," Peter countered, "when patients ask questions because of seeing ads, it seems they really want to have a conversation. To me, they seem more motivated to understand and participate in their care than to ride roughshod over me. I can't tell you how many times those 'pesky' questions led me to pay more attention to their symptoms; I probably made a quicker diagnosis too, which means they got on with their treatment more quickly and didn't have to come back a second or third time. You can bet the HMOs like *that*!"

"I know those advertising questions can seem annoying," Bob agreed, "but I also think we have to resist changing how we prescribe just because a patient sees an ad or asks a question."

"Sometimes they may just want to get information or understand why a drug *isn't* the right thing for them. I think it's a *good* thing when patients show interest in their care, even if we don't agree with what they may propose. We just need to stick to our guns when they ask for something we know isn't appropriate," Joe continued the benefits argument. "And of course, if we diagnose more accurately and more quickly, and if the patients themselves feel like they've had a say, then we end up with healthier patients who are costing the health care system less. That's just good business sense."

George sensed the conversation had gotten away from recognizing problems with the ads themselves. "Wait a minute, though," he said, "we're talking about the patients, but the ads really *cause* those problems. They're misleading and inaccurate; they leave out a lot of the risks or make them sound like minor issues but make the drug seem effective; that's unrealistic and is simply false advertising."

"I think what happens then," said Bob, "is we get all of these questions about drugs, often not suited to the particular patient, and then we feel pressured to prescribe what they seem to be 'demanding.' I know I sometimes feel conflict between what patients say they want and what I know is good medicine."

George added, "And *that*, my friends, is the crux of the matter. We may not be able to practice good medicine without running the risk that patients will be disappointed or go find another doctor who *will* prescribe what they want."

"But one way to look at those ads," countered Peter, "is that they really do inform and educate our patients. Because of the ads, and some other factors too, like the Internet, they often know a great deal more when they come to see us than they used to. I think it's easier to explain our medical reasoning to informed patients who *want* to play a role in their care than to the patients we see who don't offer up relevant information or ask questions; then we feel like we're trying to solve a medical mystery without some of the clues we depend on our patients to give us."

Peter suddenly realized that the men had been vocal but that Katherine hadn't said a word; he knew from an earlier conversation that she actually knew quite a bit about DTCA, how it works and the effects it has. Turning to her, he said, "You know, you're really the expert here. I understand that you have researched drug advertising and spoken at many meetings. What's your take on advertising drugs directly to patients?"

Katherine paused, "Well, you should know that all of you have made the same points that have been debated in major medical journals over the past couple of years. There's a lot of conflict on this issue, so it's not surprising that you don't all agree. Plus this is a relatively new thing for us as doctors. As we all know, the pharmaceutical companies used to rely entirely on drug reps and ads in medical journals as a way of letting us know about new products and trying to persuade us to use them. It seems like the economics of health care means those companies have figured out that they may be able to have even *greater* influence on us by advertising directly to consumers, especially at a time managed care is trying to keep costs down."

"Don't you think," George jumped in, "that this is just an economic boon to the industry and really has nothing to do with good medicine?"

"Yeah," said Joe, "and in the course of things, we're losing our authority as doctors!"

"Hang on a second, fellows, let's hear what Katherine has to say. She really knows this stuff better than we do," Peter said.

Bob jumped in too and said, "Yes, I'd really like to know more. We all have opinions but, like medicine itself, there must be some evidence about advertising's actual effects. Tell us what you know, Katherine."

"OK guys, just understand that we really don't have a lot of direct evidence yet about DTCA's effects. We all know that the ad companies have figured out some ways to try to influence consumers. They give consumers information about medical conditions and drugs for treating those conditions, as Peter said; those ads do some other important things too. Drug ads are chock full of cues that attract patients to the ads and then to the particular drugs. Some research shows that the ads repeatedly make connections between the drug and things people value, especially two things. Through the pictures and text in the ads, the drug companies connect taking a particular drug to being the kind of person the consumer wants to be, such as healthy, active, and happy. Those ads also imply that patients gain some relational benefits by using the particular drug. The pictures show people interacting with family, friends, or coworkers. So the ads seem to be saying that patients can have better self-images and better social lives by using the advertised drugs. Besides that, I bet you've noticed that the ads actually tell patients what to say or how to talk to their doctors. It's no wonder we think communication with patients has changed. In most ads, you'll see several statements telling patients to ask certain questions about the drug or talk to their doctors about certain symptoms."

George responded impatiently, "OK, that's all fine and dandy; they've figured out how to market products successfully. But what about the effects on how patients act when they see us?"

"That's the big question of course," Katharine replied. "We do know that patients pay attention to DTCA and that they are using information from the ads as a way to start conversations with their doctors. I saw one study that said that the majority of patients think DTCA contains the information they need to talk with their doctors; of course, that's what they *think*, not necessarily actually the case! Ironically, although many doctors really *hate* these ads, most of us docs agree that the advertising is encouraging patients to be more active in their health care. So, it may come down to whether we think that is a good thing or not." There was a pause as the group digested this last point.

Bob returned to the quality of prescribing issue. "We've talked a lot about the effects of the ads on patients' communication. But do you know anything about how docs' prescribing behavior might ultimately be affected? That's what concerns me, that we not trade off good medicine just to satisfy our patients."

"Again," replied Katharine, "the research doesn't show a direct effect. But it does say that doctors have become more willing to prescribe what patients request, or at least to consider those requests seriously. I know, in my own practice, I try to use those requests and questions as a basis for understanding my patients' concerns. It gives them a way of interacting more with me; after all, being a patient with folks like us really can be intimidating!" They laughed as they recognized that while they were feeling vulnerable to the effects of DTCA, their patients routinely feel vulnerable in their health care conversations.

"After all," concluded Bob, "we are the ones in control of prescriptions. No matter how pushy patients are, *we* are the only ones who can prescribe."

"Well, gentlemen, it's been an enjoyable evening," said Katherine.

"You have some good insights about these issues; thanks for sharing them," offered Bob.

"You've given us some things to think about," admitted George; Joe nodded in agreement. Although these doctors disagreed about the role of DTCA in health care, they had aired significant issues found not only among their individual practice experiences, but also in debates published in major medical journals.

THE CASES: DTCA AND PHYSICIAN–PATIENT COMMUNICATION

Executive "Orders"?

John Nixon, a 55-year-old white male, is an executive officer of a top Fortune 500 business. His major responsibilities involve overseeing day-to-day operations that are vital to the success of the company. John's job is extremely stressful and time consuming; however, he enjoys his work, as well as the power and status that accompany his position. John's personality fits the stereotype of a "driven" executive; he is domineering and controlling, in both his professional and personal lives.

Background.   During a flight while traveling for business, Mr. Nixon briefly flips through the latest issue of *Time*. While scanning the magazine, he sees an advertisement for the prescription medication Viagra and pauses for a second, thinking to himself, "I heard that this stuff spices up your love life." The ad shows a man and a woman, dressed in evening attire, dancing in what appears to be a ballroom. Both are smiling broadly and appear joyful and animated. The advertisement states only the name of the medication, "Viagra (sildenafil citrate) tablets," and "Let the dance begin."

Glancing at the Viagra advertisement, Mr. Nixon thinks that lately his sex life with his wife hasn't been as fulfilling as he would like and that Viagra may be the perfect remedy. He decides to see his physician for a prescription. As soon as his flight permits telephone use, Mr. Nixon contacts his secretary to make an appointment with his doctor for the next day.

The Doctor Visit.   A few minutes after being seen by the nurse, Dr. Robert Nelson walks into the examination room and says, "Mr. Nixon, how are you today?"

"Just fine, Dr. Nelson," Mr. Nixon replies.

"That's good. So, what brings you in today?"

In a concerned but somewhat demanding tone, Mr. Nixon says, "Dr. Nelson, after 30 years of marriage, I need a little something extra; I want a prescription for Viagra."

Dr. Nelson responds, "Many men are using Viagra for erectile dysfunction. I know this can be a difficult problem to talk about. But I have to ask, can you achieve an erection?"

Sounding indignant and authoritarian, Mr. Nixon responds, "Yes! *I am in control of my body.* My *only* problem is that my sex life has lost some of its luster; it's just not what it used to be and Viagra should help. I don't have any other health problems, so if you'll just give me the prescription we both can get on to more important matters."

Dr. Nelson replies calmly, although feeling somewhat taken aback, "Mr. Nixon, Viagra is used to treat erectile dysfunction. From what you have told me, fortunately you do not have problems attaining an erection; therefore, this drug would not help you."

Mr. Nixon raises his voice, "Look, Dr. Nelson, I know what I need. Just give me a prescription for Viagra!"

Dr. Nelson pauses to gather his thoughts, noting that his patient is not going to be happy with his decision. "I would be irresponsible if I gave you a prescription for a medication that I have no reason to believe will be beneficial. All medications have the potential for side effects and can be harmful. It's inappropriate to use a medication without a valid indicator. I'm sorry."

After arguing with Dr. Nelson briefly, Mr. Nixon storms out of the office without a prescription and begins thinking about making an appointment with another doctor.

Heartburn and Professional Heartache?

Anna Klowicky is a 32-year-old restaurant critic for a major newspaper in a large metropolitan area. She suffers from heartburn. This poses a serious problem, as Anna's job requires her to sample a variety of ethnic cuisines that often are inappropriate for her medical condition. Currently, Anna is taking Prilosec, which recently changed from a prescription to an over-the-counter medication. It provides her with excellent relief. She had obtained her prescription for Prilosec after seeing several specialists and finally finding one who gave her the medication she wanted.

Background.   After work, Anna enjoys relaxing on her porch and talking with her neighbor, Flo Johnson. One evening, Flo asked, "Anna, how's your heartburn doing?"

Anna replied, "Oh, its all right, I haven't had many problems lately. And yours?"

Flo said, "No problem at all, not since I tried that new drug. I think it's called Nexium. Seems to work better for me than Prilosec did."

Anna perks up, "Really? I've been taking Prilosec awhile; maybe I should try the stuff you are on."

Thumbing through an issue of *Better Homes and Gardens* a few minutes later, Flo says, "Look, here it is; yep, it's Nexium" and showed Anna an advertisement. The headline of the advertisement says, "Today's purple pill is Nexium, from the makers of Prilosec." The advertisement depicts a woman with a slight smile holding a Nexium pill. The body of the advertisement reads, "Relieve the heartburn. Heal the damage. For many, it's possible with Nexium. If you suffer from persistent heartburn 2 or more days a week, even though you've treated it and changed your diet, it may be due to acid reflux disease. And that can be serious. Because, over time, acid reflux can erode or wear away the delicate lining of your esophagus (erosive esophagitis). Only a doctor can determine if you have this damage. Control heartburn for 24 hours. For many people, prescription Nexium—once daily—provides complete resolution of heartburn symptoms and heals damaging erosions of the esophagus caused by acid reflux disease. Your results may vary. Talk with your doctor or health care professional to see if Nexium is right for you. Most erosions heal in 4 to 8 weeks with Nexium. The most common side effects of Nexium and Prilosec are headache, diarrhea, and abdominal pain. Symptom relief does not rule out serious stomach conditions. For a FREE Trial Offer call 1-888-PURPLEPILL. purplepill.com." After seeing the ad, Anna decided to visit her physician.

The Doctor Visit.   "Good afternoon Anna, how are you doing today?" Dr. Joseph Capel says as he enters the examination room.

Anna replies, "I'm doing just fine."

"What can I do for you today?"

"Well, Dr. Capel, my neighbor has heartburn like I do and she's taking this new drug, Nexium and she says it's better than Prilosec. She even showed me an advertisement that said that I should talk to you to see if Nexium is right for me. So, here I am. I would like to try it."

Dr. Capel asks, "Well Anna, how are you doing with the Prilosec? Is it relieving your heartburn?"

Anna replies, dismissively, "Oh, it's fine. It's taking care of my acid reflux too."

"Are you experiencing any problems due to taking Prilosec?" Dr. Capel asks.

"No, I'm not having any problems with Prilosec. I just want to take the best medication available so my heartburn doesn't get worse."

"Anna," says Dr. Capel, "you're doing fine with Prilosec; it seems to be taking care of your heartburn. There's no need to change your medication if it's working well."

"But Dr. Capel," Anna pleaded, "Nexium is working *great* for my neighbor; she has the exact same thing I do! I want to try it."

Flustered, Dr. Capel pauses for a second and ponders. He reminds himself that business is not going as well as it should, the economy continues to get worse, and he doesn't want to risk losing any more patients. Just last week a patient who asked for an inappropriate prescription threatened to "find a better doctor." Dr. Capel says, while writing, "All right, I'll write a script for Nexium. Take one pill a day as needed." He hands the prescription to Anna as he questions whether he has done the right thing.

An Easy Fix vs. Lifestyle Changes?

Clarence Powell is a 48-year-old African American. He is 5 feet, 11 inches tall and weighs about 250 pounds. Mr. Powell is a manager of a telemarketing firm. His job entails overseeing 35 employees, reviewing telephone logs, and negotiating contracts with potential clients. Mr. Powell spends the majority of his time at work behind a desk, with very little physical activity.

Background.   After work, Clarence relaxes at home by sitting on his couch, eating a continuous meal, reading sports magazines (he occasionally makes friendly wagers on sports teams with people at work), and watching television. Clarence's continuous meals often begin with a snack of pretzels or potato chips while waiting for dinner. Later, Clarence enjoys a big dinner. His wife, Mary, is an excellent soul-food cook. She likes to prepare Clarence's favorite foods often, deep-fried chicken, pork chops or stewed oxtails. Clarence ends the evening with dessert, typically huge pieces of cake or pie.

Recently, Mr. Powell was required to have a physical examination for his job's new insurance program. He received a written report indicating that his cholesterol levels were slightly elevated. A cautionary note on the report said that high cholesterol could lead to serious health problems and advised Clarence to consult with his personal physician about how to reduce his cholesterol levels. Clarence's first thought was, "But I feel fine!" But he decided to see his doctor anyway just to be sure, hoping to take care of this problem before it got worse. The next day, Clarence made a doctor's appointment for the following Tuesday at 3:00 p.m.

The night before his doctor's appointment, Clarence engaged in his usual routine, enjoying an after-dinner snack, inattentively watching television, and skimming through the latest issue of *Sports Illustrated*. Clarence's attention was captured by an advertisement for Lipitor, a prescription medication that lowers cholesterol levels.

Clarence noticed that the advertisement said something about talking to your doctor to get more information about Lipitor. The ad actually contained four separate references to communicating with a doctor about Lipitor, including a large heading, featured over a picture of a pair of dice that showed the numbers 290 and 220. The heading read, "If You're Trying to Lower Your Cholesterol, But Your Numbers Still Come Up High . . . Ask Your Doctor for the Lowdown On Lipitor." The advertisement stated that Lipitor, "in combination with diet and exercise, was proven in clinical studies to reduce LDL 'bad' cholesterol by 39%–60%," and that "Lipitor is prescribed more than any other cholesterol medication." The advertisement also contained a graph showing that Lipitor lowers total cholesterol, LDL ("bad" cholesterol), and triglycerides. Clarence decided to talk to his physician about taking Lipitor.

The Doctor Visit.   Clarence arrived for his appointment at his physician's office 5 minutes early. Clarence's physician, Dr. Peter Smith, is usually prompt in seeing patients at appointed times. Clarence has been seeing Dr. Smith for about 20 years, and they have established a pleasant and open relationship. Both are big sports fans and they usually spend the first couple of minutes of each appointment talking about the latest sports news.

Shortly after the nurse finished taking Clarence's vitals, Dr. Smith entered the examination room. "Clarence, how about those Buccaneers?"

"They were just too strong. The Bucs' defense totally dominated the game. I knew they were good, but I didn't know they were that good."

Nodding his head in agreement, Dr. Smith replied, "You said it. And it was the head coach's first year with the team; what a job he did!" After a couple of minutes of sports banter, Dr. Smith said, "Enough about football, Clarence, what brings you in today?"

"Well, Doc, my job just changed insurance companies and the new insurance program required us to take a physical to get on the insurance plan. We had to go to their clinic for the physicals, that's why I didn't see you. I got this report in the mail that says I have high cholesterol and that I should see you to get some help to reduce my cholesterol before something bad happens."

"Oh, I see." replied Dr. Smith. "Let me take some blood so I can run some tests to find out how high your cholesterol levels are, and we'll go from there."

"Doc, maybe there's no need," Clarence said confidently. "I saw an ad in a magazine for a drug called Lipitor. It said that I can take my 'Bad cholesterol numbers to new lows' by using Lipitor."

"Yes, Lipitor can help reduce your cholesterol levels," Dr. Smith answered in a calm tone. "However, before we start you on any medication, we need to know more about your cholesterol levels."

Bewildered, Clarence asked, "What else do you need to know, Doc? The tests said that my cholesterol was slightly high, and that if I didn't take care of it, something bad might happen."

"This is true. *High* cholesterol levels *can* lead to major health problems. But first, I need to see your test results. Depending on the levels, we can devise a plan to help reduce your cholesterol. You said that the tests indicated that your cholesterol levels were slightly high. If the levels aren't too high, we could probably control your cholesterol just by changing your diet and exercise. That way you could avoid using prescription medications and still reduce risks associated with high cholesterol."

"Great!" Clarence said aloud. He thought to himself, "Maybe I can take care of this problem without spending money on prescription drugs; our budget has been tight enough lately."

"So Clarence, if it's ok with you, I will have you come back in the morning so we can draw some blood so we can get those test results."

"Sure, Doc. No problem," Clarence replied.

I Want to Crawl Again: A Question Perceived as a Demand?

Ruth Fairchild is a 65-year-old Caucasian female and a retired physical education teacher. When Ruth decided to retire at age 55, she was concerned about what her life would be like without work. Ruth soon found a variety of things to keep her busy. She became active in her community, participating in programs like Habitat for Humanity and Meals on Wheels.

Background.   When Ruth turned 61 years old, her daughter Cathy had a beautiful baby girl named Cynthia. Ruth fell head-over-heels in love with Cynthia the moment she laid eyes on her. From that point on, Ruth decided that Cynthia would be her first concern. For the next few months, Ruth spent night and day with Cathy and the baby, sharing her experience as a mother and providing Cathy with day-to-day help taking care of the baby.

When Cathy returned to work, Ruth offered to care for the baby during the day. This saved Cathy from paying for day care and gave Ruth great satisfaction. While the baby was still quite young, Ruth spent the day reading books to her and taking her on walks through the local neighborhood park, first in a stroller and later in a little red wagon. When Cynthia began to walk and, all too soon, to run, Ruth began to do more activities with Cynthia that required greater physical strength and endurance. However, at age 63, Ruth's own body had changed as well. Her knee joints began to ache, bothering her to the point of preventing her from engaging in the physical activities she had done routinely until recently. Ruth had begun experiencing stiffness in her knees after sitting with the baby for long periods of time and soon began to have trouble keeping up with the active child. Ruth discussed her condition with her neighbor, a nurse by profession. Ruth's neighbor told her that she might be experiencing the early stages of osteoarthritis and advised her to see a doctor. All of her life, Ruth hated going to the doctor, so two years have passed since Ruth began having problems with her knees, and her condition has deteriorated. Ruth frequently experiences swelling, pain, and loss of motion in her knees, severely limiting her ability to engage in physical activities with her granddaughter. Sometimes, Ruth feels helpless as well as depressed by her condition. Finally, she decides to seek medical attention.

The Doctor Visit.   Ruth arrived at the doctor's office early and sat in the waiting room. A few minutes later, a nurse informed Ruth that Dr. Joseph Callahan was backed up and would see her in about 20 minutes. Waiting anxiously, Ruth picks up an issue of *Reader's Digest.*

Flipping through the pages, Ruth sees a picture of an older woman on her hands and knees, giving her young grandson a ride on her back. A quote in large type reads, "I can crawl again!" A statement at the top of the picture says, "The remarkable treatment for the pain of osteoarthritis of the knee." Ruth thinks, "I used to be able to do that. Maybe this is what I need." The rest of the ad reads, "Now you can get up to 12 months of pain relief with just 1 month of treatment. No pills to take—just five injections into the knee, spaced over a single month. Makes daily living easier and more comfortable—contains a natural substance that acts like an 'oil' to help cushion and lubricate your knee joint. Easy on your system—avoids the side effects of prescription-strength arthritis drugs. [In small print] Available only from your doctor. As with any injection, you may feel temporary mild pain at the injection site. You may also have swelling, heat and/or redness, rash, itching or bruising around the joint. These reactions are generally mild and usually do not last long. Duration and degree of pain relief will vary; not all patients will experience relief. HYALGAN is used to relieve pain due to osteoarthritis of the knee in patients who do not get adequate relief from simple pain killers and physical therapy, including exercise. HYALGAN should not be used in patients with known hypersensitivity to hyaluronate preparations." After reading the advertisement, Ruth decides to take the ad in with her just in case she wants to show it to Dr. Callahan.

The nurse calls Ruth in and takes her vitals. A few minutes later Dr. Callahan enters the examination room.

"Good to see you, Mrs. Fairchild, it's been a long time."

"Yes, Dr. Callahan. You may not remember, but I don't enjoy going to see doctors, only when I really need help."

"So what's going on?"

"Well, about two years ago, the joints in my knees began giving me problems, and now my knees are so bad that my daily activities are extremely limited."

Dr. Callahan takes a clinical history, performs a physical examination, and decides to take x-rays to do a full evaluation of the knee area. After looking at the x-ray films, he says, "It looks like you've developed osteoarthritis. That's a common type of arthritis also called degenerative joint disease. It has affected the cartilage in your knees. Cartilage is the slippery tissue that covers the ends on bones. Osteoarthritis breaks down and wears away cartilage, causing the bones to rub together. That's what is causing the pain, swelling, and loss of motion in your knee."

"Well, Dr. Callahan, can you treat it?"

"Yes, osteoarthritis treatment involves exercise, weight control, rest and joint care, pain relief techniques, medicines, alternative therapies, and, in the worst case scenario, surgery."

"You mentioned medications. I have this advertisement here." Ruth pulls out the issue of *Reader's Digest* and shows Dr. Callahan the advertisement for Hyalgan. "What do you think about this drug?"

Dr. Callahan reads the advertisement quickly. From previous experience with patients and DTCA, Dr. Callahan assumes that Ruth is asking for a prescription for Hyalgan. He thinks, "I'm so tired of these advertisements pushing my patients to demand drugs from me. I'm the one who has to deal with them; they are such an interference." Dr. Callahan says, "Mrs. Fairchild,

I know that some of these ads can be very persuasive; however, not all of the drugs are right for all situations. I'm sorry, but I cannot give you a prescription for this drug. We'll start with an exercise program and some pain killers."

"Dr. Callahan, I'm sorry if I offended you. I wasn't *asking* for a prescription for this drug. I just wanted to know what you thought. I saw this ad while waiting to see you and remembered that the drug treats osteoarthritis. I thought this might give you some ideas about what I can use to treat my knees. All I wanted was to know is if this or some other drug might help me so I can do the things I really want to do."

Researcher Meets Physician

Jessica Carter, a 53-year-old Caucasian female, is a university professor in health communication. She has studied physician–patient communication and is dedicated to being in a partnership with her providers. Dr. Carter has conducted research about DTCA for several years and knows that requesting a specific drug may not be appreciated by the doctor. What she does not know is that her physician also has a professional interest in DTCA.

Background. Dr. Carter has been experiencing migraine headaches, associated with her menstrual cycle, for several years. They have become increasingly severe, lasting from 3 to 5 days, and often are debilitating when they coincide with other stressors. Otherwise healthy, she has seen Dr. Katherine Wallace primarily for routine checkups. Jessica mentioned the headaches in the past, and Dr. Wallace suggested stress-management techniques and, most recently, prescribed an estrogen patch for Jessica to use during the "off week" of her oral contraceptives, when the headaches predictably occur. These efforts have gone for naught; the headaches persist. Jessica is desperate for a solution. She talks with a colleague who experiences similar headaches; they discuss things they have tried. The colleague suggests a supplement; Jessica tries that and it alleviates the headache somewhat, but only for a couple of hours; the headache returns later in the day. The colleague later tells Jessica that she might try Imitrex, a drug she has found helpful. One day at work, Jessica has a headache that is rapidly increasing in severity. The colleague offers her a sample of Imitrex. Jessica checks out Imitrex on a federal health website before taking it. She finds no contraindications that apply to her. Miraculously, the headache disappears within the hour and does not return in the remaining days when typically it would persist or recur. Jessica determines that she will ask her doctor for a prescription for Imitrex.

In the intervening weeks, Jessica notices an advertisement for Imitrex in *Time* magazine. The large print reads, "Break through migraine pain with IMITREX. Stay alert and active. Most prescribed migraine medicine in the U.S." Further on, the text explains the benefits of the drug as "nonsedating" and says "Ask your doctor if IMITREX is right for you." The ad also explains, "You should not take IMITREX if you have certain types of heart or blood vessel disease, a history of strokes or TIAs, or uncontrolled blood pressure. Very rarely, certain people, even some without heart disease, have had serious heart-related problems." But the ad also includes a toll-free number the reader can call for a "free trial" of IMITREX. Jessica knows that the ads are required to identify risks and, because she has no history of the mentioned contraindications, remains confident that IMITREX is the solution for her migraines. Jessica also noticed the drug being advertised on television; that ad reinforced her view that Imitrex was both effective and safe.

The Doctor Visit. Jessica's office visit is routine. As she typically does, following the examination, Dr. Wallace sits down for a couple of minutes of what always seems to Jessica more like a conversation with a friend than a medical consultation.

Dr. Wallace says, "Everything seems fine. We'll run your routine blood tests and let you know the results. What else should we be talking about today?"

"You know," Jessica replied, "I have been having these menstrual migraine headaches over the past few years. Last time you prescribed an estrogen patch. Unfortunately, that hasn't helped. I really am ready to try something stronger. These headaches have been debilitating several times in the past six months and I'm getting desperate."

"Let me do some checking about some possible drugs for you, OK?" asked Dr. Wallace.

Jessica stopped her and said, "Well, I hate to admit this because I know it's not a good idea generally, but I got a sample of Imitrex from a friend who has the same problem."

"Oh, everyone does that," Dr. Wallace said reassuringly. "Did it help?"

"Did it ever! Not only did my headache go away, it didn't return over the next few days. Just one dose took it out completely. I checked Imitrex out on Healthfinder before I took it; I didn't see anything that sounded problematic."

"Wow! That's great!" said Dr. Wallace. "Just let me check my PDR and see if there is anything we should be concerned about."

Dr. Wallace left the room for a few minutes; she returned with a slight frown on her face. She said, "You aren't going to believe this! I don't think I've ever seen this for another drug. The *PDR* recommends a cardiovascular evaluation *before* prescribing Imitrex and suggests that the first dose should be taken *in the doctor's office*!"

Jessica, crestfallen, says, "Oh, no, and I checked for problems."

"Yea, this sucks, doesn't it?" said Dr. Wallace sympathetically. "But it says there have been some problems with strokes and we don't want you stroking-out over just a headache."

"But these aren't *just* headaches! They are debilitating for several days several times a year," explained Jessica, sounding frustrated.

"Well, this *is* the *PDR*, which is going to be cautious, but I think this means we need to get you a cardiovascular checkup. You probably ought to have one about now anyway," offered Dr. Wallace.

"I know," admitted Jessica. "I just hoped we had a solution." Then she chuckled and explained, "You know why I laughed? I *study* this stuff! Some of my research is on direct-to-consumer prescription drug advertising,"

"Really?" asked Dr. Wallace.

Jessica continued, "This drug is advertised on television! And I *know* they don't say those kinds of things in the ads!"

Dr. Wallace retorted, "Yep. If they can't get the docs to prescribe a drug, they go straight to the patient!"

"One thing I just remembered," said Jessica. "The only other thing that ever worked for me was a sample of a drug my previous doctor gave me one day when I was going out the door. They didn't even put it in my records but I remember that it contained both caffeine and a barbiturate. I used it sparingly, a fraction of a pill at a time, because I can be pretty sensitive to drugs and I knew this was a serious drug. That worked. But I never was able to get the drug's name from that doctor," sighed Jessica.

"Well, I'm pretty sure I know what drug that is; let me check, but I think it's Fiorinal; that's a common treatment for stress headaches. I'll check, but I think we could give you a small amount to get you through the next couple of cycles until we have time to get that cardiovascular evaluation."

"Great, I've really been suffering," said Jessica, relieved.

"How long have you been having these now, several years right? I think if I were you I'd be ready to string my doctors up by now," said Dr. Wallace. "I *am* comfortable giving you *this* drug."

Jessica admitted she wasn't so sure she wanted Imitrex, given what the *PDR* said, but Dr. Wallace assured her that "Imitrex is a good drug; we just want to be careful about risk factors."

"Maybe this other drug will work and I won't need Imitrex anyway, but I'll get that cardiovascular evaluation anyway," reasoned Jessica. "I really appreciate you trying less drastic treatments first; I've just gotten to the point that I can't *take* these headaches anymore. I'm glad you're willing to work with me on this."

THE DEBATE CONTINUES

The physicians' debate and the five cases involving patients reflect the potential for DTCA to influence the physician–patient relationship and their communication. Although the ads themselves have been studied and research notes changing patterns both in communication between physicians and their patients regarding advertised drugs and in the nature of the health care relationship, future research needs to study the direct links between DTCA and those changes. Meanwhile, the debate continues.

RELEVANT CONCEPTS

Consumerism: A model of the physician–patient relationship in which the patient (consumer) takes a business orientation and holds the primary decision-making authority; the doctor's role consists of an expert being consulted by the patient.

Direct-to-consumer advertising: A marketing strategy by which the pharmaceutical industry promotes prescription drugs directly to consumers.

Health care relationship models: Prototypes of the relationship between health care providers and their clients (often labeled doctor–patient relationships).

Identity appeals/motivators: Persuasive cues that may appeal to or motivate behavior on the basis of how an individual sees himself or herself or would like to be seen by others (self-presentation; e.g., enhance perception of being friendly, likeable, attractive).

Instrumental appeals/motivators: Persuasive cues that may appeal to or motivate behavior on the basis of a task orientation, that is, provide a rational task-based reason for action (e.g., improve health, reduce symptoms).

Modeling: Behavior change that results from imitating others' behavior observed to result in rewards or avoidance of punishment.

Participatory health care model: Also called mutual participation model. A model of the physician–patient relationship in which the provider and the patient share control of decision making.

Paternalism: A model of the physician–patient relationship in which the provider holds primary control of decision making; the patient's role is to cooperate with the doctor's decisions.

Relational appeals/motivators: Persuasive cues that may appeal to or motivate behavior on the basis of desired relational outcomes (e.g., trust, intimacy, connectedness).

Relational control: Holding definitional authority within the relationship.

Social cognitive theory: A social influence theory developed by Albert Bandura that explains behavior change in terms of rewards associated with observed behavior that, in turn, become motivators for imitating (modeling) that behavior.

DISCUSSION QUESTIONS

1. Discuss how the cases might be understood and explained using social cognitive theory. Identify examples of motivators (identity, relational, and instrumental) and modeling cues from the specific advertisements, and consider (a) how these might have influenced the patients' behavior in the cases, and (b) how such cues might influences consumers' behavior in general.

2. Discuss ways in which the dynamics of relational control and the nature of the specific doctor–patient relationship (a) were potentially altered by the patients' exposure to DTCA in the cases, and (b) might be altered in general as consumers are exposed repeatedly over time to a large number of prescription drug advertisements. Consider differences in physicians' responses to drug requests based on the relationship model preferred by the physician (i.e., paternalism, participatory, consumerism).

3. How might differences in patients' ways of approaching physicians about advertised drugs influence both the physician's response and the physician–patient relationship? Consider how physicians might interpret (or misinterpret, for example, as "demanding" a prescription) patients' approaches resulting from DTCA and alter their responses accordingly.

4. What opinions, if any, did you have about DTCA prior to reading this chapter? Have your views changed about the value of DTCA in the larger health care system? If so, how?

5. If you saw an advertisement for a prescription drug that seemed relevant to a medical condition you experience, how do you think you would approach the physician about the drug? How might your previous relationship with that physician influence your approach? Consider how the reactions and approaches of older patients, with established relationships with their doctors, might differ from those of the often-healthy traditional college student, who often does not have an established relationship with a doctor.

REFERENCES/SUGGESTED READINGS

Bandura, A. (1994). Social cognitive theory of mass communication. In J. Bryant & D. Zillman (Eds.), *Media effects: Advances in theory and research* (pp. 61–90). Hillsdale, NJ: Lawrence Erlbaum Associates.

Bradley, L. R., & Zito, J. M. (1997). Direct-to-consumer prescription drug advertising. *Medical Care, 35*(1), 86–92.

Cline, R. J. W., & Young, H. N. (2004). Marketing drugs, marketing health care relationships: A content analysis of visual cues in direct-to-consumer prescription drug advertising. *Health Communication, 16*, 131–157.

Hollon, M. F. (1999). Direct-to-consumer marketing of prescription drugs: Creating consumer demand. *Journal of the American Medical Association, 281*, 382–384.

Holmer, A. F. (1999). Direct-to-consumer prescription drug advertising builds bridges between patients and physicians. *Journal of the American Medical Association, 281*, 380–382.

II

Issues in Decision Making

6

Communication and Shared Decision Making in Context: Choosing Between Reasonable Options

Carma L. Bylund
Columbia University Medical Center

Rebecca S. Imes
University of Iowa

People make all types of medical decisions on an individual level as a part of their health care processes—whether to go to the physician when feeling ill, whether to take medication prescribed by a physician, or whether to attend a follow-up visit. In many cases, though, medical decisions are made between a physician (or other health care provider) and a patient; this is often called *shared decision making*. Shared decision making in the physician–patient encounter is generally thought to happen when the physician and patient are both involved in the decision by sharing information, taking steps to build consensus about the preferred action, and finally, reaching an agreement (Charles, Gafni, & Whelan, 1997).

To truly understand the shared decision-making process, it is important to look at the *contexts* in which these shared decisions occur. In other words, when examining shared decision making in the medical encounter, you should consider three questions about context. First, what is the medical context of the decision? The medical context strongly impacts the nature of shared decision making. For instance, shared decision making about managing diabetes will likely be quite different from shared decision making during acute care in the emergency room. Second, what is the physician–patient relational context of the decision? For example, when a patient has gone to the same physician for several years, they may develop a sense of trust and liking that would affect the shared decision-making process and would consequently make their relationship different from that of a patient and physician who have a very limited history. Additionally, that patient's and physician's beliefs about who has the power in the physician–patient relationship may also influence shared decision making. Third, what is the patient's personal context for making the decision? Each patient has a unique personal context; he or she is embedded in multiple systems, such as families, friends, cultures, organizations, and societies. Within each of these systems, health communication occurs that affects and is affected by the physician–patient talk. All of these contexts can have important implications on the shared decision-making process.

It is especially interesting to look at shared decision making when the decision is about a controversial issue that is important to the patient and the patient's family. The following cases illustrate two sets of patients and physicians making shared decisions about these types of issues, although in very different ways.

CASE ONE

Marianne Stewart sat on the cold, hard chair in the examination room next to her husband Josh, who was engrossed in a *Time* magazine article. *Where is the doctor?* she thought impatiently, looking at her watch again. She'd already been weighed, had given her urine sample, and had her physical exam. A wave of panic came over her—*She never made me wait like this after an exam during my last pregnancy. I hope this doesn't mean anything's wrong. Why else would she have asked us to stay after I got dressed?* She tried to dismiss the thought. She'd made it past the crucial first 12 weeks; in fact, she was 14 weeks along now, and Dr. McKinley had found the heart beat with no problem today; everything had to be fine. So far, it had been an uneventful pregnancy. She'd had less morning sickness than she'd had with her previous pregnancy. In fact, everything seemed easier than before; perhaps this was simply because she knew what to expect this time around.

Her pregnancy with now three-year-old Nicholas hadn't been bad; she'd had friends who'd had a much worse time with pregnancy than she had. Sure, she'd had some nausea, heartburn, and headaches, but it didn't seem so bad compared with what others had dealt with. Labor was the only area where Marianne felt she still didn't know what to expect. Early in her ninth month of pregnancy with Nicholas, Marianne had awoken one morning to feel something very uncomfortable under her ribs. She'd always heard that babies kick you in the ribs, so she'd figured it was his feet. A couple of weeks later, Marianne's mother had put her hand on Marianne's belly and felt the baby. "That's got to be the baby's bottom," she'd said. It did feel kind of round, Marianne remembered thinking.

At her next appointment, Dr. McKinley had felt the baby's position and said that everything seemed fine. Marianne had hesitated, and then had told Dr. McKinley how she'd been feeling something uncomfortable under her ribs. Dr. McKinley had replied that she was pretty sure the baby was in the right position, but that an ultrasound scan would let them know for sure. The ultrasound technician had confirmed Marianne's suspicion—the baby was not in the right position. But that wasn't the baby's bottom she was feeling under her ribs—it was his head. Dr. McKinley had explained that if the baby didn't turn around by about a week before her due date, she could try to turn the baby. If Marianne and Josh chose not to try that, or if the baby wouldn't turn, Marianne would need to have a caesarean section (C-section). After researching their options, Marianne and Josh had decided to let the doctor try to turn the baby about five days before her due date, and when that didn't work, they agreed to the C-section.

Even as she thought back on it now, Marianne didn't regret having the C-section. The recovery wasn't that bad, and she actually thought the extra recovery time in the hospital was nice. Still, sometimes when she looked at other mothers, she somehow felt left out of the club—she'd had a baby, but still had no idea what it was like to go through labor. Other women she knew would talk about their labors: when they decided to go to the hospital, how far dilated they were, how painful it was, what choices they made about pain medication, how supportive (or not) their husbands were, and on and on. What could she say? *I got drugged up, they cut me open and pulled him out.* Oh well, she thought. I can't expect much different this time. Her mother-in-law, who had been an obstetric nurse for 20 years, had repeatedly told her, "Once a C-section, always a C-section."

Dr. McKinley's knock at the door jolted Marianne back into the present. "Sorry to keep you waiting," Dr. McKinley said, smiling as she entered the room and sat down at the desk. Josh put away the magazine, and Marianne took a deep breath. "Is everything okay?"

"Yes, everything is fine," Dr. McKinley said reassuringly. "I asked you to stay because I wanted to take a little more time to talk to you about your options for delivery. I know it may seem like a long way down the road still, but you have a big decision ahead of you, so I wanted to make sure you had plenty of time to think about it."

Marianne looked puzzled, "What do you mean? I thought I had to have another C-section."

"If it were 20 years ago, that would probably be what most doctors would suggest to you. But now, we deliver babies vaginally after a previous C-section nearly every day. It's called a VBAC, which stands for vaginal birth after caesarean. You're really a good candidate for one," Dr. McKinley added.

"Wait," said Josh. "Does she have to have a VBAC?"

"Absolutely not. In fact, in most cases like Marianne's, it is up to the woman—and her husband—whether or not to have one. Either decision you make will be respected by me and the other doctors here in the practice," Dr. McKinley assured Josh. She looked at both of them. "You have some time to think about this, and I would be happy if we could talk about it some more during your next visits. I'm sure that as the weeks go by you will have questions."

Marianne nodded. "Okay," was all she really could think of to say. This possibility had come as a shock to her. On one hand, it was welcome news— she could have the vaginal birth she'd wanted and prepared for last time. On the other hand, it also scared her. The stories she'd heard from her friends made labor sound like no picnic. Besides, what would Josh's mother say?

"All right." Dr. McKinley stood up. "See you next time."

20 Weeks

A few weeks later, Marianne and Josh were back in Dr. McKinley's office, this time for the ultrasound scan. When the technician told them that they were adding a daughter to their family, they were delighted and started talking about names while waiting for Dr. McKinley to come in. After the ultrasound scan, Dr. McKinley measured Marianne's growth, and they talked about how Marianne had been feeling. Then Dr. McKinley asked, "Have you thought much about the VBAC? Do you have any questions about it?"

Marianne looked hesitantly at Josh. "Well, we've talked a little bit about it." She paused.

"My mom was a nurse on the obstetrics floor of County Hospital for 20 years—she's retired now—and she keeps telling us that it's not a good idea," Josh added.

"When did she retire?"

"Well, she left the hospital, oh, in about 1990. Then she spent five years in a pediatrician's office before actually retiring," Josh said.

Dr. McKinley nodded. "It makes sense that she's telling you that. The time that she left the hospital is about the time that the medical community started talking more and more about the safety of VBACs. Has she told you why she thinks you shouldn't have a VBAC?"

Marianne nodded. "She mentioned something about uterine rupture. I looked it up on the Internet and found that there's about a 1–3% chance of that occurring, which doesn't seem like a lot to me."

"That's about right," Dr. McKinley said, "although some evidence indicates the risk is on the higher end of that range if you are induced than if you go into labor naturally. But let me assure you, and you can assure her, that if you decide to try a VBAC, we will definitely be monitoring you for uterine rupture."

"I also read something on the Internet about the VBAC being better if you want to have more children," Marianne said.

"Yes, often the issue of wanting more children is a factor in women's decisions. In fact, I just did a repeat C-section on a woman yesterday who had decided that since this was her second and last child, she didn't want to worry about trying the VBAC."

"Okay. Well, I'm sure we'll have more questions over the next few weeks," Marianne said.

"That's what I'm here for," Dr. McKinley said, smiling, and prepared to leave.

"Thanks," said Marianne. "See you soon."

28 Weeks

Marianne was glad she was seeing Dr. McKinley this visit. Dr. McKinley had been out of town right before her last visit, so she'd seen a new doctor in the practice instead. Josh wasn't with her this time. Although he had diligently come to all of her appointments the first time she was pregnant, she'd told him she didn't think he needed to come after the heartbeat was heard and the ultrasound scan was performed this pregnancy, as the visits seemed pretty routine at this point. After the physical exam was done, Marianne raised the issue of the VBAC again.

"When we first talked about VBAC, you said that you thought I was a good candidate for it. I've read some more things on the Internet and talked to a friend who had to make a similar decision about having a VBAC, and I think I know what you mean by me being a good candidate, but I want to make sure."

"Sure, go ahead," Dr. McKinley nodded and sat down.

"From what I found out, it sounds like I'm a good candidate because I didn't have a problem with labor or anything—my baby was just breech."

"Right. If you'd gone through 36 hours of labor, and we'd found out the baby was in distress and had to do an emergency C-section, it would be a bit of a different story," Dr. McKinley replied. "I'd probably still encourage you to consider it, but there would be more risk. You're also a good candidate because you're young, and when I did the C-section last time I didn't notice anything abnormal about your uterus."

"You seem to think I should try the VBAC," Marianne said.

Dr. McKinley smiled. "I'm sorry if it seems like I'm trying to pressure you," she said. "You are right. I would like to see you try a VBAC. But," she paused and looked straight at Marianne, "if you aren't comfortable with it, then I will have no problem scheduling the C-section for you."

"Yeah, I just think my mother-in-law will have a problem if I *don't* schedule the C-section!" Marianne said.

Dr. McKinley laughed. "Well, grandparents can be pretty concerned about their grandchildren's births. And I know your mother-in-law means well—you just have to remember that she is operating under a different set of facts and assumptions. Have you and Josh talked to her about what we've talked about?"

"Yes," Marianne sighed. "But it doesn't seem to change her mind. She's pretty stubborn."

"Well, you still have a few weeks to make your decision. And remember, it is *your* decision, not hers. But try not to get too stressed over it. The most important thing right now is to make sure you are taking good care of yourself and this baby," Dr. McKinley stood up to go. "Don't forget—I want to start seeing you every two weeks now that you're in the third trimester."

"Wow—it's that time already," Marianne said. "Okay, see you in a couple of weeks!"

34 Weeks

Marianne's 30- and 32-week visits with Dr. McKinley were short. In fact, they hadn't talked at all about the VBAC decision, which was fine with Marianne because she and Josh still hadn't decided what to do. Marianne was leaning toward trying the VBAC, whereas Josh wanted her to just have the C-section. But today, Marianne had some more questions.

After the physical exam, Marianne told Dr. McKinley, "I read something in the paper sometime last week about VBACs. Did you see it?"

"Yes, you mean the article about the medical study?"

"Yeah, that's right. It said that VBACs are only successful about 65% of the time. That doesn't seem like a very good success rate."

"I can see why that could be a little disheartening," Dr. McKinley replied. "Let me say a couple of things about that statistic, though. First, as I think we've already talked about, you are a good candidate for VBAC. That success rate takes into account other people who aren't as good candidates—people who've had distress during labor before, who are older, and so forth. So, I'd give you a better-than-average chance of success. Second, you need to think about what the word *success* means in this case. Let's say that, for some reason, you aren't successful in having a VBAC. We'll do a repeat C-section delivery, and you will, in all likelihood, have a healthy baby and recover from the C-section just fine, just like you did with your first one. Now, I'd call *that* a successful birth."

Marianne nodded. "That makes sense." She took a deep breath. "This is a really hard decision for me. I keep thinking that I've made up my mind, but it only lasts for a little while and then I change it again."

"I can tell it's a tough decision for you—it is for a lot of people," Dr. McKinley said. "I'm glad that you are giving it a lot of consideration."

"I suppose I need to decide soon, though."

"How is Josh feeling about it?"

"Well, he was pretty adamant against it—because of his mother—and then a woman he knows at work had a VBAC a few weeks ago. He talked to her a little bit when she came into the office to show off the baby yesterday, and she only had good things to say about it—how much better the recovery was, how she liked being completely aware of what was going on, rather than under anesthesia, and stuff like that," Marianne replied. "So now, he says he would be okay with the VBAC if that's what I want to do."

"That's good!" Dr. McKinley said, then added, "But it sounds like you're still not sure."

"No, but I've told myself I'm going to make a decision by my next visit, so I'll tell you then."

"Fair enough," Dr. McKinley said. "See you then."

"Bye."

36 Weeks

Marianne sat waiting for Dr. McKinley in exam room, with Josh next to her. He'd come this time because she'd been having what she thought were some intermittent, light contractions since the night before. She really didn't know what a contraction felt like, though, because she'd never had one. Josh had wanted her to page the on-call doctor last night, but because she'd had an appointment scheduled already for today, she just figured she'd wait to see Dr. McKinley.

Dr. McKinley came in and checked Marianne. "You aren't dilated yet," she said. "Those are probably just Braxton Hicks contractions—just think of them as 'practice' contractions. Your uterus is getting warmed up for the real thing!"

Marianne smiled. "That's right. I remember hearing about those when we took the birthing class the first time I was pregnant. Good. I was starting to think that it wouldn't matter if I'd decided to try the VBAC or not if I was already in labor."

Dr. McKinley laughed, "That has been known to happen. Someone is determined to have a repeat C-section and then shows up in labor and delivery pretty far along in labor and changes her mind and decides to have a VBAC!" She paused. "Speaking of which—at our last visit, you said you'd have a decision by today."

Marianne took a deep breath. "Yes. I guess it really wouldn't have mattered if I was in labor because we've decided to try the VBAC. I know that I still might end up with a C-section, but it seems to me that the risk is pretty low, all things considered. I feel comfortable that you and the others will make sure I'm doing okay. Also, we're not sure this is the last child we want to have, so we would rather not have another C-section."

Dr. McKinley looked at Josh. "You're okay with this?"

"Yes," he nodded.

"And your mother?" she asked.

"Well, I told her that either she better start supporting us in this decision or else she wouldn't be seeing this grandchild!" He laughed. "Actually, I wasn't that harsh, but I did explain to her that this is what we wanted to do, and she agreed to keep her doubts to herself."

"Great. I'm glad to hear it. Now let's talk a bit about what you should look for and what you should do when Marianne starts having real contractions."

CASE TWO

Jim Cooper sat down in the living room to await the weekly call from his son, Ryan. Sure, he'd call back if Jim didn't answer the phone right away, but Jim's two granddaughters, Ryan's girls, could only be corralled for so long, and Ryan always had them ready to get on the phone first to tell Grandpa about their week. Jim and his son had always been close, but ever since Jim's wife, Irene, passed away three years ago, Ryan never missed his weekly phone call to his now 72-year-old father. The phone rang.

"Hey, Dad, how are you? Hold on a sec . . . yes Vicki, you are first . . . Dad, here are the girls."

Jim talked to his granddaughters, Vicki and Maya, about biology, basketball, and boys—their favorite subjects, although not in that order! They wanted to know if he would be flying down to see their spring concerts for band and ballet. Ryan's wife, Sheila, got on the phone for a few minutes to invite Jim to go on the family trip over Memorial Day. When Ryan got back on the phone, Jim was still chuckling over the southern accent he could hear in the girls' voices. After Irene died, Ryan had suggested that Jim move to Texas to live near them, but Jim said that Ohio was his home. Besides, this was where his golf buddies were from his old advertising agency, and his Kiwanis club was always busy with projects in which Jim still took an active role.

Jim and Ryan chatted about developments in Ryan's job as a software engineer, and after hearing about the Kiwanis fundraiser, Ryan turned the conversation back to his father.

"Dad, did you see the doctor this week like you said you would? Was it about your heart? Is that why you went?"

Jim hesitated a second before answering. He had never liked discussing his medical issues with anyone but his wife—Irene had always known which questions to ask. Plus, she told him that she loved him and she felt it was important to know what was going on with his health. About six months after she died, Ryan started asking health questions of his father as well. Ryan wasn't as skilled at the questioning as Irene had been, but after a few months, Jim understood why Ryan felt he needed to ask and he tried to be truthful, even when it was embarrassing.

"Yeah, I saw Doc. But it wasn't about my heart. I've been taking my medicine and golfing more just like I said I would. This was for something else. Doc says . . . uh, well, he says that my problem going to, going to, um, going to the bathroom probably is just because of an enlarged prostate. I'm supposed to see him again in two months or sooner if I have any more pain or serious discomfort."

"Well, Dad, I'm glad you saw him. You've been seeing Dr. Willett for how long?"

"Hmm . . . I don't need to see Doc very often, but I'd guess he's been my doctor for more than 30 years now."

"I'm just glad you went. Well, Dad, I need to help the girls with some homework so I'll talk to you soon. I love you!"

"I love you too, Ryan. Give the girls a kiss goodnight for me!"

A couple of days later, Jim was working on a fundraising letter for his Kiwanis group when the phone rang.

"Ryan! What a pleasure to hear from you twice in one week! Did we forget something Sunday?"

"No, Dad, but something you said worried me, and I wanted to talk to you about it. Remember what you said about the enlarged prostate? Could you tell me exactly what you remember about your doctor's visit?"

"Just what I said on Sunday. I saw Doc, he made me do my business in a cup and give it to the lab lady, and then later he said that I probably just have an enlarged prostate and that it wasn't anything to worry about. He said that is what happens when guys get old and it may not be very comfortable at times, but I shouldn't worry about it and come back and see him in a couple of months."

"What about the results of your PSA test? Didn't he do a PSA?"

"A public service announcement? Ryan, what are you talking about? I only did the pee in the cup test. Oh, and he did that, well, he did that exam on me with his finger. Is that what you mean?"

"No, Dad. That was what I was worried about. This morning while I was driving to work, I saw a billboard that said older people should see their doctor regularly and do preventative checkups for cancer."

"Cancer? What? Doc never said anything about cancer."

"Well, Dad, the billboard got me to thinking and I looked up prostate problems on the Internet. I didn't think this was going to be a big deal but what I read really scared me. I think you need to have this PSA test—that means *prostate-specific antigen* test, Dad, not public service announcement. Anyway, I think you should do it right away! A PSA test is a blood test that can tell you if you have prostate cancer. What if *that* is the reason you are having trouble going to the bathroom? I'm really worried, Dad. If it is cancer, then I don't think you want to 'wait and see' for a few months, do you? This information on the Internet says that PSA tests can help find cancer, and I don't understand why Dr. Willett wouldn't give you the test. I want you to promise me that you will go back to see Dr. Willett *this week* and if he won't give you the test, then we should find you a different doctor."

"But I've been with Doc for 30–"

Ryan interrupted him. "Just promise me you'll go, Dad. Please? And call me right after."

Two days later, Jim sat in one of Dr. Willett's exam rooms.

"Jim! What a surprise. I thought I wouldn't see you for another few months. Is something else wrong? What can I do for you today?"

"Doc, well, I'm a little embarrassed about this. You see, um, well, my son wanted me to come back and see you."

"Ryan is worried? What? Did he think I missed something?" Dr. Willett said jokingly.

"Well, he doesn't think you missed something, but that you didn't do something he thought you should have done."

"Oh? And what was that?" Dr. Willett didn't appear to be joking anymore.

"It is about this prostate thing. He says that I need to have a P . . . a PS . . . a . . ."

"A PSA test?"

"Yeah . . . that's the one. Now, you know I don't like needles, but if it will make Ryan feel better, we'd just as well do it. He says I need this right away. I'm ready now, but could you get that nice nurse I always like? I barely feel the needle when she does it." Jim rolled up his sleeve as he spoke.

Dr. Willett perched on a stool next to the exam table where Jim was seated. "Now, Jim, I didn't forget about the PSA test. I just didn't tell you about it because I didn't think there was any reason to do so. Like you said, I know how you hate needles so I thought we'd wait a few months to see if we even needed to do this test."

"But Doc, how can we wait? What if it is cancer? You never said anything about cancer before, but Ryan says we need to do this now, before the cancer gets any worse. He read all about it on the Internet, and he sounds really worried. Then yesterday, I started thinking about Irene's stroke and how hard her death was on me and the kids and then I got worried. I say if there is a test that can tell us about the cancer, let's do it!"

"Jim, let's take just a minute and talk about this test. I know you and Ryan are worried, and I commend you for being willing to take the blood test to help Ryan to feel better. I wonder what Ryan told you about the PSA test."

"Just that there is a blood test that can tell me if I have prostate cancer."

"I wish it were that simple. Why don't I tell you some more about this test and why I decided you don't need it right now? Then, after we've talked about it, you can decide whether or not you want to do this. Here, why don't you pull up a chair rather than sit up there? I need to grab a brochure for you, and I'll be right back."

Dr. Willett came back with an informational brochure and a chart. "Here you go, Jim. Some information to take home with you. We'll talk about what's in there, but I want you to have them anyway. You and Ryan were right, the PSA test is a blood test that we sometimes use to help look for prostate cancer. Sometimes, if a person has this cancer, we can discover traces in the blood of what is called prostate-specific antigen. However, this test is just one tool that helps us look for cancer. Unfortunately, the PSA test isn't accurate enough to tell us, by itself, if you have cancer."

Jim looked up from the brochure. "I don't understand. A blood test is a blood test, right? If the stuff you are looking for is in there, then I have cancer. Isn't that how it works?"

"Like I said, Jim, this test isn't always accurate. Let's look at that chart you are holding. You see, what we look for when we do a PSA test is a level. Any level above 4 is considered elevated. But now—and this is the part about why I didn't want to give you the test yet—only 20–30% of men who have a level above 4 actually have prostate cancer. In fact, as many as half of men who do have prostate cancer have a level that is *lower* than 4. Do you see what I mean?"

"I think so. You're telling me that this blood test might tell me if I had an elevated level, but knowing that level might not tell us if I have cancer? So why did Ryan want me to have this test?"

"You are exactly right about the level, Jim. In fact, not even the experts agree about when to use this test. There just is no clear-cut answer for this one. Now, the test isn't useless, but I decide to use it on patients only if their other risk factors are high. Your risk factors are low, your digital rectal exam did not seem abnormal, and so I decided that we should wait a few months and see. You should also know that most prostate cancers are very slow growers, and for men over the age of 70, like yourself, it may not be necessary to treat an enlarged prostate at all. You are in good company, though. Like it says right here in your brochure, over half of men 50 and older have an enlarged prostate. Now, what questions do you have for me, Jim?"

"So you think that we should wait on this test? I think that might be best, if you agree. If the test doesn't tell us much and my other exams look good, I think this PSA test might just worry me for no reason. If you say I'm fine to keep golfing and go down to visit the kids next month, I think that is fine with me. What do I tell Ryan? I'm not sure I'll be able to remember all this, and he is the one who does the Internet research."

"Tell Ryan that his research was good, but there are some parts of it he needs to read a little more closely. Sometimes, after people read the word 'cancer,' they forget all the rest. He's just a good son, trying to look out for his father. Be sure to tell him that! I'll get you some extra brochures, if you want. And if you and he still have questions, be sure to call. Also, remember this doesn't mean that we'll never do the test. If things change, or if you change your mind, we can do this test at any time. How does that sound?"

"I think it sounds good. I guess I'll just come back if anything changes, but no needles today! And I would like some extra brochures, if that is OK. I'm going to need to send some to Ryan so he doesn't worry too much."

DISCUSSION

Both of these cases illustrate how shared decision making is affected by context. Let's start with the definition of shared decision making and see if the criteria were met in the cases, and then we will examine issues of context in these cases and how context made these cases different.

Shared Decision Making

Remember that we defined shared decision making as having the following elements—both the physician and patient are involved in the decision, they share information, they take steps to build consensus about the preferred action, and they reach an agreement. Marianne and Dr. McKinley were both actively involved in discussion about the VBAC decision during several of the medical visits. They also shared a great deal of information with each other. Dr. McKinley shared medical information about VBAC with Marianne, including information about the procedure, risks, benefits, and chances of success. Marianne also shared information with Dr. McKinley—medical information that she found, as well as information about the decision-making process she and Josh were going through. In addition, Marianne and Dr. McKinley used a variety of techniques during these visits to build consensus. At the beginning of the case, Dr. McKinley presented the options to Marianne and Josh, and by stating that they could talk about the decision over the course of the next few visits, she created an environment conducive to open communication. Marianne also participated in taking steps toward consensus by finding out information on her own and then discussing it with Dr. McKinley. It seems clear that both Marianne and Dr. McKinley were working in partnership with each other on this decision. Finally, when Marianne stated she wanted to try the VBAC, Dr. McKinley agreed that this was a good decision (although she had been clear with Marianne that she would have agreed with either decision).

Jim Cooper and Dr. Willet also participated in a shared decision, although different in many ways from Marianne and Dr. McKinley. Actually, the first real decision was not a shared decision—Dr. Willet made his own decision to not offer the PSA blood test to Jim the first time. The PSA decision had to be made a second time after Jim brought up the issue of the PSA test with Dr. Willet, and then it became a shared decision. This time, both Jim and Dr. Willet were involved in making the decision. Jim shared information that he had received from his son about the test and why he thought he should get it, and Dr. Willet shared information with Jim about some of the problems with the test. They worked together to build consensus by each being open to the other's opinion and wishes. Finally, Jim decided that he agreed with Dr. Willet's choice to not offer Jim the PSA test in the first place.

Context

The medical contexts in these two cases differed significantly and played an important role in the decision-making process. For Marianne, because the decision regarded a birthing procedure, it was necessary that one of the two choices were made. Marianne and Josh had to consider the consequences of both decisions—including health risks and benefits, personal preferences, and family pressures. Jim's situation was different in that his decision was not which procedure to have, but whether or not to have a procedure, in this case, a screening test. For Jim, primary outcomes to consider seemed to be balancing the unnecessary anxiety that may result in the case of a false-positive test with his son's anxiety about the possibility of cancer.

As mentioned earlier, both of these decisions were about issues that had some controversy surrounding them. The issues' controversial nature played a part in the decision-making process. There were no easy answers; in fact, different doctors may have encouraged each of these patients to make different decisions, with either decision being considered reasonable in each case. In Marianne's case, it was a difficult decision, one that took a few conversations with the doctor and several months to make. Jim's decision didn't take months, but it still took some time for Dr. Willet and him to discuss. In both cases, the doctors were willing to honor the patients' preferences.

The second type of context to consider is the context of the physician–patient relationship. In any interpersonal relationship, the parties operate under the norms, expectations, and beliefs they have developed in interacting with each other. Both sets of patients and doctors were operating in a context of a previous relationship that had been established over time. For Marianne and Dr. McKinley, this relationship included working together during a previous birth, whereas Jim had seen Dr. Willet for 30 years. Certainly, the histories these patients and doctors had played a role in how they interacted during the decision-making process. For example, Dr. McKinley probably remembered from Marianne's first birth that Marianne and Josh took a very active role in making the decision of whether or not to try to turn Nicholas before agreeing to a C-section. This knowledge of Marianne and Josh may have led Dr. McKinley to interact with them differently than she might have with a patient who has been unwilling to participate in decisions in the past. Because Dr. Willet had known Irene before she died, and also knew Jim's son Ryan, he was able to better understand Jim's situation for this decision, trying to make his son happy, while still doing what was best for him.

In examining the physician–patient relationships present in these two cases, we can also see how shared decision making can happen in medical relationships with different power structures. Marianne and Dr. McKinley's relationship, at least in this decision, allowed Marianne to have much of the power of making the decision. This relationship was co-constructed by Marianne and Dr. McKinley. Marianne took an active role, asked questions, and sought information both from Dr. McKinley and from other sources. Dr. McKinley encouraged Marianne to make the decision and provided information and input when asked. The power structure of Jim and Dr. Willet's relationship was markedly different. Dr. Willet had made the first decision to not give Jim the PSA test—or even the option of having the PSA test. It was only because of Ryan's insistence that Jim even approached Dr. Willet about making a different decision. Even though Dr. Willet told Jim he could decide what to do, after Dr. Willet explained to Jim his reasons for not giving him the PSA test, Jim was convinced and willing to go along with what Dr. Willet believed to be best. Clearly, these power structures had been created by both participants in both cases over time.

Finally, it is clear that the patients' personal contexts played a large role in the decision-making process. For both Marianne and Jim, being part of a larger family system was significant. Josh's mother's opposition to the VBAC affected both Marianne and Josh's feelings about trying to have a VBAC and their conversations with Dr. McKinley. In the end, when they decided to try to have the VBAC, it was necessary for Josh to explain this decision to his mother. In Jim's case, his son was the reason that the decision-making visit was initiated in the first place. In both cases, the doctors were sensitive to the patients' family contexts and discussed these contexts with their patients. They also pointed out that the family members were concerned about the patients' well-being.

It isn't only family members, however, that can affect the decision-making process. In Marianne and Josh's case, it was clear that a friend and coworker also had influence on the decision-making process. Marianne mentions a friend that she had spoken to who also went through a VBAC, whereas Josh's talk with a coworker who had a successful VBAC seems to be the eventual turning point for him to think they should try the VBAC.

The mass media's influence on Marianne's and Jim's decision-making process was also evident in these cases. Marianne searched the Internet for information about VBACs and read an article in the newspaper. In both cases, she shared the information she found with Dr. McKinley, which became part of the decision-making process. Jim's son was also influenced by the mass media—the initial billboard that he saw grabbed his attention and made him think more about his recent conversation with his father. He then used the Internet to further his search into prostate cancer testing. Although Ryan did not understand all the conditions surrounding the screening test, his information search convinced him that his father needed to return to Dr. Willet. That visit resulted in a more correct understanding of the situation.

These cases illustrate how important it is to look at the various contexts of the decision making process in order to better understand why and how it happens. By considering the medical context, the physician–patient relational context, and the patient's personal context, we are able to gain a better understanding of how and why medical decisions are made in certain ways.

RELEVANT CONCEPTS

Medical context: The reason for the patient seeing the physician. This could be an illness, a disease, or preventive care.

Patient participation: The level to which a patient participates in the medical encounter and/or the decision-making processes.

Patient's personal context: Systems in which the patient is embedded, including families, social networks, organizations, and societies.

Physician–patient relational context: The relationship that the physician and patient have created; affected by length of time of relationship and each person's perceptions of power, liking, and trust in the relationship.

Physician reliance: Relying on a doctor to make choices about medical options and to keep oneself healthy.

Self-reliance: Relying on oneself to make choices about medical options and to keep oneself healthy.

Shared decision making: When the physician and patient are both involved in the decision by sharing information, taking steps to build consensus about the preferred action, and, finally, reaching an agreement.

DISCUSSION QUESTIONS

1. In each of these cases, which elements of the physician–patient relational context seem most important to the decision that was made? Which elements of the patient's personal context seem most important?
2. As you read in these cases, power in the physician–patient relationship is not unchanging. What are some medical contexts in which the power structure might be balanced differently for Marianne and Dr. McKinley or Jim and Dr. Willet?
3. What other factors (beyond those discussed here) in a patient's personal context might influence the medical decision-making process?

4. Do you think shared decision making is always the best model? Is it the physician's respon-
    sibility to try to engage the patient in shared decision making? What if the patient doesn't
    want to be involved in the decision?

REFERENCES/SUGGESTED READINGS

Beisecker, A. E., & Beisecker, T. D. (1993). Using metaphors to characterize doctor-patient relationships: Paternalism
    versus consumerism. *Health Communication, 5*(1), 41–58.
Charles, C., Gafni, A., & Whelan, T. (1997). Shared decision-making in the medical encounter: What does it mean?
    (or it takes at least two to tango). *Social Science and Medicine, 44*(5), 681–692.
Makoul, G. (1998). Perpetuating passivity: Reliance and reciprocal determinism in physician-patient interaction.
    Journal of Health Communication, 3, 233–259.
Street, R. L. (2003). Communication in medical encounters: An ecological perspective. In T. L. Thompson, A. M.
    Dorsey, K. I. Miller, & R. Parrott (Eds.), *The handbook of health communication* (pp. 63–93). Mahwah, NJ:
    Lawrence Erlbaum Associates.

7

Negotiating Cancer Care Through Communication

Dan O'Hair
Sharlene R. Thompson
University of Oklahoma

Lisa Sparks
George Mason University

"I should have just bought the flowers for myself," Ann Benton said under her breath, repeating words from the movie, *The Hours*. While Ann was waiting for her lab results, she could hear that obnoxious show *Montel* playing on a television in the dark, windowless waiting room. Montel was talking to young women about their torrid relational traumas. As Ann stared blankly at the television, she shifted her thoughts back to the meaning of her life. She had just seen the blockbuster movie, *The Hours* and thus, was inspired to read Virginia Woolf's *Mrs. Dalloway*. She began making a list of all the things she wanted to do, from reading more of the classics, to learning to speak Spanish, to spending more time with true friends, to just taking care of herself. As she looked around at the other people in the waiting room, she heard whispers of other patients talking about adjuvant therapy, Whipple procedure, and ECRP. What she heard sounded like a new language, but not a beautiful romance language that she had once studied. After waiting for nearly 2 hours, she is called to the sterile examination room.

Almost 9 million people in the United States have been diagnosed with cancer, and over 1 million new cases are diagnosed each year (National Cancer Institute [NCI], 2001a). After heart disease, cancer ranks as the second leading cause of death in this country. It is not surprising that cancer continues to be the greatest health concern among Americans (Carlson, 2001). Medical research has enjoyed substantial success in reducing the cancer burden, especially in areas where funding has been targeted. It is heartening to know that cancer patients are overcoming this dreaded disease in record numbers (National Cancer Institute, 2001b).

Despite such encouraging trends, cancer survivorship is a difficult process. Cancer patients face a multitude of challenges as they access care for their disease. The first challenge confronting cancer patients is the sense of shock and inevitable change in self-identity. Following close behind these feelings are endless decisions that patients must make about their care. To make the situation even more complex, patients and their families face a health care delivery system that is often incompatible with the goals of patient care. To fully understand the

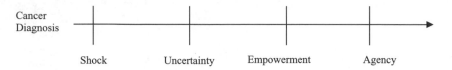

FIG. 7.1. Cancer Survivorship and Agency Model. (Adapted from O'Hair et al., 2003)

problems of how social life can be perceived as a whole on the basis of a single case, case studies must provide a holistic view of modern social life. Hence, this case study follows Le Play's method, which "... presumes that society cannot be studied as a single entity or unit. The focus must be on some key element" (Hamel, 1993, p. 7).

This case study focuses on Ann Benton, who is diagnosed with pancreatic cancer. As the case unfolds, it will become clear that Ann and her family must become actively involved in information management and communication strategies with her physicians and other providers as well as the managed care system. Thus, the social unit of analysis for the following case study is the cancer patient and the navigation and adaptation to her rapidly changing social world. As in the tradition of Le Play, it is "a social unit intentionally selected to provide a better understanding of the characteristic traits of society as whole" (Hamel, 1993, p. 7).

THE CANCER SURVIVORSHIP AND AGENCY MODEL

The Cancer Survivorship and Agency Model (CSAM; O'Hair et al., 2003) will serve as an explanatory mechanism for charting how and why Ann and her family made decisions about her medical care. CSAM involves four steps that occur in a rather sequential manner: (1) shock, (2) uncertainty, (3) empowerment, and (4) agency (Fig. 7.1).

Shock

In the first stage of this model, a patient learns of the cancer diagnosis. It is termed *shock* because of the bewildering and often terrifying feelings that patients experience. Patients are all at once forced to enter a new world where they must learn a new language and new norms, and navigate a new environment. Within this new environment, they must quickly make decisions that are going to affect the rest of their lives.

Uncertainty

The second stage is one of *uncertainty*. Once patients get over the shock of the cancer diagnosis, they develop dozens of questions that need answering. Some of the answers create even more uncertainty among patients. In this stage, patients must face the reality of their diagnosis and learn the language and norms of the cancer world.

Empowerment

The third stage is termed *empowerment*. This is a place where patients begin to understand how to assert themselves in the process of cancer care. In this stage, patients have become fluent in the language and norms of the cancer world and begin to "take the wheel" and start making strategic choices to ensure their health. Patients may begin doing their own research, calling the American Cancer Society and asking questions, and possibly joining a chat room with others who are currently suffering from cancer.

Agency

In the fourth stage, *agency*, patients begin making choices about their lives and exerting the type of control that helps them to find a quality of life that they desire. When patients reach the agency stage, they start asserting their right to live the rest of their lives the way that they choose. This may mean that patients decide not to do a painful and risky surgical procedure to preserve their quality of life.

THE PATIENT AND FAMILY

Ann Benton is a 64-year-old mother of three who continues to work in her lifelong career as an advertising executive. She is part owner of the ad agency and feels a great deal of pride in helping to build the business into one that stands as the second largest in her community. Ann is known for her strength of character and her strong will. She is active in her community and church and takes great interest in her family. Ann's first husband, and the father of her three children, died from a heart attack about 10 years ago. She married Alex 7 years ago. Alex gets along reasonably well with Ann's children, Clarise (31), Jack (28), and Erica (27), all of whom are married. Ann does not have grandchildren yet. However, she is looking forward to the day when she will have the opportunity to spoil her own grandchildren.

The Diagnosis

Ann had been experiencing some pain in her midsection accompanied with a slight burning sensation when she urinated. She had also been feeling very tired lately, but chalked that up to some overtime work she was putting in on a special advertising project. She thinks she remembers this happening in the past, but this time the symptoms didn't go away. She was scheduled for her biannual appointment with her obstetrician-gynecologist in about a month, but thought that maybe she ought to have herself looked at right away. She was able to get an earlier appointment and explained to her physician, Dr. Meese, the symptoms she had been experiencing.

Dr. Meese: Any other symptoms you noticed besides the burning, abdominal discomfort, and fatigue?

Ann: Just nervousness. Do you think this has anything to do with my ovarian operation four years ago?

Dr. Meese: I can't be certain until we run some tests. I am going to send you to the lab, and they'll take blood and urine samples. I should know something in a couple of days.

After going to the lab, Ann returned home feeling anxious and tense. She wanted to know the results of the lab test immediately and hated having to wait. She decided not to tell Alex or her children anything about this until she learned of the lab results.

Alex: Hi, I'm home. How was your day? I see that the neighbors finally decided to call the landscapers we suggested. (Silence) Is there something wrong, honey? You seem really tense. Why don't we go out for a nice dinner, and maybe catch a movie tonight. If you don't feel up to it we could order in, how about Chinese?

Ann: I'm not hungry.

Alex: Ann, what is wrong, you seem . . . ?

Ann: I'm fine. I'm just busy. I just want to finish this work.

As promised, Dr. Meese called Ann at work two days later. She asked that Ann come in to discuss the lab results. When they met, Dr. Meese told Ann that the results were suspiciously similar to results she has seen before of patients who developed chronic pancreatitis.

Dr. Meese: I want you to have a CT scan some time this week. We just need to see if there's something else.

Ann: Like what?

Dr. Meese: It is too early to say at this point, you have early signs of jaundice, you have an unusual enzyme count sometimes associated with diabetes, and you appear to be anemic. I just want to cover all bases.

Ann went to the radiology department of a large outpatient clinic near her home and had the CT scan test performed. Dr. Meese called once again and asked Ann to come in the next day. Ann wasn't having any of it.

Ann: No! I want to know now what the CT scan found.

Dr. Meese: I don't like doing this on the phone, but you are a friend and I know how strong willed you can be. There is a mass or spot on the head of your pancreas 2 cm by 4 cm. We need to have another test done to determine if it's cancerous.

Ann was speechless. The word *cancer* coming from the phone totally unnerved her. Her grandmother had died of breast cancer, her best friend from high school had died of colon cancer, and her pastor from church had died of lung cancer.

Dr. Meese: Ann . . . Ann . . . I know this is rough especially coming over the phone, that is why I wanted to see you. We can't jump to conclusions, it may simply be a cyst or even a benign form of cancer. But we really need to conduct an advanced imaging procedure called endoscopic retrograde cholangiopancreatogram or ERCP. It takes pictures of the pancreas and is more detailed and accurate than a CT scan. I also need to have you see a gastroenterologist, a GI, who is a specialist for diseases of the pancreas. His name is Dr. Vendi and he will interpret the ERCP images along with the radiologist who conducts the ERCP.

Ann: Pancreatic cancer? Isn't that what Michael Landon from Little House on the Prairie died from? Are you sure taking more pictures is the right thing. Don't they do a biopsy or something to make sure?

Dr. Meese: Ann, we don't know that the mass is cancerous or, even if it is, that it's malignant. Biopsies are where a needle is run into your pancreas and cells are taken out for a pathologist to test. With a biopsy you run the risk of breaking the tumor capsule and spreading malignant cells throughout the abdominal area. The imaging test is just as good without the risk. I've already set up an appointment with the radiologist and the GI. Here are the details. . . .

Ann went back to the radiology department and had the ERCP imaging test conducted. The following day, she went for her appointment with the GI, Dr. Vendi. This time, she asked her husband, Alex to go with her. She decided not to tell him much except that she had some tests done and would like to have him there to help her understand what the doctors would say.

Dr. Vendi: Ann, I consulted with your radiologist, Dr. Westmore, and we both agree that the mass on the head of your pancreas is adenocarcinoma of the pancreas . . .

Ann: Cancer, right?

Dr. Vendi: Yes, we are almost certain. Unfortunately, the tumor is larger than what the CT revealed and it may be in a stage where it is metastasizing. We hope that is not the case.

Alex: What is metastasizing? Spreading?

Dr. Vendi: That is often the case in advanced stages of pancreatic cancer. If it is spreading to other parts, such as the liver or lymph nodes, we wouldn't be able to do surgery. If the cancer is not stable, surgery will make it spread even more. We need to get you in to see Dr. Lewis, who is a leading oncological surgeon specializing in the pancreas.

Ann: Why a surgeon? Don't most people with cancer get chemo or radiation treatments? I know that is what happened with my pastor.

Dr. Vendi: Actually, surgery is the best possible treatment for adenocarcinoma of the pancreas. Chemo and radiation may be recommended after surgery, this is called adjuvant therapy, but life expectancy goes way up if you can have the tumorous tissue removed.

Ann: So, what is life expectancy for pancreatic cancer?

Dr. Vendi: Obviously that depends on the nature of the tumor, its size, the extent to which it has metastasized, and other factors. Some patients have lived for several years after diagnosis, but I have to be honest with you, Ann, pancreatic cancer is a very difficult disease to manage. Some patients only have 3–6 months. We hope your prognosis will be much better.

Ann was indeed a strong-willed woman, but hearing all of this talk of cancerous tissue and death completely stunned her. The rest of the appointment and the ride home was just a daze for Ann. She remembers little of what else was said. After going into their bedroom, she finally said to Alex, "How am I going to tell the kids? They have always looked at me as the strong one in the family, the role model, especially after Jerry's death." "We'll do it together," Alex smiled weakly.

Ann decided to call each of her children separately on the phone to break the news. After each call, Ann began to feel detached from life. She had cancer and others did not. She was now different from them and could almost hear it in their voices when they expressed their concern. She wondered if all cancer patients felt this alone.

The following day, Ann arranged an appointment with the surgeon, Dr. Lewis. When she met him, he gave Ann the impression that he knew all about her disease and about her specific case.

Dr. Lewis: Ann, from all of the tests, I am certain that the mass identified on the CT scan and the ERCP is a tumor and is malignant. It would not be wise to have surgery at this time. We will need to have you see a radiologist who will use radiation therapy to help contain, stabilize, and hopefully shrink the tumor. This is what we call neoadjuvant therapy, or treatments before surgery. If it shrinks, we can then do the Whipple procedure—the surgery to resect or remove the cancerous tissue.

Ann: Is this Whipple procedure the only way I will be able to live longer?

Dr. Lewis: It is the best treatment we know of at this time. It's a very difficult procedure, but if it's successful it can extend life for the patient.

Ann: What is your best guess of my life expectancy?

Dr. Lewis: That's impossible to say at this point. We will begin monitoring your blood levels and enzyme counts, and that will tell us many things such as metastatic rate and whether the tumor in your pancreas is communicating to nearby organs and vessels such as your liver and intestines. We hope it doesn't get into the lymph nodes because they're connected to so many other organs in the body.

Once again, Ann felt completely numb. How could this happen? Why her? She ate right and she exercised regularly. There was cancer in her family but not pancreatic cancer, as far as she knew. The more she thought about her situation, the feelings of loneliness, humiliation, and fear turned to anger. This was not fair. After Ann returned home, she decided to call her regular doctor, Dr. Meese.

Ann: Dr. Meese, do you think I ought to have a second opinion about this. Dr. Lewis and Dr. Vendi were fine, but this is my life we're talking about.
Dr. Meese: Sure, if you want to. Do you want me to recommend other physicians?
Ann: Let me get back to you.

Uncertainty

Ann received a call from one of her friends, Judy, who knew someone who died from pancreatic cancer. Ann mentioned her thoughts about getting second opinions.

Judy: Paul, my friend who had pancreatic cancer was impressed with the American Cancer Society's website. His wife gave me all his printouts, let's see, yes, there's a special section on "second opinions." Do you want the website address? It's www.cancer.org.
Ann: Yes, I'll take a look.

Ann examined the material from the American Cancer Society's website about second opinions. After thinking it over a while, she decided that she really didn't know what to do. If she waited to get second opinions, it would delay her treatment. On the other hand, it might ease her mind that she was certain that the first set of doctors was correct in their diagnosis and treatment plan. She asked Alex what to do, and he thought that it was best for her to get treatment right away. He also thought that she should consult her daughter, Clarise. Clarise agreed with Alex, and Ann decided to move forward with her treatment.

Although Ann did not feel completely alone and helpless, she really wasn't sure where to turn. Alex and her children only made her feel guilty about having cancer. Her pastor was soothing in his style, but he didn't build much confidence in Ann. By her very nature, Ann felt that she ought to be doing something about the situation, but what? Her feelings of uncertainty seemed to increase as she talked to people who knew others who had died from pancreatic cancer. One suggestion from a friend was to attend support group sessions at the local American Cancer Society office. This was not particularly appealing to Ann. At the same time, Ann was beginning to feel more tired, feelings of nausea were almost constant, and the pain in her upper abdominal area was getting more intense. She wasn't sure if it was the cancer or the radiation treatments she had begun. She decided against getting a second opinion. She knew that she was supposed to maintain a healthy diet, but food was not a priority for her; she simply had no appetite.

Ann received a call from Dr. Lewis and was told that the radiation treatments were working and that she was a good candidate for surgery, a Whipple procedure. Because her tumor was now localized to the head of the pancreas and the nearby cells had not been substantially affected, she should have the operation immediately. Dr. Lewis seemed reassuring that with follow-up chemotherapy, Ann would have a chance of extending her life expectancy. How much, Dr. Lewis would not commit to.

For the first time since her diagnosis, Ann felt that she had a goal to pursue. She got on a search engine on the Internet and typed in pancreatic cancer. She was stunned by the number of hits her search returned. When she found the National Cancer Institute, she navigated the Web site, found the Whipple procedure, and read that this surgical procedure was the best way to extend life for pancreatic cancer patients. She also learned that the Whipple procedure is among the most complicated and demanding types of surgery, often taking 3 to 4 hours to perform. Most of the information she found mentioned that survival rates from the Whipple were dramatically increased if the surgeon (a) was experienced with the procedure (performing more than 40 per year) and (b) performed the surgery at a major research medical hospital that was also familiar with the procedure. She visited a number of other websites and learned many other things about the disease. She learned that few cancers are more fatal, that many people who are diagnosed are encouraged to immediately enter a hospice program for the terminally ill, and that it was a painful disease. Ann was once again taken aback. She was conflicted—on one hand, she was encouraged with the optimism she thought she heard in Dr. Lewis's voice. On the other hand, she was disillusioned with the doomsday news she was reading on the Internet.

After her conversation with Clarise, Ann phoned Dr. Lewis and asked about his experience with Whipple procedures. He said that he usually does about one to two a month in the local hospital. This made Ann very nervous, and she got in touch with Dr. Meese, expressing her concern about Dr. Lewis's level of experience. Dr. Meese did some research and called Ann back.

Dr. Meese: I determined that an oncological surgeon in Oklahoma City, a Dr. Postier, is a leading pancreatic surgeon. I even talked with him about your case. He performs his surgery at the University of Oklahoma Health Sciences Center hospital, where he does over 50 Whipple procedures a year. He publishes several articles a year about his work in the leading surgical journals.

Ann: Let me think about it.

Again, Ann was conflicted. Oklahoma City was 300 hundred miles away and that would be inconvenient for her, Alex, and everyone else. She decided to call Dr. Postier herself, and after a few minutes on the phone, she felt completely relieved with his confident and reassuring tone. He even mentioned the names of some of his patients whom she could call and ask about their experiences. He did mention that from the information he has seen about her tumor, it was important that she have the surgery within a week regardless of who did it.

Dr. Postier: Ann, right now, your tumor is a stage II, which means it is only affecting your pancreas and is only 2 cm in diameter. This makes you a strong candidate for the Whipple. You may not realize it, but your situation is much better than most. Only about 15–20% of pancreatic patients are eligible for the Whipple. It's your best chance.

Ann did call two of Dr. Postier's patients, and they were highly complimentary of his style and the progress they made during recovery. Ann decided to have Dr. Postier perform the surgery.

Empowerment

As is typical with adenocarcinoma of the pancreas, Ann's GI recommended that she undergo a round of chemotherapy after her surgery to ensure the elimination of all cancer cells. Four weeks after having the Whipple procedure, Ann was told that she would begin chemotherapy. Before they could administer the chemo to Ann, they had to insert a port into her chest, as the chemicals are so toxic that giving them intravenously proves to be uncomfortable and difficult. Ann asked her oncologist what types of drugs he was planning to use.

> *Dr. Kim:* With adjuvant therapy, or post-surgical therapy, the standard treatment is a drug called 5-FU. We will use that and monitor your progress through a tumor marker blood test. It's called CA 19-9. This will tell us if the tumor cells are growing, stagnating, or declining over the period of your treatment.

CA 19-9, 5-FU, adjuvant therapy? Ann began to wonder if everything associated with her now had to have a sterile sounding name. Maybe she would just call herself, *Pancre-Ann*, after the disease she had.

After successfully making it through the surgery, Ann had a renewed sense of hope but felt reluctant and nervous about her treatment regimen. She became anxious and wondered how well she would cope with the side effects of hair loss, nausea, weight loss, and fatigue that often accompanied this treatment and felt uncertain about the process. The night before her first treatment, she decided to start a journal to reflect on her experiences dealing with her cancer. When she survived this cancer (she never thought to herself, *if* I survive), Ann told herself, she wanted to remember this experience and never forget how precious life really was. This experience had, in some way, given her a renewed sense of what life was really about, what was really important in life. In her diary, she wrote, "I am looking forward to a future that is cancer free, one that no longer involves the words chemotherapy, radiation, 5-FU or Whipple procedure. I dread tomorrow and remain uncertain about my future, but I am going to fight back and, despite the sadness, despair, and discomfort, I will prevail, I will survive."

> *Ann:* Alex, I feel so defeated. Having pancreatic cancer is like climbing a mountain without mountaineering equipment or even a guide. I can see the top (healing and recovery) but I often wonder how or if I will get there. I have also begun to feel like a stranger in my own body. I feel like I have become a bunch of parts and less of a whole human being.
> *Alex:* Ann, I don't know what to say. I can't imagine what you must feel like but we are beating this . . . things are moving forward.

That morning, Ann woke before her alarm and began to get dressed in their large walk-in closet. She made sure to wear the appropriate shirt so that they could easily reach her chemotherapy port. Nervously, she marched down the stairs to the kitchen and began her day as she had so many days before, reading her daily meditation and the newspaper while she drank a cup of coffee.

When Ann and Alex walked into the hospital, they were immediately greeted by the head nurse. The head nurse introduced herself as Karla and began explaining the procedure to Ann. She directed her to pick a chair and have a seat. Throughout the room, there were several leather recliner chairs, and Ann proceeded toward one in the far back corner. She noticed right away that, in the middle of the room, there was a large fish tank with 50 or 60 brightly colored tropical fish. As she settled into the chair, her nerves calmed as she gazed at the fish swimming in and out of the castles and rock formations in the tank. Alex sat next to her as they both acclimated to their new surroundings. Ann noticed that this place was not as she had imagined it, that there were even patients sitting with family and friends laughing and idly chatting as they received their chemo treatments. A different nurse came to give her the first drug, an anti-nausea medication. The nurse told her to settle in, as this would take a while to drip in, and offered her a couple of magazines while she waited.

As the medication began to slowly drip, she noticed that the room was cheerful and bright, with many magazines, two televisions, and a table full of puzzles. The nurse's station was at the front of the room behind a glass window, and she observed that the nurses were very friendly and supportive. After receiving her anti-nausea medication, she was ready to begin her first treatment, but before this happened, Karla began discussing with her the way that this drug would make her feel. She recommended that Ann begin drinking a dietary supplement, such as Ensure. Karla asked if she had felt anything different or unusual in the last few days and took her vital signs. Ann commented that she had felt really fatigued since the surgery, and Karla made a note and told her that she would discuss this with her doctor. Karla offered them both something to drink, a soda for Alex and an Ensure for Ann. The treatment itself was relatively painless, and Ann just lay back in her chair while the toxic chemicals entered her system. Ann began to realize that she wanted and needed to learn more about her cancer and this treatment procedure so that she could be more involved in her own care.

After the treatment, the nurse scheduled her next appointment and told Ann to call if she had questions or needed help. As they were leaving, Ann thought to herself, it is so odd that everyone treats this as though it were a routine procedure, forgetting that, for me, this is a life-changing experience. At the same time, it began to feel like a routine experience, and she was finding herself familiar with cancer terminology and was beginning to adapt to being a cancer patient. After this first treatment, Ann began to think differently about her experience with cancer and began to realize that she could play a powerful role in her recovery. She realized that she had a voice in her own recovery.

The next morning, she began reading through the myriad of pamphlets and books she had been given about pancreatic cancer, cancer treatment, and pain management. She made a list of her questions and called the nurses at the hospital for advice on nutrition, alternative therapies, and pain management. She followed their advice and called her doctor to ask him some pertinent questions about alternative therapies she had been considering.

Throughout this process, Ann's children had different reactions to their mother's cancer. Although Jack and Erica had been very supportive by emailing their mother new research they found on pancreatic cancer and by coming to visit and help take care of her, Clarise had a much harder time coping with her mother's illness and had been somewhat unsupportive. Ann began to feel like she was letting down her family, especially Clarise. Ann was afraid that she wouldn't be able to be there for her daughter when she really needed her. Clarise had just learned that she was pregnant, and she was really concerned that her mother survive so that she could be there for the birth of her grandchild. Clarise became very unemotional about the cancer and spoke with her mother in a very matter-of-fact way about the decisions she felt she should make. Ann did not understand Clarise's reaction to her illness and felt hurt when her daughter was not there to emotionally support her throughout her illness.

When Ann was not feeling sick as a result of the chemo treatments and not working at her advertising agency, she did her own research on cancer to find alternative treatments. Ann joined an online support group called ACOR.org and began to regularly share her experiences with other pancreatic cancer patients. She began to realize that if she wanted to get better, she was going to have to become her own advocate so that she could do what was best for her. Ann sent the following message to her pancreatic online support group:

> *Ann:* Does anyone know anything about a new chemo drug called gemcitibine? Or cisplatin?

After a day, Ann received a number of responses:

> *Jack:* Ann, gemcitibine and cisplatin aren't really new drugs; they are relatively new treatments for pancreatic cancer. Specialists at Johns Hopkins think it is best to combine the two. They have been doing clinical trials on it.

Joyce: When my father became stage IV, they put him on gemcitibine, and his CA 19-9 levels came down for a while, but it made him more nauseous than 5-FU.

Patrice: My husband was put on gemcitibine and radiotherapy, and that worked for a while, but when his CA 19-9 went up, the oncologist put him back on 5-FU.

At her next visit, Ann took printouts of the comments made by her support groups and asked Dr. Kim about them. Dr. Kim assured Ann that he was very familiar with all of these drugs and a lot depends on how the patient is faring with the treatment. Then, out of the blue, Dr. Kim asked Ann if she would be interested in enrolling in a clinical trial.

Ann: What is a clinical trial, exactly?

Dr. Kim: Clinical trials are carefully controlled experiments in which new agents or a new combination of agents are administered to patients to see the results. Although you might think of it as being used as a guinea pig, if it works, it has a chance to prolong your life.

Ann: From the little I've read, some patients get no treatment but they don't know it?

Dr. Kim: A placebo? No, not these days; if you are in the control group, and you won't know which group you are in, you will get the standard treatment for pancreatic cancer. Probably 5-FU. You won't be any worse off than you are now.

Ann: Let me think about it.

When Ann returned home, she went to ACOR.org and asked her support group what they knew about clinical trials near her. No one had much to offer, except Jack mentioned that a website call pancreatica.org specialized in knowing where all the clinical trials were being conducted in the country. Ann visited pancratica.org and learning that a Phase II clinical trial was recruiting patients in a medical clinic in Tulsa, only 80 miles from her home. Ann forwarded the information to Dr. Kim and asked what she thought. Dr. Kim responded that this sounded like a good trial and would request that Ann be considered. In the meantime, one of Ann's support group members sent Ann an email saying that not all clinical trials are covered by insurance companies and that Ann might want to check on this. When Ann called her case worker at the insurance company, she was shocked to learn that the experimental drug being used in the clinical trial was not covered as a treatment protocol.

Ann: Why not? Are you denying my right to the best care I can get?

Case Worker: It's not that simple. Many of these drugs are worthless and actually do more harm than good. This one has no track record with pancreatic cancer.

Ann went back to her online support group with her news and received a response from Sam, someone she had never heard from before.

Sam: Ann, there is an organization that helps patients and their families stand up to insurance companies. It is called the Patient Advocate Foundation. Their Internet address is http://www.patientadvocate.org/.

Ann was feeling so nauseous and tired, she called Clarise and asked her to check on it for her. Clarise acted almost privileged that her mother was entrusting her with an important detail of her life. Clarise contacted the foundation, and a case worker was assigned. As it turned out, the insurance company capitulated and allowed Ann to enroll in the clinical trial. Clarise and Alex took turns taking Ann to Tulsa for the treatments, which were five sets of four times a week for six weeks, with two weeks off to assess the CA 19-9 levels. The daily trips, the sickness from the treatments, the sterile environment, and the uncertainty of not knowing if she was getting the real drug were draining on Ann. Yet, she still felt that she was doing all she could to beat her disease. Both Alex and Clarise expressed a great deal of enthusiasm for the trial process.

At the end of the trial, Ann's oncologist told her that she had indeed been receiving the new agent, RFS 2000. Ann didn't feel any different after the treatment than she did before it started. She was usually tired, nauseous, and had abdominal pain, although the itching she had had with 5-FU wasn't as bad.

> *Dr. Bolder:* Your CA 19-9 levels have remained constant during the trial. That is good news in the sense that no new tumor growth is indicated. It is disappointing news in that we are not seeing any drop in those levels either. In your case, we are not sure if the new agent is any better for you than what you were using before. We don't think it's worth the risk to enroll you in Phase III of this trial.

In a way, Ann was relieved because she was tired of the daily 80-mile trips to get the same infusion she could get in her hometown. On the other hand, Ann began to worry that she was coming to a critical junction in the road of her life. For the first time, Ann rationally considered the possibility of dying from pancreatic cancer.

Agency

Ann went back to her oncologist, Dr. Kim, and they began follow-up treatments. Ann had made a list of her concerns prior to this meeting and went in more prepared than she had ever been. Ann decided to lay it all out on the table.

> *Ann:* Dr. Kim, you've been straight with me throughout this whole ordeal and I appreciate how you put aside your own treatment to help me get enrolled in the clinical trial—even though that may not have been our best option. One of my online buddies made a comment a few days earlier that oncologists have a tendency to treat patients right up to the last minute because they don't want to give up. They do so even if the patient is dying and could live a much better life with palliative treatment (pain management) and hospice care (end of life). I have already beat the odds by living 14 months since the diagnosis. What's in store for me in the next 6 months? Three months? What are you going to recommend as a treatment regimen now that the clinical trial is over?
>
> *Dr. Kim* (pausing): It really is the patient who has to make these decisions. If given a choice, oncologists always want to do everything they can to prolong life. You mentioned palliative care; well, often times, chemotherapy is a form of palliative care. It can help keep cancer cells in check so that new tumors do not block the bile duct, making you feel even worse. It's impossible to say that you will have the same quality of life in 3 years or even 3 months. Pancreatic cancer is difficult to predict. I do agree that you are beyond the norm for survivorship and would hate to see you give up treatment.
>
> *Ann:* Well, you have given me something to think about.
>
> *Dr. Kim:* I think I have a pretty good idea of when you are likely to progress to stage IV of the disease. When I think you are getting close, I will let you know so that you and your family can make these decisions with me. I do agree, at any point you decide to discontinue adjuvant therapy, you should immediately get involved in a hospice program. Do you already have all of your affairs in order, just in case?

Ann: Not everything, I've been putting off some of it because of my
    reluctance to give up.
Dr. Kim: I hope you never give up, Ann.

Being a cancer patient had changed the way that Ann looked at her life, causing her to question her past beliefs, values, and goals. Ann made the decision that she would reduce her work hours and telecommute to spend more time with her husband, her family, and by herself. She began to make lists of all of the things that she wanted to accomplish and do in her lifetime and made plans to accomplish them. She had always wanted to visit her friend in Italy and decided that if she was well enough, she would make that journey the following year.

Along with a journal, Ann also began to keep a notebook full of medical articles and research on pancreatic cancer. She joined other pancreatic cancer Web sites, such as PANCAN.COM, and regularly read the sites for updates. Ann kept in contact with her providers and regularly questioned them when she found articles that conflicted with their advice. Ann sought to reduce her uncertainty and raise her self-efficacy through many means, including her local support group, her online support groups, and sharing her feelings with her family. At one point, Ann received a phone call from Dr. Bolder, the oncologist who treated her during the clinical trial in Tulsa.

Dr. Bolder: Ann, I just wanted you to know that even though your trial wasn't particularly
    effective for you and your disease state, the results from that experiment have
    lead to some very exciting possibilities for combining varying doses of the
    new agents with some old ones. We wouldn't have been able to do that without
    your participation in our clinical trial. A lot of pancreatic cancer patients in the
    future will owe you and the others in the trial a debt of gratitude. I'm pretty
    certain that you would be eligible for our new trial, but whether you enroll or
    not, you have made a meaningful contribution for controlling pancreatic
    cancer.
Ann: Thanks for saying so. I may be in touch.

Later that night, Ann relayed the oncologist's message to her local support group. She was asked if she would try to get enrolled in the new trial that was mentioned. Ann paused—she thought of the disappointment from the last one, she thought of the hassle of traveling so often, she thought of the potential side effects of new drugs, she thought of what she might miss in life by participating. Ann smiled and said, "I'm not sure, but at least I have a choice, and that's what matters most."

EPILOGUE

The CSAM (O'Hair et al., 2003) served as an explanatory mechanism for charting how Ann navigated her way through the cancer experience. Her experience of living with cancer involved the four stages of CSAM: (1) shock, (2) uncertainty, (3) empowerment, and (4) agency.

In the shock stage, Ann simultaneously negotiated and renegotiated her own adaptation to the new cultural world of cancer (Sparks, 2003). At the same time, she had to negotiate and renegotiate her social identity of living with cancer with those whom she cared about (Harwood & Sparks, 2003). She had to deal with her own "shock" over the diagnosis and implications, but had to then break this news to loved ones and cope with their responses to it.

In the uncertainty stage, Ann continues to deal with the information overload and conflicting information she receives from various health care providers. In addition, she continues to struggle with decisions about when and to whom to communicate her diagnosis, and in how much depth. For example, when conversing with Alex, Ann has learned that he is most comfortable with discussion related to the cognitive aspects of the disease. In other word Alex would rather discuss chemotherapy regimens, blood counts, and protocols than Ann's feelings about living with the disease.

In the third stage (empowerment), Ann begins to think differently about her diagnosis and finds ways to integrate it more seamlessly into the various aspects of her life. Thus, Ann begins to negotiate the aspects of her treatment with health care providers, family, and friends. For example, she moves some of her appointment times around to fit her schedule rather than the schedule of the health care providers or her family members.

In the agency stage, Ann actively and assertively becomes involved in her treatment. For instance, she began to keep a journal of current research articles on pancreatic cancer, frequented the National Cancer Institute website, and began to eat healthier.

Ann's experiences as a pancreatic cancer patient are not atypical for most cancer patients. The grim and gruesome details of cancer and its almost equally deleterious treatment side effects were purposely muted to focus more clearly on the communication aspects of cancer care. Cancer care is a common part of everyday life, and as life expectancy continues to grow, more people will live long enough to get cancer. The National Cancer Institute has recognized the powerful effects that communication processes can bring to bear on the care of cancer. They are clear in their message that few other processes have the chance to positively influence care in such a cost-effective way. Ann's case illustrates how communication is an essential aspect in all four phases of cancer care: shock, uncertainty, empowerment, and agency. Cancer communication research carried out in the future will be instrumental in filling the gaps between what we know now and what we desperately need to understand to deliver better care for cancer patients in the future.

RELEVANT CONCEPTS

Agency: Process where patients understand the choices they have and can employ competence to act on these choices.
Chemotherapy: The treatment of cancer through chemicals.
Clinical trial: Research study conducted with patients to evaluate a new treatment or drug.
CT scan: Computed tomography. A special radiographic technique that uses a computer to display x-ray images into a two-dimensional cross-sectional image.
Disease staging: Staging of cancer is based on a system that classifies the size, site, and spread of the cancer. The numbers I, II, III, and IV are used to denote stages.
Empowerment: Processes of exerting control and influence in one's life.
Gastroenterologist: A medical specialist in internal medicine who treats diseases of the digestive system.
Hospice: A program of palliative and supportive services to dying persons and their families in the form of physical, psychological, social, and spiritual care.
Metastatic: Spread of a disease from the point of origin to another part of the body.
Oncologist: Medical doctor with a speciality in treating cancer.
Online support groups: An interactive computer network designed for special circumstances.
Palliative care: Treatment designed to reduce symptoms and pain rather than to find a cure.
Radiologist: A specialist who uses imaging techniques (x-rays, ultrasound, CT, magnetic resonance imaging, fine-needle biopsy, etc.) for diagnosis (diagnostic radiologist) or treatment.

Whipple procedure: Surgical procedure to resect (remove) the (cancerous) head of the pancreas to prevent the cancer from spreading.

DISCUSSION QUESTIONS

1. In the diagnosis stage, was Dr. Meese right in telling Ann over the phone that she might have cancer? Is it better to have made her wait with nervous expectations? Is the phone an appropriate communication channel for discussing medical issues? When would it be and when would it not be?
2. How can cancer support groups be more effective in helping its members cope with cancer care? Do you think online groups are the best place to start, as Ann did? What do you think are the communication differences between face-to-face and online support groups?
3. What would you identify as effective communication strategies that cancer patients can pursue to communicate more openly and directly with family members and significant others? What stands in the way of healthy communication? How does a family member developing cancer affect family communication, especially if communication problems existed prior to cancer entering the family?
4. For cancer patients, is more information always a good thing? When would more information actually be counterproductive for cancer patients?
5. What is the best method for evaluating health information you get from the Internet? Which sources are you more likely to trust? Why might physicians not be open to discussing information that patients bring with them from the Internet?

REFERENCES/SUGGESTED READINGS

Carlson, D. K. (2001, June). AIDS ranks third among American's most urgent health problems. *Gallup Poll News Service*. Retrieved August 31, 2001, from http://www.gallup.com/poll/releases/pr010625b.asp.

Hamel, J. (1993). *Case study methods: Qualitative research methods series 32*. Newbury Park, CA: Sage.

Murphy, G. P., Morris, L. B., & Lange, D. (1997). *Informed decisions: The complete book of cancer diagnosis, treatment, and recovery*. New York: Penguin.

National Cancer Institute. (2001a). Key cancer statistics. Retrieved August 31, 2001, from http://cra.nci.nih.gov /3_types_cancer/index.htm

National Cancer Institute. (2001b). Cancer survivorship. Retrieved August 31, 2001, from http://cra.nci.nih.gov /3_types_cancer/cancer_survivorship.htm

O'Hair, H. D., Villagran, M. M., Wittenberg, E., Brown, K., Ferguson, M., Hall, H. T., & Doty, T. (2003). Cancer survivorship and agency model (CSAM): Implications for patient choice, decision-making, and influence. *Health Communication, 15*(2), 195–202.

Sparks, L. (2003). An introduction to cancer communication and aging: Theoretical and research insights. *Health Communication, 15*(2),123–132.

Harwood, J., & Sparks, L. (2003). Social identity and health: An intergroup communication approach to cancer. *Health Communication, 15*(2), 145–170.

O'Reilly, E., & Kelvin, J. (2003). *100 questions and answers about pancreatic cancer*. Boston: Jones and Bartlett Publishers.

Additional Resource

On-line Medical Dictionary: http://cancerweb.ncl.ac.uk

8

Explanations of Illness: A Bridge to Understanding

Timothy M. Edgar
Emerson College

Dawn W. Satterfield
Centers for Disease Control and Prevention

Bryan B. Whaley
University of San Francisco

As frequent and integral a communicative practice as explaining illness is in health practitioner–patient interaction, relatively little is known about the most effective method(s) for explicating illness-related information. This state of affairs is problematic in that understanding the nature of one's illness is considered to be a vital component to reducing illness-related stress, increasing adherence to the medical regimen, and self-management. However, recent research has begun to determine a few of the intricacies involved in explaining illness.

For instance, the use of figurative language (i.e., analogies, metaphors, and similes) is an intuitive and frequently employed illness explanation device. However, investigations have found that children process figurative forms differently than adults and that even medical students' understanding of medical-related information can be hampered with the use of a less-than-appropriate comparison. In addition to age, effective illness explanation strategies can vary as a result of culture. Storytelling among some peoples is a powerful method of interacting about illness, but less effective among other cultures. There are many more concerns to be considered when creating and articulating illness explanation messages.

The following scenarios use diabetes as the health-related topic to exemplify many of the issues and variables to be considered (e.g., audience/culture, message content, and structure) in designing messages to explain illness. As you read the cases below, pay attention to the many nuances involved in explaining illness.

PROLOGUE

On a sunny Saturday morning in June in the Minneapolis–St. Paul area, a Twin Cities community group sponsored an event called "Walk for Life: A Bridge to a Healthy Tomorrow" to promote the idea that walking is an effective way to lower blood glucose levels (Fritz & Rosenquist, 2003), to reduce the risk of certain complications of diabetes (Gregg, Gerzoff,

Caspersen, Williamson, & Narayan, 2003), and to help prevent diabetes (Diabetes Prevention Program Research Group, 2001). The walk organizers chose a 5-kilometer route that began in St. Paul and headed west through the smaller of the two cities toward Minneapolis. The plan called for the band of approximately 300 participants to follow a path that would lead them across the Mississippi River via the Stone Arch Bridge to Mill Ruins Park, where the walk would end.

As they prepared to cross the bridge that morning, all of the hundreds of people who chose to take part in the walk carried with them personal stories and motives for being there that day. Some walked to honor the memory of a loved one who had lost the battle with diabetes, whereas others walked in support of family and friends still facing the challenges of the disease. Many in the crowd walked for themselves in an effort to manage an illness that already affected their lives or to prevent the onset of diabetes because they knew they were at greater risk.

For many, type 2 diabetes was a long-time nemesis, but for others, the personal confrontation began only recently. Two people at the walk coincidentally came face-to-face with the realities of the disease on the same day in April only two months before. Prior to the early spring, type 2 diabetes had touched the lives of both Charlene Byrd and Victor Cardoso to varying degrees. Because several members of Charlene's family battled the illness, she knew how serious type 2 diabetes could be, but her knowledge of the reality of the disease was limited. Family members made reference, at times, to their "condition," and sometimes, "this diabetes"; she witnessed the physical struggles they endured when complications arose, but she realized she had much more to learn. Victor, who is a teenager, also knew that members of his family had something called "diabetes," but it always seemed to him to be a problem that only affected old people.

On the afternoon of April 3, the lives of Charlene and Victor changed when their respective physicians delivered diabetes-related diagnoses to them. Charlene's doctor told her that she had pre-diabetes, whereas Victor's pediatrician explained to him and his parents that he would have to begin treatment immediately for type 2 diabetes. Shortly after their diagnoses, both Charlene and Victor learned about the June walk.

As the walkers saw the finish line just over the bridge, Victor and his mother stepped onto the structure at the same moment as Charlene. Without speaking, Charlene and Victor's gaze met as they propelled themselves toward the waving banner and cheering supporters. Feeling a similar sense of accomplishment, they had no idea they shared a history of receiving news about diabetes on the same day. The two began their walk across the river armed with hope and less intense feelings of anxiety than those they experienced back in April when their doctors first revealed their test results to them. In each case, Charlene and Victor had the good fortune of having their new health conditions explained to them in understandable terms by gifted communicators who chose appropriate strategies for telling them about the most relevant aspects of diabetes for their lives. Though information was communicated to them in different ways, both gained knowledge crucial to a healthy emotional response, and the experts they encountered provided them with targeted frameworks for making sense out of their new situations.

VICTOR'S STORY

Victor Cardoso, 15, lives in St. Paul with his family where he is completing his first year of high school. Victor, who currently stands 5 feet 7 inches and weighs 190 pounds, has struggled with his weight most of his life. He had been a large baby, and many people described him as "chubby" when he was a toddler. When friends and extended family members made comments about Victor's weight, his parents would just say that he still had "baby fat" that he needed to lose. Throughout his life, Victor has not been very physically active, but his parents, especially his father, encouraged him, in earlier years, in baseball. He liked the sport, especially to watch the Minnesota Twins on TV and to go to games occasionally with his dad. He played some in elementary school, but when he tried out for his middle school team in sixth grade, he found he got very tired and winded in practice, so he gave it up. In addition to getting little physical activity, Victor's weight also is the result of his high-fat diet. He loves fried foods for his main meals and often snacks with a bag of fried cheese snacks and a soda while playing video games or working on the family computer in the evening.

School is a very mixed experience for Victor. He always has been a good student, excelling in most subjects but especially math. Ever since he was very young, he has been absorbed in learning and reading. In some ways, school has been an environment that has built Victor's self-esteem because of the praise he has received from teachers and his parents for his consistently high grades. At the same time, going to school often causes Victor to feel very anxious. Because of his weight, many of the kids at school, especially the other boys, tease him about his size. During his freshman year in high school, the most dreaded period of the day was gym class. Not only did he have a difficult time keeping up with the activities, but also his classmates frequently harassed him in the locker room about his weight when he had to get undressed to take a shower at the end of the period.

Rico and Angela Cardoso—ages 37 and 36, respectively—are Victor's parents. They were born in the United States, the children of Mexican immigrants. Rico and Angela, who were high school sweethearts, grew up in Texas, where they got married right after their senior year. They moved to the Twin Cities a few years after getting married when a friend of Rico's helped him get a job as a construction worker. Victor was born the following year, and his sister, Helenita, was born two years later. For the last 7 years, Angela has worked as a checkout clerk at a grocery store.

Despite his weight problem, Victor has been relatively healthy for most of his life. Like most kids, he had the typical childhood illnesses like, chickenpox and bouts with the flu, but he has avoided serious health problems. However, in the late winter, his mother became concerned when she noticed that Victor had an unusual darkening of the skin around his neck.[1] She tried to scrub it off at one point, but soon realized that it was not dirt but some type of skin change from within the body. When his parents realized that the discoloration was not going to go away on its own, they decided that Victor should pay a visit to his pediatrician.

Within a few days, Angela Cardoso was able to get an appointment to see Dr. Nancy Price, 51, who has been Victor's pediatrician for the last 3 years. Dr. Price has been practicing for over 20 years. At Victor's afternoon appointment, his mother mentioned to Dr. Price the strange dark patch on the back of Victor's neck that alerted Dr. Price to the likelihood that he had pre-diabetes or had progressed to type 2 diabetes. In recent years, type 2 diabetes, long considered a "middle-aged disease" (Mazur, Joe, & Young, 1998) has become increasingly common among younger populations, particularly among those already disproportionately affected by diabetes (Fagot-Campagna et al., 2000). While gathering information for Victor's history, Dr. Price learned that one of Victor's uncles on his mother's side was diagnosed with diabetes in his 40s, and his maternal grandmother has had diabetes for many years and has taken insulin. Recently, his grandmother had to have her foot amputated. Dr. Price performed a complete physical examination and had blood work drawn to include a random blood glucose. The lab reported on the phone to Dr. Price a glucose value of 208 mg/dl, diagnostic for type 2 diabetes.

The doctor asked Angela Cardoso to meet with her in her office while Victor stayed in the waiting room. When she entered the consultation room, Dr. Price said, "Mrs. Cardoso, I'm glad you brought Victor in to be checked out. The dark coloring on Victor's neck is not, in itself, harmful or infectious, but it is an outward sign that his body is not able to use insulin as it should—we call it insulin resistance. This goes along with type 2 diabetes, which is a disease we have started to see in some young people, particularly when they tend to be overweight and not very active. Diabetes occurs when someone has too much sugar in the blood, and that is what Victor's lab report tells us, but I would like to ask you to bring him back first thing in the morning to do another blood test, just to make sure."

Angela, who was stunned to hear the news, told Dr. Price that she knew that kids can get diabetes because a child in their neighborhood developed diabetes when she was just 4 years old.

Dr. Price replied, "The little girl to whom you are referring probably has what we call type 1 diabetes. People used to call it juvenile diabetes because we most often saw it in children. Those who have type 1 diabetes have to take insulin shots because their body no longer produces insulin. I believe, however, that Victor's body makes insulin but his body is not responding to it as it should."

Angela exclaimed, "But that is what my mother and my oldest brother have. How could this be?"

Dr. Price offered her hand to Mrs. Cardoso who clung to it for a moment, "I know this is hard to hear and believe. When I was in medical school, we called type 2 diabetes "adult-onset diabetes" because it appeared in some adults as they got older. In the last few years, though, we've started to see type 2 diabetes among younger people, including teenagers like Victor who struggle with their weight. It's also becoming more common among Hispanic kids."

Dr. Price said to Angela, "I'm sure that this is a lot to take in right now. If this is diabetes, as I suspect, there is a lot Victor and your family can do to take charge of this. We'll have more time to talk about it tomorrow. Don't allow Victor to eat after midnight before coming to the office at 8 a.m. He can only drink water."

Angela agreed to Dr. Price's recommendation and said that she would return the next morning. When they got to the car, Victor, of course, wanted to know what the doctor said. His mother simply told him that there were different possibilities and that he should not worry. When he got home from work that evening, Rico Cardoso questioned his wife about what had happened at the doctor's office that day. Angela recounted the conversation she had with Dr. Price and the things the doctor said about the possibility of Victor having diabetes. Rico simply said, "I'll go with you tomorrow."

The next morning, Dr. Price got the results very shortly after the laboratory technician drew blood from Victor and saw that his fasting glucose was 138 mg/dl.[2] The results she saw on the printout confirmed her suspicions from yesterday, and she knew she was now going to have to tell Victor and his parents the news. Although Dr. Price had been treating children of all ages for many years, talking to children and their parents about type 2 diabetes was not something with which she had extensive experience. She had diagnosed five teenagers with diabetes in the past year and one the previous year, but she was not completely happy with her communication about it to children and their parents. Looking for new ways of communicating this complex disease to children, Dr. Price engaged a pediatric diabetes educator in discussions. Together, they built a strategy for using easy-to-understand illustrations and analogies for youngsters just learning they have diabetes. Their main goals were to make things understandable, memorable, and relevant to day-to-day life.

After Victor and his parents entered the consultation room, Dr. Price introduced herself to Mr. Cardoso, thanking him for coming that morning. She then began, "Victor, when you were here yesterday, the dark spot on your neck and the results of your blood test made me think that you probably have a condition called type 2 diabetes. After getting the results of the blood test we did this morning, I now know for sure that's what you have. I know this might sound a bit scary, but it doesn't have to be. It's something that I can help you with."

Dr. Price knew from recent experience that it did not make sense to go directly into explanations of the difference between type 2 and type 1 diabetes or to try to explain in detail the causes of the disease. She said, "Now I would like to make sure you understand the basics about diabetes—just so the next steps we take will make sense to you. I want you to promise me that if I'm going too fast or you want me to explain something again, then you will stop me. Can you promise me that?"

Feeling a bit shocked and not knowing what else to say, Victor looked at his mom and simply said, "OK." He knew that his grandmother who lived in Texas has diabetes, but he only saw her a few times a year and never asked that many questions about it. He assumed it was something that happened to people when they got old, like having heart trouble or difficulty remembering things. He knew that his grandmother had her foot removed and that it had something to do with diabetes, but again, he thought it happened primarily because she was elderly. When he first heard Dr. Price say that he had diabetes, he could not imagine how this was relevant to him.

Dr. Price started by saying, "Victor, in science class at school, you might remember your teacher talking at some point about how every cell in our body gets energy to do its work from the food that we eat. It's kind of like fuel to run a car. That energy comes from what we call glucose or blood sugar. We all have an organ called a pancreas that is located about here." Dr. Price then gently took her hand and placed it on Victor's abdomen. As she pointed to a picture of the human anatomy on her wall, she continued, "You can see a picture of what it looks like right here. What the pancreas does is to make something called insulin, which helps sugar from food get into your body's cells. When a person has the type of diabetes that you have, your body makes insulin, but it doesn't do the job it should. So, sugar builds up in your blood and can't get into your cells the way it is supposed to. Here is another way to think of it."

Dr. Price then pulled from her desk an old black-and-white photograph of logs floating down a river. She continued, "I saw this picture not too long ago in a bookstore here in the city and thought it would be a good way to talk to kids about diabetes. You might also have talked in school about how when people cut down trees in forests to make into wood to build houses, they have to have some way to get the logs from the forest to the place where they cut up the logs. So they would float them down the river to the sawmill. Workers on the shores had to grab the logs to get them in the place they needed to be. If the supply of logs floating down into the river was too great for the workers to keep up with, or if the workers are not doing their job, the river would get jammed with logs. Picture for a minute your bloodstream as a river and the sugar as logs. As the sugar, or think of the logs, floats down the river, or through your bloodstream, it has to be transported by insulin where it belongs—into the cells. If the workers aren't working efficiently, the logs remain in the river and get jammed together. That's what happens with type 2 diabetes. The insulin is there to do the job, which is to transport the sugar to the cells as needed, but it's not able to do a good enough job, so glucose builds up in the bloodstream. Just like having a logjam is not a good thing for the river, having too much sugar in your blood is not good for your body and can make you sick."

Victor understood the illustration, but like other children his age who Dr. Price had diagnosed with type 2 diabetes, he had other concerns. His immediate questions were, "So, am I going to be really sick? Will I have to stay home from school?"

Dr. Price answered, "If you do some very important things for yourself, then you should feel good most of the time. What I want to try at the beginning is to have you eat good foods and get more exercise. If it's hard for you to do really strenuous exercise at first, then I suggest that you begin by walking each day. Maybe your parents and your sister can take turns going for walks with you. Or maybe some of your friends can walk places with you as well. At some point, you also might have to take a pill, too, but let's try it without the pill for right now. When you talk to people about having diabetes, some people might ask if you have to take shots. Your mom told me yesterday, for instance, that your grandma takes shots for her diabetes. That probably sounds a little frightening, but I think we also can avoid shots for right now—maybe for a *very* long time."

Victor then asked, "What about this dark stuff on my neck? When is this going to go away? Some kid sitting behind me in English class saw it the other day at school and then told some guys that I don't take showers."

Dr. Price replied, "If you do the things we just talked about, like exercising and eating better foods, you should notice it start to disappear soon."

Dr. Price continued by explaining what she wanted Victor to do next. "First," she said, "I want you and your mom to make an appointment this next week with a terrific dietitian here at the office who will talk to you about good food choices for you to eat. Our receptionist will help you make that appointment. Second, I want you to start getting more exercise."

"To show you what good foods and exercise will do for you, I want to give you another mental picture." She went over to a cabinet and pulled out a brightly colored round object and handed it to Victor. She continued, "You probably have seen one of these before in a store or maybe one of your friends has one. They're actually called Hoberman spheres (Satterfield et al., in press), but," she laughed, "I like to just refer to them as 'those weird looking balls that grow.' They look strange, but I think they're great for talking about diabetes. Glucose isn't able to get into your cells because insulin isn't able to get the cells to open up like they should. Well, what happens when you choose healthy foods and start getting exercise is that your own insulin starts to do a better job. Now, pull on the ball with your fingers, and you'll see what happens."

As Victor pulled, he saw the sphere expand in volume 10 times. "Now," said Dr. Price, "think of your cells allowing in the glucose to make energy." Victor contracted and expanded the globe a few more times, and then said to his dad, "We have to get one of these."

Dr. Price replied, "I think it's a good idea to get one too. They're not that expensive, and it's a great reminder. After you walk, open it up and think about what your body is doing." Dr. Price then explained to Victor and his parents the importance of monitoring his blood glucose on a regular basis. The doctor showed them a meter and said that when they finished with their meeting, her nurse would demonstrate to them how to use it, how to keep track of readings, and tell them where they could buy their own. "At first," she said, "people are a little nervous about having to stick their finger to do the blood test, but they make meters these days so that you can barely feel it. When the nurse gives you instructions on the appropriate level you want to reach, you can then turn it into a game for yourself to see each day how good of a job you're doing. Think of it like keeping score for a baseball game."

Before Victor and his parents left, Dr. Price discussed one more thing with them. She said, "I know that what I've told you will give you quite a bit to think about. You're probably going to have lots of questions about how diabetes will affect your life that you can't think of right how. Instead of pressuring you into coming up with all of your questions now, I want you to come back in about 10 days from now so that I can see how you're progressing. During that time, I want you to take this with you." At that point, Dr. Price reached into a drawer and pulled out a small, blank notepad. On the cover in big letters, she wrote: VICTOR'S QUESTIONS. "Before I see you again," she continued, "I want you to use this pad to write down whatever questions come to your mind. Maybe your family can help you think of things. Bring the pad and your questions with you when you come next time."

After talking to the nurse about how to use the monitor and making an appointment to see the dietitian, Victor and his parents headed home. During the next 10 days, his parents worked with him to get him started on the things he would have to do to stay healthy. For instance, they began by alternating days that they would take walks with him to get him exercising. For variety, sometimes they would walk to the park, whereas other times, they would go to a local mall to walk. Angela and Rico also talked about ways they could start to change the meals they prepared so that Victor would eat more of the types of foods the dietitian recommended. Rico, who enjoyed working on computers like his son, helped Victor set up a spreadsheet so that Victor could record his glucose levels each day. Because he liked math so much, Victor then figured out a way to do printouts that showed his progress on charts.

As Dr. Price predicted, a number of questions did come to Victor's mind during the time that he was waiting to see her again, and, as she encouraged him to do, he wrote down the major questions in the notebook she gave him. As she learned over the years in her practice, kids are more concerned with how an illness is going to affect their lifestyle than they are with the medical details of the health problem. As Victor thought about what he wanted to ask her, most of his questions focused on changes he might or might not see in his daily life. When he and his mom arrived at Dr. Price's office for the follow-up, he brought along one of his charts with his glucose readings and showed her his scores. She congratulated him for keeping such good track. The levels were not yet where she wanted them to be consistently, but she encouraged him for heading in the right direction.

Dr. Price then asked Victor if he had more questions for her, at which point he tore a sheet from his notepad and handed it to her. She saw the following five questions scribbled on the paper:

- Will other kids be able to tell that I have diabetes?
- If I do all the right things, is there a chance that the diabetes will just go away?
- If I have to start taking medicine, will it give me bad breath?
- Will I ever have to have my foot taken off like my grandmother?
- Will I ever be able to be thin as long as I have diabetes?

After reading the questions, Dr. Price gave him answers to each that were honest but hopeful. The answers were not necessarily the ones he wanted to hear as, for instance, when she told him that the diabetes would not just go away, but Dr. Price was able to respond in a way that eased some of his anxieties.

When she finished answering his questions, Dr. Price said, "When you were here the last time, I didn't want to overwhelm you with too much information about the future, but we need to talk about how often you should come to see me from now on. As we talked about, it is very important that you monitor your blood sugar each day, but in order for me to know for sure that your glucose is in the right range, I want you to come in every 3 months to take an important blood test. That will better help me to know what's going on with your blood sugar over a longer period of time instead of just looking at the day-to-day readings that your monitor will give you. The best way to think about the test is to compare it to figuring out how well a baseball player is doing. I remember that you told me one time when you were in here for a checkup that you're a Twins fan, and I know you're good at math. Is that right?"

Victor acknowledged that he loved the Twins and that Torii Hunter was his favorite player. He also told her that he had received straight As in math all year.

"Ever since I was a little girl, I've been a Twins fan too. When I was young, a player named Tony Oliva was my favorite, and he was one of the best hitters in the game. I remember, when I was about 12, my father took me to a Twins game early in the season, and Tony went 0-for-5 that day. I was so upset because I thought that meant he would have a terrible average that season and wouldn't win the batting title. But my father said to me, 'You can't judge the way a player hits by what he does on one day. You have to look at the average for the whole season.' That's what this test will do. It will help to me to see not just how you're doing at that particular time on that certain day like your monitor does. What is more helpful is to have an idea of how well your glucose is being controlled over a whole season, like the summer or winter."

Finally, Dr. Price looked up on her wall where the diabetes educator had posted a sign for the "Walk for Life" to be held in June. "This might be something good for you and your family to do, Victor," she said. "It would be a good way to get in some fun walking that day, and you might meet other kids going through the same thing. If you don't feel comfortable telling people that you're doing it for yourself, then just say that you're walking for your grandma."

"That would mean a lot to her," Mrs. Cardoso added.

"When I see you at your next visit," Dr. Price continued, "maybe you can tell me all about it."

CHARLENE'S STORY

Charlene Byrd, 44, a Lakota Sioux woman who grew up on a reservation in South Dakota, moved to the Twin Cities area when she was 24 because her husband, Marlin, had gotten a job with his uncle's small independent moving company. The Byrds now have a 17-year-old daughter and a 14-year-old son. Charlene works part time as a dispatcher with the same moving company that employs Marlin and has a part-time job a few evenings a week at a large discount department store in the deli department. Charlene is 5 feet 5 inches and weighs about 180 pounds.

Charlene has been reasonably healthy for most of her adult life, but this past winter has been difficult. In January, she developed a case of bronchitis that she could not completely shake. She still had bouts of coughing and fatigue, causing her to miss several days of work. Her husband finally convinced her to see a doctor, something she rarely does. Charlene has no health insurance with either one of her part-time jobs, and the insurance that Marlin has from his job provides very minimal coverage. As a result, if the Byrds need health care, they usually go to a local clinic or sometimes home to the reservation.

On March 23, Charlene walked into a new clinic that had recently opened in their neighborhood and waited for 2 hours. When her turn finally came, the nurse escorted her to an examining room, where she met with Dr. James Foran, 56, a general practitioner at the clinic, who had retired to the Twin Cities area after his career as a physician in the U.S. Air Force was complete. Because it was Charlene's first visit to the clinic, Dr. Foran took a thorough medical history. After auscultating her lungs and getting a chest x-ray that ruled out serious lung problems, Dr. Foran decided to prescribe an antibiotic and a bronchodilator to resolve the bronchitis.

Noting that she was also overweight, he asked Charlene if anyone had ever talked to her about diabetes. She had never discussed diabetes with a health care professional, she said, but her father had died 2 years ago from kidney failure after having been on dialysis for six years. She added that an aunt and an uncle on her father's side have diabetes, and her uncle was recovering from a heart attack, which the doctor said was related to his diabetes. Her maternal grandmother also had diabetes before she died, and Charlene remembered her discomfort as a teenager at having to watch her take insulin shots. Charlene had no symptoms of diabetes, and a fingerstick blood glucose reading at her afternoon appointment was 145 mg/dl, not particularly remarkable, but Dr. Foran felt that Charlene was at risk for diabetes.

Shortly before starting at the clinic, Dr. Foran had been intrigued by a series of clinical trials that confirmed his hunch based on his observations over the years—type 2 diabetes can be prevented, or at least held at bay, for years by regular physical activity and taking and keeping off just a modest amount of weight (Diabetes Prevention Program Research Group, 2001). He had followed in the medical literature the heightened interest in lifestyle interventions for people with impaired glucose tolerance or impaired fasting glucose, now called pre-diabetes by many professionals (Benjamin, Rolka, Valdez, Narayan, & Geiss, 2003). He maintained that the glucose tolerance test, based on his experience, was the best way to figure out what was going on.

Dr. Foran sensed that Charlene was concerned about her health, and he thought that she might be willing to take some preventive action against diabetes, considering her family's history with the disease. He asked her to come in the following week for a test in the morning after fasting the previous night.

She said to the doctor, "I can't really afford to take off more time from work to come back next week. Are the other tests really necessary?"

Dr. Foran replied, "I think this test might tell us important information that you can do something about. Just come one morning next week and make sure that you've had nothing to eat since midnight the night before. The lab technician will take some blood, and then you will wait 2 hours before they take blood again."

Charlene had more questions, but other people were waiting at the busy clinic, and there was no more time. She reluctantly went to the laboratory on the morning of April 1 for the additional test. When she arrived, a technician drew a fasting glucose from a vein in her arm and then poured a sugary, orange beverage over ice for her to drink. Two hours later, the technician drew another sample of blood from Charlene. When Dr. Foran got the results in his office that afternoon, he saw that Charlene indeed had pre-diabetes according to the standard published in the literature. Her fasting glucose was 118 mg/dl, and her blood glucose, after a 75-gram glucose beverage, was 185 mg/dl.[3]

Two days later, when they sat down in his office to discuss the results, Dr. Foran began, "Mrs. Byrd, based on your family history and the fact that you are a little overweight, I ran a test to tell me whether or you not you are significantly at risk for diabetes. Although you do not have diabetes itself, the results show that you have impaired glucose tolerance. We've just started calling this pre-diabetes. Is that something you have ever heard of? Most people haven't."

Struggling to grasp his meaning, Mrs. Byrd said, "You said I don't have diabetes, but I have something like it?"

"Well," the doctor continued, "you don't have diabetes now, but many people who have pre-diabetes go on to develop type 2 diabetes. It means that the glucose is higher in your blood than it should be, but it has not moved to the stage we would definitely say is diabetes. What I suggest that you do is lose some weight and try to exercise more, and you might be able to do something about it. If you do these things, you should probably be OK for now. Come back in 6 months, and we can check your progress then. Any questions?"

Questions were forming in Charlene's mind, but she was too stunned to articulate them, so she just replied, "Not right now." As she rose to leave, she had a sick feeling in her stomach as she saw in her mind the image of her father lying in bed as he died—a once-large man who was small and dwarfed by the dialysis and heart equipment and intravenous lines surrounding him. The doctor had said she did not actually have diabetes, but she immediately assumed that she was destined for the same fate that her father, grandmother, and so many other American Indian people faced.[4]

As she walked home from the clinic, the tears trickled down her cheeks, a mixture of grief for her father and fear for her own future. That evening, as she told her husband about her interaction, he asked questions she was not able to answer. She realized that she left the office without really understanding what the doctor was telling her. She was not clear on the difference between diabetes and pre-diabetes, nor did she know what kind of exercise she should do, how to lose weight, or how much weight to lose. As busy as her life was already, she felt tired, overwhelmed, and resigned to the fact that she, too, would get diabetes. It would be good to be back home the following week for a family celebration. Right now, she needed the support of people from home.

When the Byrds arrived at her family's home in South Dakota on Friday evening, they stayed with Charlene's mother at the house where she grew up. The next morning, Charlene and her mother drove to visit her sister, Brenda, at her home 20 miles away. When her sister asked Charlene how things were going, Charlene choked back tears as she told her them about her visit with Dr. Foran. Like Charlene's husband, her mother and sister asked questions because they had not heard of pre-diabetes. Again, Charlene had few answers. Since talking with Dr. Foran, she had not really known where to turn for more information.

Charlene's sister quickly said, "Let's call Mary Keeps Eagle while you're here. I saw Mary a few weeks ago at the grocery store, and she looks so good. You know she used to be big and she has lost weight, and I saw her walking on that path by the reservoir several days ago. She told me that she just took a course to be able to talk to people here in the community about diabetes. She goes to homes, and they've had a few community meetings, too."

Eager to talk to someone about her diagnosis, Charlene took her sister's advice and called Mary at her home that day. Charlene explained to Mary that a doctor told her recently that she has pre-diabetes, but she does not really understand what it means or what she should do. Mary offered to meet Charlene at her mother's house on Sunday to talk to her about diabetes.

On Sunday, as she drove her pick-up to the home of Charlene's mother, Mary reflected on how she first became involved in diabetes work. Mary, who is 42 and grew up on a nearby reservation, had stayed at home with her four children for most of her adult life. Over a year ago, her husband had a car accident that put him in the hospital for weeks and permanently injured his leg. His recovery has been very slow, in part, because of his diabetes. Mary needed to work to help support the family and heard about opportunities to train as a community health representative (CHR), part of a program that receives special funds for diabetes prevention and control. Friends and family members encouraged her to take this job because of her people skills and the reputation she has as an excellent storyteller. Nine months ago, she went through a 3-week training course funded through the Indian Health Service to become a CHR. In the class, she learned a great deal about health, and for the entire three weeks enjoyed the healthy choices offered in the classes, including sugar-free drinks and pudding, fruit, and an endless supply of non-fat popcorn. The class went for a walk every afternoon about two, which she had looked forward to after sitting in class, and the class members all received a blood glucose meter and learned to test their own glucose. When the class talked of ways to communicate effectively and nonjudgmentally with their clients, Mary's thoughts turned to the legacy of storytelling passed on to her from her mother and grandmother. She believed that this Indian way of teaching—so that things are remembered and are not threatening to people—can help create a new, positive vision of things that otherwise might seem hopeless, like diabetes (Carter, Perez, & Gilliland, 1999).

When Mary got to the home of Charlene's mother, Charlene thanked her for coming and invited her in. After sitting at the kitchen table talking with Charlene and her mother for a while, Mary said to them, "I try to get some walking in almost every day. Would you like to come with me, Charlene?" Charlene agreed, and they walked to a nearby path together.

Charlene said, "When I called you, I told you that the doctor said that I have a condition—a long name I can't remember, but it's like having 'pre-diabetes.' He said that I may not go on to develop diabetes, but I'm very afraid that I will. You know what diabetes has done to my family. He also said I needed to exercise and lose some weight, but I don't know if that will do any good."

From her training and her several months of experience, Mary knew that diabetes can be frightening for people who had witnessed the devastation it can cause among people they love. She had learned many facts in the course, but did not want to overwhelm Charlene with these. Small steps are the key. She talked about how, just by the walking they were doing then, their bodies were enjoying the benefits. Mary explained, "When we eat, the insulin in our bodies needs to do its work to take blood sugar to our cells for energy. Just by moving our muscles, like we are doing now, allows the insulin to open up the cells and allow glucose or blood sugar to get in rather than stay in the bloodstream. We don't want that to happen." Mary then opened her hands as she said this to illustrate symbolically for Charlene the effect walking could have for her, especially if it became a routine. She added that dropping some weight can complement the effect. Mary said, "Taking off just 10 pounds can be a big help."[5] Charlene was encouraged because these steps seemed like simple ones she could take.

As they walked further, Mary said to Charlene, "I have a story I'd like to try out on you, if you don't mind. I think stories might help people—different stories for different people." Mary began, "You might already know this story. A young Indian man was on a quest for vision and preparation for adulthood when he set off to climb a mountain peak. When he reached the top, his heart swelled with joy at the beauty of all that lay before him. Then he saw a snake who spoke to him that said, 'I am about to die. It is too cold for me up here, and I am freezing. There is no food, and I am starving. I beg you to put me under your shirt and take me down to the valley.' 'No,' said the young man. 'I know your kind. You are a snake. If I pick you up, you will bite and kill me.' 'Not so,' said the snake, 'I will treat you differently. If you do this for me, I will not harm you.' The young man resisted, but finally, he tucked the snake under his shirt and carried it down to the valley. There, as the young man lay gently on the grass, the snake suddenly coiled and leapt, biting him on the leg. 'But you promised,' cried the young man as he lay dying. And the snake said, 'You knew what I was when you picked me up. I am what I am.'"

Mary then added, "Charlene, that snake is like diabetes. We know what it is, and it can't be trusted. Just like with the young man, it strikes at Indian people without mercy." Mary continued, "But we can't give up hope. I don't like ending the story with the snake winning. So, I want to tell you another story about the same snake. The snake, basking in the sun at the foot of the mountain, suddenly got trapped by a rock that fell on him. A kind-hearted rabbit that heard his cries responded and rolled the rock off of him. However, the snake surprised him by saying that he wanted to 'reward' the rabbit by eating him for dinner. A wise coyote, which knew the character of both the snake and the rabbit, came along just in time and said she would be the judge. The coyote listened to both their stories, and then tricked the snake by telling him that he could best judge the truth if she could see the snake's exact, former position under the rock. Once the snake was trapped back under the rock, the coyote announced that the snake's reward for trying to eat the kind rabbit was to stay under the rock." Mary laughed, "That snake is our enemy. It's diabetes, after all, and we know what it does, but I think we can put it under a rock. We should not ignore it, like it's not there, but we should be clever enough to outsmart it. And maybe we can learn something from diabetes, too. It's an enemy, but it's also a teacher" (Creeden, 1994; Satterfield, 2001).

"I like the stories," Charlene said. "Do you mean that maybe there are some things we need to learn from diabetes? Like about why so many people are getting it?" Charlene asked.

"Yes," Mary replied, "that's what I've been thinking. That we can learn something from it—like remembering the good ways of our people and trying to keep them in the picture, even now. We can eat good foods and stay active so we can avoid diabetes."

"Can you explain, Mary, what exactly the doctor meant when he said that I have pre-diabetes?" Charlene asked. "That means you're at a stage where you could go on to get diabetes, but it doesn't always have to happen."

Mary replied. "A little can be a lot. Like what we're doing now—walking. She added, "We can keep the snake under the rock by taking small steps. Do you have a place to walk where you live in Minneapolis?"

"Well," said Charlene, "I don't like to go out alone, but as long as one of my kids will go with me, we can walk around the neighborhood. I think they both would help me, but it's not going to be easy. I'm just not sure that I can find the time. It could become a burden."

Mary responded, "I know that it's not easy, but try not to think of it as a burden. Instead, I want you to think of it as a gift. It is a gift you can give to yourself. It is a gift you can give to your husband, your two children, and the grandchildren that your children will give you someday. Your husband needs his wife, your children need their mother, and your grandchildren someday will need you for your wisdom. By taking care of your health, you will give them a great gift. You might have to be clever to find ways to fit walking into to your life, but it'll be worth it. When you get back to Minnesota and go for your first walk, you should say to yourself, 'Today I'm walking for the future. Today I'm walking for my grandchildren who are not yet born so that they will have a healthy grandmother who will love them and teach them about our ways the same way that my grandmother taught me.'"

"The food part won't be easy either," Charlene continued. "I'm working two part-time jobs and I have about 20 minutes to get home and change clothes before going to my second job. I pick up food at the deli where I work. Who has time to cook? You also know what it's like when you visit people—you eat."

"Yes," Mary nodded. "But I think that's where we can sort of let diabetes teach us. Our people didn't get this disease before our grandparents' time. What did they do that kept them from getting diabetes? It had to be partly the foods they ate, and they worked so hard. I've been making soups like my grandmother still keeps on the stove, and I take that and a pot of Indian beans to feasts. People always say those bring back good memories."

"That's a good thought," Charlene responded. "I want my kids to have those 'memory foods,' too. I think I'll talk to my mother about cooking up some beans and things and maybe take back a little of her soup."

As they headed back to the home of Charlene's mother, Charlene felt less anxious than she had before. She took comfort in Mary's words and the walk felt good. As they parted ways, Charlene thanked Mary, and Charlene asked Mary if she could call her the next week if she had more questions. Mary encouraged her to do so. The following week, after arriving back in the Twin Cities, Charlene called Mary to proudly tell her that she and her kids were walking almost every day, and they were trying to eat good foods, like the ones she remembered from her childhood. Charlene's mother had even packed up some frozen soup and beans they were using. Mary was thrilled and said they should celebrate soon. She added she had seen a poster on a walk for health in the Twin Cities called "Walk for Life: A Bridge to a Healthy Tomorrow" on June 3. "Why don't you go?" she said. "We're going to have one here on the same day, so I'll be thinking of you. I'll be walking at the same time."

EPILOGUE

When Victor and Charlene crossed the bridge at the end of the walk, they were greeted with shouts of encouragement, handshakes, and cold water to drink. Feeling a sense of accomplishment, their private thoughts turned to the resistance each was putting up against diabetes. Victor still felt somewhat angry about his diagnosis. "Why should a kid like me have to deal with an old person's disease?" he thought at times since Dr. Price first told him he had diabetes. But as he walked and saw other kids at the event, he started picturing that weird-looking ball opening to let the glucose in, and he already seemed to have energy. His body was not resisting the insulin as it had. His muscles were moving, and that made it possible for glucose to get in its place in his cells to give him energy, not sitting around in his bloodstream like a logjam in a river. Maybe he and his dad could hit some balls later that day.

As Victor downed his water, he saw Charlene getting a refill herself. She smiled at him and his mother. "What brought you here today?" she asked.

"We're here because of my son's diabetes. He just found out he has it," his mother said.

"That's too bad," Charlene said. "I just found out I have pre-diabetes. I'm trying to outsmart it." She smiled to herself as she thought of the coyote and the snake.

"Me, too" said Victor.

"Do you want to hear a story a friend told me?" Charlene asked.

RELEVANT CONCEPTS

Age of interactant: Number of years lived of persons involved in the discussion of illness.
Comparisons: Illustrating a point through a form of similitude (e.g., analogy, metaphor).
Content of illness explanation: The "what" of a message designed to explicate illness.
Culture: A body of meanings, beliefs, norms, values, and practices that are learned, transmitted, and shared through a communication.
Illness explanation strategies: Communicative methods or tactics to make the nature of illness and its implications understood.
Storytelling: The practice of using the narrative form for communicative purposes.

DISCUSSION QUESTIONS

1. Think back to a time when you had an experience with a health care provider who did an excellent job of explaining a medical condition or health threat to either you or to a member of your family. Describe that health care provider's approach to sharing illness-related information. What did he or she do or say that made you feel that you received a satisfactory explanation?
2. Discuss the appropriateness of Dr. Price taking two sessions to convey needed information to Victor and his parents. Should she have tried to tell them everything when she first diagnosed him with type 2 diabetes?
3. How might Dr. Price alter her explanatory strategy if she had to talk about a serious health condition with a child 3–5 years younger than Victor?
4. How could Dr. Foran have been more effective in the way that he explained Charlene's medical condition to her?
5. When Mary talked to Charlene about diabetes, she relied heavily on her culture's oral tradition in her use of the snake story. How effective would storytelling be in explaining illness to an individual who comes from your own culture or ethnic heritage?
6. Discuss the role visual presentations of illness (e.g., drawings, videos) might play in enhancing an illness explanation expressed orally.

ACKNOWLEDGMENTS

The authors wish to thank Gwen Hosey and Kris Ernst of the Centers for Disease Control and Prevention for reviewing an earlier draft of this case study. Partial funding for the preparation of this chapter came from the Office of the Dean, Emerson College, School of Communication, Health Communication Research Fund, established by Dr. and Mrs. Donald B. Giddon.

ENDNOTES

[1] This is a condition known as acanthosis nigricans, which is a symptom of type 2 diabetes for about 90% of children who develop the illness. In addition to the appearance of dark, shiny patches on the back of the neck, many children with type 2 diabetes have similar patterns of discoloration between the fingers and toes and axillary creases (Children with Diabetes, n.d.). For more information on how to diagnose children with type 2 diabetes, see American Diabetes Association (2000).

[2] The criteria for the diagnosis of type 2 diabetes are: symptoms of diabetes plus casual plasma glucose concentration ≥ 200 mg/dl (11.1 mmol/l). Casual is defined as any time of day without regard to time since last meal. The classic symptoms of diabetes include polyuria, polydipsia, and unexplained weight loss, or fasting plasma glucose

≥126 mg/dl (7.0 mmol/l). Fasting is defined as no caloric intake for at least 8 hours. Or two-hour plasma glucose ≥200 mg/dl (11.1 mmol/l) during an oral glucose tolerance test. The test should be performed using a glucose load (75 g).

[3] Nondiabetic individuals with a fasting plasma glucose (FPG) ≥110 mg/dl (6.1 mmol/l) but <126 mg/dl (7.0 mmol/l) are considered to have impaired fasting glucose (IFG), and those with 2-hour values in the oral glucose tolerance test (OGTT) ≥140 mg/dl (7.8 mmol/l) but <200 mg/dl (11.1 mmol/l) are defined as having impaired glucose tolerance (IGT). Both IFG and IGT are risk factors for future diabetes. Normoglycemia is defined as plasma glucose levels <110 mg/dl (6.1 mmol/l) in the FPG test and a 2-hour postload value <140 mg/dl (7.8 mmol/l) in the OGTT (American Diabetes Association, 2003).

[4] In the past 50 years, diabetes has become one of the most common and serious illnesses among American Indians and Alaska Natives (Narayan, 1997). The age-adjusted prevalence of diabetes among American Indians and Alaska Native adults (15.3%) is more than twice that of the overall U.S. population (7.3%) (Centers for Disease Control and Prevention, 2003).

[5] Recent studies have provided scientific evidence confirming the feasibility of preventing or delaying the onset of type 2 diabetes. In this country, the Diabetes Prevention Program (DPP) was a randomized clinical trial involving 3,234 adults, including 171 American Indians (Diabetes Prevention Program Research Group, 2001). The DPP found that an intensive lifestyle intervention, which involved achieving and maintaining about 7% of their weight and 150 minutes of physical activity a week for about three years, reduced the risk of developing type 2 diabetes by 58%. An arm of the trial that included administration of a drug, metformin, demonstrated a 31% reduced risk. The Centers for Disease Control and Prevention (CDC) estimates that 12 million overweight Americans, aged 45 to 74 years, have pre-diabetes, a vast audience for messages about the potential for prevention or delay of diabetes.

REFERENCES/SUGGESTED READINGS

American Diabetes Association. (2003). Screening for type 2 diabetes: Position statement. *Diabetes Care, 26*, S21–S24.

American Diabetes Association. (2000). Type 2 diabetes in children and adolescents. *Diabetes Care, 23*, 381–389.

Benjamin, S. M., Rolka, D. B., Valdez, R., Narayan, K. M. V., & Geiss, L. S. (2003). Estimated number of adults with prediabetes in the U.S. in 2000: Opportunities for prevention. *Diabetes Care, 26*, 645–649.

Carter, J. S., Perez, G. E., & Gilliland, S. S. (1999). Communicating through stories: Experience of the Native American Diabetes Project. *Diabetes Educator, 25(2)*, 179–187.

Centers for Disease Control and Prevention. (2003). Diabetes prevalence among American Indians and Alaska Natives and the overall population—United States, 1994–2002. *Morbidity and Mortality Weekly Report, 52*, 702–704.

Children with Diabetes. (n.d.). Type 2 diabetes in children. Retrieved May 22, 2003, from http://www.childrenwithdiabetes.com/d_on d00.html

Creeden, S. (1994). *Fair is fair: World folktales of justice.* Little Rock, AR: August House.

Diabetes Prevention Program Research Group. (2001). The Diabetes Prevention Program: Reduction in the incidence of type 2 diabetes. *New England Journal of Medicine, 344*, 393–403.

Fagot-Campagna, A., Pettit, D. J., Engelgau, M. M., Burrows, N. R., Geiss, L. S., Valdez, R. et al. (2000). Type 2 diabetes mellitus among North American children and adolescents: An epidemiologic review and a public health perspective. *The Journal of Pediatrics, 136*, 644–672.

Fritz, T., & Rosenquist, U. (2003). Walking for exercise: Immediate effect on blood glucose levels in type 2 diabetes. *Scandinavian Journal of Primary Health Care, 19*, 31–33.

Gregg, E. W., Gerzoff, R. B., Caspersen, C. J., Williamson, D. F., & Narayan, K. M. V. (2003). Relationship of walking to mortality among U.S. adults with diabetes. *Archives of Internal Medicine, 163*, 1440–1447.

Mazur, M., Joe, J., & Young, R. S. (1998, December). Why are children being diagnosed with a "middle-aged" disease? *Diabetes Forecast,* 47–48.

Narayan, K. M. V. (1997). Diabetes mellitus in Native Americans: The problem and its implications. *Population Research and Policy Review, 16*, 169–192.

Satterfield, D. (2001). Stories connect science to souls. *Diabetes Educator, 27*, 176–178.

Satterfield, D. W., Lofton, T., May, J. E., Bowman, B., Alfaro-Correa, A., Benjamin, C. et al. (in press). Learning from listening: Common concerns and perceptions about diabetes prevention among diverse American populations. *Public Health Management and Practices.*

Whaley, B. B. (Ed.). (2000). *Explaining illness: Research, theory, and strategies.* Mahwah, NJ: Lawrence Erlbaum Associates.

Additional Resources

Diabetes: Disabling, Deadly, and On the Rise: At a Glance 2003 http://www.cdc.gov/nccdphp/aag/aag_ddt.htm
Diabetes Risk Test http://www.diabetes.org/main/info/risk/risktest.jsp
Source: American Diabetes Association
Health for Native Life
(a magazine to help American Indians and Alaska Natives prevent and manage diabetes)
Source: Indian Health Service National Diabetes Program
Helping the Student with Diabetes Succeed: A Guide for School Personnel
http://ndep.nih.gov/materials/pubs/schoolguide.pdf
Source: National Diabetes Education Program (CDC and National Institutes of Health)
Message of Hope—We Can Prevent Diabetes in Native American Communities
(video about the Diabetes Prevention Program)
Source: Indian Health Service National Diabetes Program
Sepa cuánta azúcar tiene en la sangre: Hágase la prueba para controlar el azúcar sanguíneo (NDEP-11) (also available
   in English) http://ndep.nih.gov/get-info/spanish.htm
Tome su diabetes en serio, para que no se vuelva cosa seria. Recomendaciones para sentirse mejor y estar mas saludable
   (NDEP-9) (also available in English)
Source: National Diabetes Education Program http://ndep.nih.gov/get-info/spanish.htm

Organization Listings

American Diabetes Association
1660 Duke Street
Alexandria, Virginia 22314
800-DIABETES (342-2383)
800-ADA-ORDER (236-6733-to order publications)
800-232-3472
http://www.diabetes.org

Centers for Disease Control and Prevention (CDC)
Division of Diabetes Translation
Public Inquiries and Publications
P.O. Box 8728
Silver Spring, Maryland 20910
877-CDC-DIAB (232-3422)
E-mail: diabetes@cdc.gov
http://www.cdc.gov/diabetes

Centers for Disease Control and Prevention (CDC) and National Institutes of Health (NIH)
National Diabetes Education Program
CDC and National Institutes of Health
http://ndep.nih.gov
1-800-438-5383; E-mail berryt@extra.niddk.nih.gov
Mail requests to NDEP, National Diabetes Education Clearinghouse, 1
Information Way Bethesda, Maryland 20892-3560

Indian Health Service Diabetes Program
5300 Homestead Road, N.E.
Albuquerque, New Mexico 87110
505-248-4182
http://www.ihs.gov/medicalprograms/diabetes

Juvenile Diabetes Research Foundation International
120 Wall Street, 19th Floor
New York, New York 10005-4001
800-JDF-CURE (533-2873)
800-223-1138
E-mail: info@jdrf.org
http://www.jdf.org

9

Talking to Children About Illness

Jenifer E. Kopfman
Eileen Berlin Ray
Cleveland State University

Ethan leaped out of the mini-van with his favorite Rescue Hero toy in hand, eager to begin his day at preschool. He waited impatiently on the sidewalk for his mom, Cathy, to gather the rest of his things, and as soon as she locked the door, he raced for the entrance. Cathy caught up with him while Ethan carefully pressed the four-digit code into the keypad of the security door. Once inside, Ethan urged, "Hurry up, Mom! We need to get down to my classroom!"

Even before they reached the classroom door, Cathy and Ethan were greeted with a chorus of cries from his friends. "Hey, it's Ethan!" and "Ms. Lisa, Ethan's back!" filled their ears as Ethan was surrounded by 6 four-year-olds, each trying to hug him, while the 10 other children in the room watched curiously. It was Wednesday, and Ethan had not been at preschool since the previous Friday. Cathy smiled a silent greeting to Ms. Lisa.

"Where were you Ethan? Why weren't you here yesterday?" asked his best friend Logan.

"I was sick," Ethan replied.

"Did you throw up? I threw up the last time I was sick."

"No, I had the coughs and the sword throat again," Ethan told his friend. "And I couldn't breathe good. But Mom took me to the hospital late at night, and a doctor there helped me breathe. And today I went to three doctors, and I got lotsa new medicines to make me feel better." With a quick "Oh" for a reply, Logan ran to the other side of the room with two other boys as they all called, "Come play trucks, Ethan."

Ms. Lisa made her way through the chaos and toys to talk to Cathy in a normal tone of voice. "The hospital and three doctors since Friday . . . sounds like you've been busy. Is it serious?"

"Yes and no," Cathy answered. "I think we've finally got his asthma under control, but now we're dealing with the long-term issues. Sunday night, he had a bad asthma attack. Poor kid, he could barely breathe. So I rushed him to the emergency room, and they got that under control quickly. When you have some time, I'll tell you what happened to Lucy while we were there. Nothing bad, just bizarre. Anyway, then we saw his pediatrician Monday morning, and since she felt like she hasn't been able to get a handle on what's triggering the asthma, she referred us to a pulmonologist and an allergist. We saw one that afternoon and one yesterday. So, yeah, I guess we have been busy!"

Ethan hung up his coat and put his Rescue Hero in his cubby. Turning around, he almost bumped into his friend, Sophia, who was waiting quietly for her turn to welcome him back.

"So what did all those doctors do to you?" Sophia wanted to know.

"Well, Dr. Tracy just listened to my heart and my breathing like she always does," Ethan told her. "But then she had to put a stick in my throat and make me choke. I cried when she did that, but I got a red lollipop."

"I like the purple ones," Sophia said.

Cathy, eavesdropping on the childrens' conversation, interpreted for Ms. Lisa. "Throat culture. Don't worry, it was negative for strep."

"That's good" Lisa commented, glancing around at the various groups of children playing.

Ethan continued, "Then I went to a boy doctor who made me lay on my tummy and watch cartoons. He poked my back with stuff that made me itchy, but I wasn't allowed to scratch it or even rub it."

"That's yucky. Was it boring?" Sophia commented.

"Nope. 'Cause I got to watch any show I wanted!" Ethan replied.

"That was the allergist," Cathy explained to Lisa. "They tested him for a whole slew of household allergens, as well as all the common outdoor ones like ragweed and pollen. He had these huge red welts all across his back in reaction to the testing, but we got a whole list of his allergy triggers along with information on how to prevent unnecessary exposure to some of them."

"That sounds like progress," Lisa said.

"Then, yesterday, I went to another girl doctor that's not Dr. Tracy, and she just listened to my breathing and asked me who my Rescue Hero was, and then talked to Mom for a really, really long time," Ethan told Sophia. "She's the one who gave me all the new medicines."

Cathy explained, "The last doctor was the pulmonologist. Based on the results of the allergy testing and my descriptions of his symptoms, she diagnosed him with allergy-induced asthma. She prescribed a couple of treatments for the acute attacks he gets, an antibiotic to help clear up the sinus infection that developed, and a couple of preventative medicines that should help keep things from getting as bad as they did last week."

"What kinda medicine do you hafta take?" Sophia wanted to know.

"I got four medicines now," Ethan described. "When it's bedtime, we get everything out and I sit on the counter. First, I take white medicine from the squeezy thing Mom uses to suck up the medicine. That gets rid of my green boogers."

"Antibiotic for the sinus infection," Cathy told Lisa. "He only has to take that one for 10 days as long as the infection clears up."

Ethan continued, "And after the white medicine, I always have to have a drink of water. Then I pretend to be like the guy on TV and I tell Mom 'Coming up next, it's . . . runny . . . right here on countertop!' And so Mom gives me my runny nose medicine, but I just call it my runny, and then I get another drink of water."

"That one's an antihistamine for the allergies. He knows we start to take it when his nose gets runny, so that's why he calls it his runny nose medicine," Cathy explained to Lisa.

"After that, we hafta do my nose squirts, and I take lots of deep breaths in my nose and then I wipe it with a tissue," Ethan described for Sophia.

Cathy interpreted again, "It's a nasal spray that opens up the breathing passages and also helps with the allergies. This one's got him all confused, though. After we finally taught him how to blow his nose to clear it out, we had to teach him how to breathe in to get this spray to work. Now, whenever he blows his nose, he tries to breathe in," Cathy laughed.

Ethan continued telling Sophia all about his medicine routine, "And my last one every night is my breathing medicine. First, I shake it, and then Mom puts it in this long thing that goes over my face. She does two pushes and I do lots of deep breaths. Sometimes, when I do my deep breaths I moo like a cow just to be silly, and it makes Mommy laugh." Ethan and Sophia started laughing and "moo"-ing together, which of course provoked even more laughter.

Lisa had an amused but quizzical look on her face, so Cathy explained, "It's an albuterol inhaler to treat the acute asthma. He's too young to do the inhaler by himself, so the doctor gave me what she called a spacer to help administer it. The spacer fits over his nose and mouth while the inhaler fits in the other end, and it holds the medicine in there until he can breathe enough of it into his lungs. Actually, that's where I'm going to need your help. The doctor said that we need to give Ethan the albuterol at least four times a day for the next few days and then, after that, he'll need it anytime he has trouble breathing, so I'm going to have to ask you to learn how to do this. You'll need to give him a treatment every day after snack time just for this week. Then, I'll need you to keep this handy so that he can get the medicine when he needs it. Y'know how he starts coughing and wheezing after he's been running for too long? That's when he'll need it."

"No problem," Lisa told Cathy. "My niece has asthma too, and she had one of these when she was little. I know basically how they work, but if you could show me how it needs to be done, that would be great." Cathy showed Lisa how to administer Ethan's medicine while Ethan and Sophia settled down from all the animal noises and continued their conversation.

"So that's it. White, runny, nose squirts, and breathing . . . those are all my medicines," Ethan summarized.

"My mom takes more medicine than that," Sophia said.

"How come?" Ethan wondered.

"'Cause she's sick, too.' 'Cept she doesn't get runny noses and green boogers like you do. She gots bad monsters inside her tummy that try to eat her up," Sophia explained.

It was Cathy's turn to give Lisa a quizzical look. "Didn't you know?" Lisa asked. "Cindy was diagnosed with breast cancer a couple of months ago. It sounds like it's pretty bad. At first, they didn't want Sophia to know anything was wrong, but when she decided to go ahead with chemo, they figured it was better to tell her a little about what has happening. She seems comfortable with the monster metaphor."

"What color are the monsters?" Ethan wanted to know.

Sophia thought for a few seconds, and then said, "I dunno. I haven't seen them, but I think they're orange 'cause orange's a gross color and monsters are gross."

"How did the monsters get there? Did your mommy eat something to give her monsters?"

"Nope, they just grew there."

"So does the medicine make the bad monsters go away?" Ethan asked.

"I guess so," Sophia replied.

"How many medicines does your mom have?" Ethan wanted to know.

"Lots," Sophia answered. "She has to eat a bunch of pink and white things when we eat breakfast in the morning, and then she has to eat more of them at night. She even has a special kind of medicine that she only takes at the doctor's office. She always gives me lots of hugs and kisses before she gets her medicine from the doctor 'cause she says it makes her throw up and be tired after she takes it, and I hafta be quiet and let her sleep and not ask for too many hugs and kisses until she feels better again."

"So after that, then the monsters are all gone?" Ethan asked.

"Well . . ." Sophia paused. "I thought so, but Mommy just told me this morning that she has to go back for more of the medicine next week. I don't know why the monsters aren't gone yet."

"I can make a really scary monster face," Ethan told her. "Wanna see?"

"Yeah!"

As Ethan and Sophia raced across the room making monster faces and grabbing trucks to join the other kids, Cathy and Lisa continued talking.

"Wow," Cathy exclaimed. "I'm impressed with how much she knows about what's going on. For a 4-year-old, she seems pretty comfortable with everything."

"Like I said before, they figured it was better for her to know what was going on. I know that Cindy did a lot of research before she talked with Sophia, both on explaining cancer and on talking with kids about illness. She read that kids Sophia's age tend to understand figurative language, like the monster metaphor. I actually looked up a few things on the Internet myself just so I knew what to say to Sophia if she started talking about it here at school," Lisa said.

"It's hard to figure out how much to tell them," Cathy told Lisa. "The only thing Ethan kept asking me this week was 'Why am I sick?' and I didn't really want to get into a physiological explanation that he wouldn't understand, but I didn't want to answer him with baby talk either. Finding that balance that is right for this age is difficult. What did you find when you were on the 'Net?"

"A few things," Lisa replied. "First of all, it's important to give the kids some information, because they're going to know that something is going on, but it's got to be age-appropriate information. And that you should first ask the child what they know about an illness or treatment so you know where to begin. It also said to understand what they call the child's scripts, basically finding out what the child thinks happens and the order of these things happening. Sophia wouldn't understand all the medical terminology related to Cindy's cancer, so they used the monster metaphor."

"It makes sense to me," Cathy stated. "It gives her a way to understand things in her own terms. I would think that'd help things go more smoothly. That's what I tried to do with Ethan, and you notice that his interpretation of all these doctors visits focused on the important things—TV shows and lollipops!"

"Yep, but he also knew what each doctor was doing. And he didn't seem to be scared or bothered by it." Lisa continued, "I also found that it's important to address any fears the kids might have about any illness, but to make sure to let them know that it's not their fault that someone got sick. Several of the websites talked about kids feeling like they did something bad to make their parent sick, or that the reason they got sick themselves was because of their misbehavior. Believing that can create all sorts of guilt or frustration, or even resentment."

"I know what you mean," Cathy exclaimed. "Ethan actually asked me if he got sick because of something he did. So I explained to him that people's bodies react different ways to different things. We talked about how some of the things in the air make him sneeze and cough and have trouble catching his breath but they don't do that to his sister, and that Ethan can eat peanut butter but his friend in the neighborhood gets hives if he has any. I think it makes sense to him that he didn't do anything to cause his illness but that it's just how his body behaves during certain times of the year. Sophia didn't feel like she caused her mom to get sick, did she?"

"No, not that I've seen," Lisa said. "It doesn't seem like she needs to place blame for this. In fact, she pretty much accepts the fact that her mom is sick and doesn't really look for any justification. I think that's because everything else in her life has stayed the same. She still comes to school every day, she still has Grandma pick her up from school 2 days a week, just like she did before her mom got sick. It doesn't seem like all that much has changed as far as she's concerned, except for when Cindy goes for chemo, and she even seemed pretty comfortable with that when she explained it to Ethan."

"From what I've read, that's a good thing," Cathy replied. "The experts suggest that parents should try to keep their kids' routines as consistent as possible, even when dealing with somebody's illness in the family. If you disrupt the routine, it seems to make everything else feel worse. I know Ethan hated missing school these past few days, but since we've been to so many doctors recently, we seem to have developed our 'doctor's visit routine,' which involves stopping for a treat while we wait for the prescriptions to be filled. He was so happy when I told him he could come back to school today."

"I'm so glad," Lisa said. "But speaking of routines, we should probably get our circle time started. If you want to keep talking about this, I should have more time at the end of the day."

"Thanks, I'll let you know" Cathy replied. "I'll just say a quick goodbye to Ethan and get out of here before I'm late for work. See you this afternoon."

Cathy found Ethan amidst a group of children driving trucks on a large floor map, and she picked him up for a quick hug. "I've gotta go or I'm going to be late for work, so you have a great day, OK?"

"OK," Ethan said, smiling.

"Hey, don't let Ms. Lisa forget to do your breathing medicine after snack time," Cathy reminded Ethan.

"I won't." Ethan said as he jumped down and grabbed a green truck to rejoin his friends.

"Bye," Cathy said, but Ethan already was busy driving his truck on a very crowded street.

THE DAY CONTINUES

As Cathy drove to work, she remembered an article she had read about explaining illness to children. It had talked about giving children the information they want and need to know about an illness, rather than what doctors or parents think the children should know. According to the research this author did, kids typically wanted to know about what he called the "normality" issues, rather than the "functional" issues. Instead of talking about the etiology of a disease (the functional issues), parents were encouraged to discuss the normality issues, which focus more on how a disease will affect the child, and to offer reassurance. The author said that when kids did start asking questions about the disease itself, parents should listen carefully to the question being asked and offer a simple yet specific answer that stresses the normality of the situation. It seemed like it was important to provide honest information, but that it was even more important to provide those reassurances of normality. Cathy made a mental note to herself to tell Lisa about that article when she picked Ethan up in the afternoon.

When Cathy got to work, she stopped to pick up her mail and headed to her desk to check voice mail and e-mail before beginning the morning's projects. She was already behind from missing 2 days of work taking Ethan to doctors. After working on her computer for about an hour, she got up to get a cup of coffee and saw that her friend Michelle was also filling her mug.

"Hey, Cathy, we've missed you around here. You look exhausted," Michelle said.

"Yeah, it's been a long few days. Ethan had an asthma attack again. Jeff is, of course, out of town for the rest of the week. I had to wake up Lucy Sunday night to go with us to the emergency room. We were there for 3 hours. Needless to say, none of us have been in the best of moods since then. But you won't believe what happened in the ER. While I was talking to the nurse, this woman starts telling Lucy that she should always be nice to her brother because her brother could die and then how would Lucy feel? And that she should never roughhouse with Ethan because that could set off an attack. Or if she made Ethan upset, that could do it, too. She scared Lucy to death. I gave her a piece of my mind, but I'm afraid the damage had already been done."

"What a witch! Poor Lucy. She must be petrified to move around Ethan."

"I know. I feel horrible about it," said Cathy. "When I took Ethan to his doctor this morning, I told her what happened. She was really angry, too."

"Did she have any ideas?" asked Michelle.

"First, she explained that Lucy's nine, so she just wants to play and have fun. When Ethan's having an attack, it scares her. She also thinks Lucy's afraid of "catching" Ethan's asthma. Lucy wants to believe everything's OK, so she tells Ethan to just quit it or that he's faking it."

"Sounds like a fun time at your house!"

"Yeah," said Cathy. "When Ethan first started having the attacks 2 years ago, I sat down with Lucy and explained that Ethan was sick, what asthma was, and how Ethan felt when he had an attack. All that stuff. Lucy seemed to understand, and I even heard her explaining it to her grandmother one day. And when Ethan would have an attack, Lucy would try to calm him down and be really sweet with him. But that was a couple of years ago."

"So what's changed, do you think?" Michelle asked.

"Well, she's older, she wants me to be available whenever she wants, and sometimes Ethan's attacks get in the way of that. So she gets jealous of Ethan, and that comes out as anger—at Ethan and me. And I'm sure it doesn't help that her father's out of town on business all the time. I feel like a single parent, and I'm sure she picks up on some of that stress, too."

"And then the witch in the ER made things even worse. But the pediatrician had a great idea. She has a video about asthma, and she wants to watch it with Lucy and show her some models of the lungs and what happens during an asthma attack and talk to her about being scared when her brother gets so sick. And she has some specific tasks Lucy can be responsible for if Ethan has an attack so she feels like she's helping. I'm taking her there tomorrow."

"That sounds fantastic. What a great way to handle it."

"Yeah, and I figure I'll learn something, too," replied Cathy. "By the way, before I got sidetracked with telling you about Ethan, I wanted to ask you a personal question."

"Sure," responded Michelle.

"Didn't your sister have breast cancer?" Cathy shifted topics.

"Yeah, she was diagnosed about a year ago, but right now everything seems to be in remission," said Michelle. "Why?"

"Well, when I dropped Ethan off at preschool this morning, I found out that one of the other moms is doing chemo for breast cancer. What amazed me, though, is how easy it was for this little girl to talk about everything with the other kids. She was just talking to Ethan about her mom's treatment like it's no big deal. I've been doing some reading about how to talk to kids about illness after dealing with all of Ethan and Lucy's issues this week, but I figured with something as serious as cancer, it would be more . . . I don't know . . . serious."

"How lucky for the mom," Michelle replied. "It sounds like she handled it pretty well and that her little girl has as much information as she needs. My sister didn't do such a great job with her kids, unfortunately. Her twin girls were about 14 when she was diagnosed, and she tried to hide it from them for a long time, but it obviously got harder and harder to hide. When she finally did sit them down to break the news, she tried to "educate" them with as much information about the disease as possible, but that's not what they wanted to hear. They would try to change the subject whenever the topic came up and sometimes even walk out in the middle of conversations. She thought the girls just didn't care, but it turns out they just couldn't handle the type of information she was trying to give them. There's so much uncertainty with a cancer diagnosis, and they were so scared. It made for some pretty nasty arguments for a while."

"That poor family," Cathy commented.

"Yeah, but they worked it out," Michelle continued. "When my sister finally told me what was happening, I started looking for information for her. I found some really great websites that not only gave information about the disease and how to deal with it, but also how to talk to family members and children about the disease. My favorite one is by the National Alliance of Breast Cancer Organizations or NABCO. That site and its links really helped her figure out what was going on with the girls and come up with ways to address the issues that the girls needed to discuss. Now, they can talk about the cancer without anyone leaving the room."

"That sounds great. Much better than this other woman I know," Cathy said. "When her teenage son found out that she was sick, he started misbehaving at school, staying out after curfew, his grades dropped. She just doesn't know what to do about him, which makes it harder to focus on her own recovery. Maybe I should tell her about that website you found. Could you e-mail the URL to me so I can send it to her?"

"Sure," Michelle replied. "Right away."

"Thanks," said Cathy.

ANOTHER OPINION

As Cathy was heading out to lunch, her cell phone rang. She looked at Caller ID and saw that it was her sister-in-law, Sarah. "Ugh," Cathy thought. "She's the last person I want to talk to right now." But she pushed the button to answer the call, and in a bright and cheery voice, said, "Hi Sarah, what's up?"

"Oh Cathy, I'm so glad I caught you," Sarah effused. "I wanted to find out how everything went at Ethan's doctor visit yesterday."

"It went well," Cathy told her. She wasn't about to tell her about Lucy and her reaction. "She prescribed a bunch of new medicines to help control the allergies and the asthma. I was a little concerned that Ethan wouldn't take all the medicines she wanted him to take just because there were so many, but when I talked to Ethan about it, he seemed. . . ."

"What do you mean you TALKED TO ETHAN about it??" Sarah exclaimed. "What are you thinking talking to him? He's a four-year-old kid!! He should just do what you tell him!"

Cathy sighed, but continued. "He may be a kid, but he's the one that's going to have to deal with this for the rest of his life. Of course, I talk to him about this."

"You don't mean you TOLD him what's wrong with him, do you? I mean, he doesn't know what it is that he has, does he?" ranted Sarah.

"Yes," Cathy said with forced patience. "He knows that he has allergies that will give him sneezes and coughs a couple of times a year and that sometimes those allergies will cause his asthma to kick in and give him a little trouble breathing. And he knows which medicines we take to stop each of those things from happening." Cathy winced in preparation for the tirade she knew was coming.

"I can't BELIEVE you TOLD him what was going on. Everyone knows that you're not supposed to talk to kids about things like this. Adults have enough trouble dealing with illness, but kids aren't nearly ready to have that kind of information!"

Sarah's protests continued, but Cathy pulled the phone away from her ear and took a deep breath. Cathy put the phone back to her ear only to find her sister-in-law still talking furiously. She interrupted again, "Sarah, I know you don't think I did the right thing in telling Ethan about his own illness, but based on what I've read, I think I did exactly what he needed. He seems to be coping with all the information just fine. But I have to get back to work, so I'll call you later." And with a sigh of relief, she hung up without waiting for Sarah's reply.

Cathy returned to work, finished everything for the day, and then drove to pick up Ethan from preschool. The kids were playing on the playground equipment outside, so Cathy had a chance to talk with Lisa for a few minutes.

"Boy, what a day. I managed to get everything done at work, but it seems like I spent my entire day talking about kids and illness! My coworker thinks that parents should only tell kids the information they can handle hearing about someone's illness, but my sister-in-law thinks that kids shouldn't be given any information at all, even if it's the kid that is sick!

Lisa thought for a moment and then replied "Well, I think it's like talking with kids about anything else . . . it just depends on each individual kid. Their maturity level, their age, and what they can cognitively understand, the questions they ask. Sophia was able to handle hearing about her mother being sick, and she's comfortable talking about it, but someone like Logan wouldn't be able to do that. You'd have to temper the information you gave to him so that it wouldn't upset him. When his grandfather had a stroke a few months ago, he was very worried, more than you'd think a kid his age would be. They're very close and spend a lot of time together, so he really noticed the absence. And his grandfather was in rehab for quite a while and not in great shape. Logan had nightmares, he was really aggressive, and it didn't stop until his grandfather came home. His parents tried to tell him just what he needed to know, but it didn't matter. It wasn't until Gramps was back in his own home that Logan felt OK."

"Wow, that sounds really intense," responded Cathy. "Does he have any siblings?"

"Yeah, he has a 7-year-old sister and a 12-year-old brother," said Michelle. "They both handled it very differently. Megan didn't seem to care and barely asked how he was doing. She'd go visit him with the family, but she never initiated it. Greg was sure Gramps was going to die and would barely talk or eat. He stuffed all his feelings inside. It was really tough for everyone, especially the parents. They had kids with very different reactions and very different needs for information. What they all had in common was that the outcome for Gramps was uncertain, and they each had their own ways to manage that uncertainty. And giving them information so they'd understand what was going on didn't always work. I'm just thrilled Gramps is OK and Logan is back to being happy."

"Yeah, I'm sure Logan's thrilled, too," Cathy said. "It's like this article that I meant to tell you about this morning. The author said that kids don't really need to know much about the illness itself, but they'd rather know how the illness is going to affect them personally. It doesn't matter if they're the one who is sick, or if it's a family member, as long as they find out how their own life will change because of it. He says kids just want normality."

"Don't we all!" Lisa laughed.

At that moment, Ethan finally noticed that his mom had arrived and ran over for a big hug yelling, "Mommyyyyyy!!!!"

"Hey! Did you have a good day?" Cathy asked Ethan.

"Yep."

"Did Ms. Lisa remember to give you your breathing medicine?" she asked.

"Yep," Ethan said.

As they drove to the elementary school to pick up Lucy, Cathy was excited to tell her about the doctor's appointment for the next day. Not only would Lucy learn ways to help with Ethan, she would be getting some one-on-one attention from adults without an asthma attack interfering.

"Hmmmm," she thought, "this will help Lucy be part of the solution instead of part of the problem."

RELEVANT CONCEPTS

Disease etiology: The physiological causes of an illness.

Figurative language: Using analogies, metaphors, or similes to explain illness; it is important that the figurative language used is not too advanced for the psycholinguistic competencies of children (Whaley, 1994).

Managing uncertainty: Our inability to predict what will happen; illness creates uncertainty, and information provides one way to decrease, maintain, or increase that uncertainty.

Normality vs. functional issues: Normality focuses on how an illness will affect the day-to-day life and the ability of the child to "fit in," whereas functional issues focus on the cause and likely progression and outcome of the illness

Scripts: Perceptions of the conventional sequencing of occurrences; research suggests that younger children may have more list-like scripts, whereas older children have more detailed and complex descriptions of sequential events (Eiser, Eiser, & Lang, 1989).

DISCUSSION QUESTIONS

1. Cathy and Sarah had very different ways of talking to children about illness. Which do you think is preferable? Why?
2. Jeremy, age six, has been diagnosed with leukemia. He will have to undergo chemotherapy and a possible bone marrow transplant. His chances of surviving are 60/40. What do you tell Jeremy about his illness, treatment, and prognosis? What do you tell his three-year-old brother? His 12-year-old sister? His best friend? How do you decide what to tell each of them?
3. What are some of the things you could do if a child with an illness or a sibling is not satisfied with the information you gave him or her?
4. How much information should children be given about a parent's illness? What are some of the variables that would affect your answer?

REFERENCE/SUGGESTED READINGS

Babrow, A. S., Kasch, C. R., & Ford, L. A. (1998). The many meanings of "uncertainty" in illness: Toward a systematic accounting. *Health Communication, 10,* 1–24.

Eiser, C., Eiser, J. R., & Lang, J. (1989). Scripts in children's reports of medical events. *European Journal of Psychology of Education, 4,* 377–384.

Eiser, C., & Kope, S. J. (1997). Children's perceptions of health and illness. In K. J. Petrie & J. A. Weinman (Eds.), *Perceptions of health and illness: Current research and applications* (pp. 47–76). Newark, NJ: Harwood.

Whaley, B. B. (1994). "Food is to me as gas is to cars??": Using figurative language to explain illness to children. *Health Communication, 6,* 193–204.

Whaley, B. B. (1999). Explaining illness to children: Advancing theory and research by determining message content. *Health Communication, 11,* 185–193.

Whaley, B. B. (2000). *Explaining illness: Research, theory, and strategies.* Mahwah, NJ: Lawrence Erlbaum Associates.

Additional Resources

Helping children understand cancer: Talking to children about their illness or about illness in the family: http://www.cancercare.org/EducationalPrograms/EducationalPrograms.cfm? ID= 3483&c=381

Taking to children about breast cancer: http//www.nabco.org/index.php/index.php/index.php/133

Talking with children about HD (Huntington's disease): http://endoflifecare.tripod.com/juvenilehuntingtonsdisease/id8.html

Talking to children about mental illness: http://www.aacap.org/publications/factsfam/84.htm

III

Issues in Social Identity

10

A Treatment Team Approach: The Negotiation of Rehabilitation Goals for Survivors of Traumatic Brain Injury

Kami J. Silk
Michigan State University

According to the Centers for Disease Control (2001), 1.5 million Americans sustain a traumatic brain injury (TBI) each year, and 80,000 survivors experience the onset of long-term disability. Survivors often have multiple and permanent physical, cognitive, and emotional impairments that require intensive rehabilitation and, depending on the severity of their deficits, long-term custodial or psychiatric care may be necessary (Jacobs, 1993). TBI has been defined as an insult to the brain caused by an external force that may produce a diminished or altered state of consciousness, which results in an impairment of cognitive abilities or physical functioning and possible disturbance of behavioral or emotional functioning (Brain Injury Association of America, 2001). Brain injury ranges from mild to severe and can result in three major types of impairments: (a) physical—speech, vision, hearing, and other sensory impairments, as well as mobility challenges and seizures; (b) cognitive—short-term and long-term memory deficits and slowness of thinking; and (c) emotional—mood swings, depression, anxiety, irritability, and anger (Jacobs, 1993). Because of the wide range of deficits that may occur as a result of brain injury, different models of rehabilitation may be more or less appropriate for clients.

A treatment team approach is used in this case study to demonstrate one rehabilitation model that incorporates all levels of the organization in the care and treatment of survivors of TBI. This case study documents the dialogue that often occurs within a treatment team meeting of a rehabilitation program, Progressive Rehabilitation and Independence (PRI), in Bensalem, PA.[1] PRI is an integrated community re-entry program for survivors of TBI that offers a day program with a variety of therapies, assisted residential living, and vocational training. Rehabilitative efforts of the PRI treatment team are aimed at integrating survivors back into the community and at maximizing independent living skills. Survivors of TBI are referred to as "clients" rather than "patients" by treatment team members as a strategy to respect survivors' rights as individuals. An explanation of PRI is followed by the proceedings of a treatment team meeting.

123

REHABILITATION AT P.R.I.

There are multiple types of programs that strive to meet the needs of survivors of TBI throughout their recovery and rehabilitative processes. The type of rehabilitation program addressed in this case study is a long-term one, specializing in subacute care for survivors of TBI who are minimally aroused for prolonged periods of time and have limited attention and stamina. Clients might be part of the PRI program for as little as six months to a year, or for as long as a decade or a lifetime. The length of clients' care at PRI is determined by rehabilitative goals, clients' achievement of goals, and resources (i.e., insurance settlement, health insurance, trust fund) available to fund the possible long-term care of clients. PRI integrates a variety of programs in its organization that meet the individually tailored goals of each client.

PRI provides community-based care in the forms of day treatment, community re-entry, and independent living programs. *Day treatment* provides intensive rehabilitation in a structured setting during normal work hours and allows survivors to return to their residences at night. The day treatment program at PRI offers a wide range of services (e.g., group, cognitive, physical, speech therapies, etc.), and it is part of a larger rehabilitation effort, whose goal is community re-entry and independent living. The *community re-entry* emphasis of PRI focuses on developing higher-level cognitive and motor skills to prepare survivors of brain injuries for their return to independent living and potentially to work. For example, PRI supports independent utilization of public transportation, basic numeracy skills, and/or vocational goals. The *independent living/residential* component of PRI places clients into living environments with multiple levels of support, typically within a residential setting. Clients work with direct care workers and other treatment team members to become as independent as possible with everyday living skills such as cooking, cleaning, personal hygiene, and money management. PRI integrates its day, community re-entry, and independent living programs to provide comprehensive services for survivors that address each of their respective rehabilitation goals.

REHABILITATION GOALS

Rehabilitation goals at PRI are tailored to clients' individual needs. Goals may range from diet plans and exercise regimens, to educational and vocational goals, to activities of daily living (ADL) skills and behavior management goals (Fraser & Curl, 2000). Many different stakeholders give input into what goals are set for each client of PRI, providing a unique and comprehensive picture of the needs, progress, and status of each client. Stakeholders include client, family members, therapists, psychiatrists, social workers, and/or direct care workers. The participatory goal-setting method used by stakeholders is associated with acceptance of the decided-upon goals. Intense negotiation, coordination, and communication between stakeholders are necessary for clients to successfully reap the benefits of their program and the rehabilitation treatment team. Each rehabilitation team member has a piece of evidence that is critical to the treatment and progress of a particular client.

THE CLIENT

Henry Dalton, a 33-year-old manager of a pet store, survived a head-on collision with another motor vehicle on November 28, 2000. As a result of the accident, Henry spent 3 weeks in a coma and sustained a traumatic brain injury that affected him physically as well as cognitively. Specifically, Henry experienced problems with short-term memory, exhibited behavioral control problems, was paralyzed from the waist down, and required assistance with his ADLs. He was unable to return to his management position. Also, prior to his accident, Henry had had a 3-year relationship with a woman. She left shortly after his return to the house they shared together and Henry was unable to cope independently. At this point, Henry moved in with his elderly parents. However, they quickly realized that they could not meet Henry's daily needs and decided that he needed to be in a supported living environment with professionals who could help him deal with his new circumstances.

After an examination of several recommended programs, Henry and his family chose PRI because of its integrated programs and team-oriented approach to treating survivors of brain injury. PRI offered a day program, where Henry could go to group and individual therapy sessions, and it had a residential program, where Henry could live with other survivors of brain injury and work on skills that might allow him to live independently some day. Henry's parents were especially pleased that PRI was only 2 hours from where they lived, allowing them to take an active role in Henry's life and in his rehabilitation. They were able to attend Henry's rehabilitation meetings and stayed in close contact with his case manager, Joyce Klazuck.

Henry's Rehabilitation Goals

After 3 weeks of evaluation by treatment members at PRI, Henry, his parents, and the treatment team met and decided on three goals with specific plans of action. The goals focused on use of public transportation, control of behavioral outbursts, and completion of ADLs. Henry's job was to work on each of the goals over the next 3 months, at which time all of the stakeholders would come together to evaluate Henry's progress and to reexamine his goals. Table 10.1 provides the plan of action for each of Henry's rehabilitation goals.

TABLE 10.1
Henry's Rehabilitation Goals

1. Henry will be able to take public transportation independently.
   a. Henry will obtain information regarding public transportation in his geographic area of interest.
   b. Henry will meet weekly with a cognitive therapist to discuss the process of taking public transportation.
   c. Henry will keep a journal that indicates his path of transportation.
   d. Henry will take public transportation accompanied by a staff member.
   e. Henry will be "shadowed" by a staff member as he independently navigates public transportation.
   f. Henry will successfully navigate public transportation independently.

2. Henry will complete his adult daily living skills (ADLs) independently each day.
   a. Henry will meet with an occupational therapist to complete an ADL schedule and to practice his ADL skills.
   b. Henry will take a shower each day, using soap and a washcloth to clean his body and shampoo to wash his hair.
   c. Henry will use an electric razor to shave each day.
   d. Henry will brush his teeth at least twice a day: once in the morning and once in the evening.
   e. Henry will select weather-appropriate clothing to wear each day.

3. Henry will have zero behavioral outbursts in the residential unit, day program, vocational training, and on outings with staff.
   a. Henry will be preset by staff members prior to outings and other situations where others are present (e.g, day program, vocational setting).
   b. Henry will be redirected by staff members if he begins to have a behavioral outburst.
   c. Henry will process any outbursts with a cognitive therapist or with the psychiatrist at the day program as soon as possible.
   d. Henry will keep a daily journal to record his behavior each day.
   e. Staff members at the day program, residential unit, and vocational training will record Henry's behaviors each day on an hourly basis.
   f. Henry will continue to take prescribed medications, and staff will monitor his intake of them.
   g. Henry will meet with the psychiatrist once a week.

THREE MONTHS LATER

The treatment team gathers in the conference room to discuss Henry's progress over the last 3 months. Those individuals in attendance include: Henry and his parents, Elaine and William Dalton; Dr. Francis, psychiatrist; Joyce Klazuck, social worker/case manager; Karen Stokes, director of day program; Jay Harris, residential manager; Jon Milton, vocational specialist; Ellen Liten, direct care worker; and Samuel Clark, cognitive therapist. The meeting has two primary purposes: (a) to evaluate Henry's progress related to his rehabilitation goals, and (b) to revise Henry's rehabilitation goals. Joyce facilitates the meeting.

"Thank you, everyone, for coming today for Henry Dalton's quarterly progress meeting. We last met 3 months ago. At that meeting we set up rehabilitation goals for Henry based on staff evaluations and input from Henry and his parents. We are meeting here today to discuss his progress and to reevaluate his goals. First, I'll give a case management report, and then we'll get reports from Jay and his staff and Karen and her staff. Okay?" Everyone nods in agreement and Joyce begins with her case management report.

"Henry sustained a closed head injury on November 28, 2000. He has now been with PRI for approximately 4 months. He resides at 339 Longwood Avenue in Bensalem, PA, an assisted living residence, with two male roommates. He attends the day program 5 days a week, where he meets twice a week with a cognitive therapist. He also meets once a week with an occupational therapist, works twice a week in a vocational program, and attends a series of group therapies throughout the week." The group therapies are named according to their content and include *social interaction, exercise, decision making, memory retention, and math group.* "Henry's parents have come to visit him almost every two weeks. They typically take him out to dinner at a restaurant of his choice." Henry's current medications are also indicated in Joyce's case management report.

After Joyce is done, Dr. Francis, who specializes in TBI, asks Henry how he feels he is doing on his medications. Henry responds that he often feels groggy. The direct care worker, Ellen, who assists Henry with his ADLs and is part of the residential staff at Longwood Avenue, agrees.

"Yeah. I have been having a hard time waking Henry up. Sometimes I am in there three or four times telling him, 'Get up, Henry, we are gonna' be late!' We have been late to the day program three or four times'cuz I had such a hard time getting him moving in the morning. I wasn't sure if he was just not a morning person or what."

The day program staff members also agree that Henry seems fatigued in the morning when he arrives and also in the early afternoon while attending his group therapies. Based on this information from the treatment team, Dr. Francis makes an adjustment to Henry's medications. He instructs all treatment team members to monitor any changes in Henry's behavior and to report on those changes at the weekly client update meeting. He reminds the residential staff that they are around Henry more than any other staff members, so it is vital that they play close attention to how Henry responds to the medication. Everyone makes a note to monitor Henry.

The meeting moves on to Henry's progress at his residence. Joyce asks Jay, the residential manager in charge of the staff at Longwood Avenue, to report on Henry's goal progress within the residential facility. Jay starts with a general report and then focuses specifically on Henry's rehabilitation goals.

"Overall," he begins, "Henry has been successful over the past 3 months in the residence. Like Joyce said, he lives with two roommates and seems to have positive relationships with them. They watch sports programs, eat, and go to the mall together. Initially, when Henry first moved in, we had some behavioral issues almost every day. For example, Henry got angry when someone was in the bathroom when he needed it. When the other person came out of the bathroom, Henry punched him. There were a couple of other incidents similar to that; it was as if Henry felt inconvenienced by his roommates, so he would physically act out. I consulted with Dr. Francis and other staff at the time . . . "

Henry interrupts Jay and says that he was not the cause of the problems in the residence. According to Henry, his roommates were disrespectful of him when he first moved in, and that is why he got mad. "Well, Henry, you were not necessarily being respectful when you punched James were you?" asks Jay.

Henry looks down shamefully and mumbles, "He deserved it."

"Just to add on to what Jay is saying," interjects Sam, "during your cognitive therapies, we processed how upset you were about having to move to a new residence, right?"

"Well, yeah. It's been real hard. I didn't want to move from my house—I had to sell it and I didn't want to. And then my girlfriend left me. And then I moved in with my parents and that was terrible, but I didn't want to leave, either. I don't know. I just get so mad and frustrated and . . . I didn't mean to hurt James. He's my friend now," says Henry.

"Exactly!" says Jay. "Once you got to know the guys, you realized you had a lot in common and we really haven't seen much of a problem with your behavior. You have really kept it together, man, and have been a pleasure to be around at the residence."

"It sounds like we might want to continue working on this goal, but with some modifications," says Joyce. "Although Henry has only had a few behavioral problems at PRI, I know that Henry's parents have talked with me a little bit about Henry's behavior when they have taken him out to dinner." Henry looks up quickly at his parents and his mother explains what Joyce is talking about it.

"Henry, you know how much we love to come visit and get together with you on our weekend visits," begins Henry's mother. "We wouldn't miss it for the world. But do you remember the one time recently we had to miss because your father was sick? You said that it wasn't a big deal, but the next weekend, you seemed very agitated with us. At the restaurant, you made inappropriate remarks to the waitress and threatened to beat up the host if we didn't get a table immediately. It was very upsetting for your father and me, so I mentioned it to Joyce."

"Why didn't you mention it to me?" demands Henry. "Why does everything have to go through her?" Henry jabs a finger in Joyce's direction.

"Henry, we did mention it to you—both your father and I did—at the restaurant and in the car on the way back. You insisted that you did nothing wrong. We were really concerned about the lewd comments and the threat . . ." Henry's mother shakes her head in dismay. "We just about died of embarrassment, Henry. Why would you say such things?" Henry says nothing.

After a few moments, Dr. Francis asks, "Henry, why don't you tell us what is going on here? It is hard for us to help you with this if you are defensive about it or deny it. We all have bad days, Henry, and for some people, bad days turn into bad weeks, bad months, and so on. We don't want that to happen to you. So, why don't you tell us what is going on?"

"I don't know, Dr. Francis. I really don't know," replies Henry.

Sam, the cognitive therapist, intervenes again, "Henry, do you remember talking to me in our sessions about how upset you were when your parents couldn't make it that one weekend?"

"Well, yeah. I mean—it gets long sometimes. Being here, that is. One of the only good things that I look forward to is Mom and Dad's visits, but Dad was sick. I understood. I wasn't mad at all."

"Are you sure about that, Henry?" asks Ellen. "I remember when your mom called to say that they were not going to make that weekend. You were all polite on the phone, but as soon as you hung that phone up you were in a foul mood. You went to your room and slammed the door. Heck, you wouldn't even come out for dinner." Henry is embarrassed and looks down.

"In our sessions, you mentioned how disappointed you were that they didn't come to visit," says Sam. "I know it's hard, Henry, but is that why you were so rude to those people?"

"I don't know. Maybe." Henry looks distressed and finally blurts out, "I just need to be able to count on something and they didn't come! They didn't even apologize or anything—they just came on in like it was the weekend they were supposed to be there or something. It wasn't. I knew it. They thought I wouldn't remember and that I wouldn't notice. Get serious! I am not stupid!" Henry's parents are shocked and taken aback at Henry's outburst. Other than the restaurant incident, they had never been present for one of his verbal or behavioral outbursts. And now it was directed at them.

"Henry, it's wonderful that you look forward to your parents' visits. They clearly love to visit with you, too," says Dr. Francis. "But let's look at this in another way. Your parents aren't getting any younger," Dr. Francis winks at Mr. and Mrs. Dalton, "and that's got to worry you a bit. Your father was sick. You were worried. You missed them both. These are good things. You can't blame your parents because they come down with the flu, can you? And certainly, you don't want to risk them not coming because they are afraid you might have a behavioral or verbal outburst while they are out with you, right?"

Henry's eyes grow wide with the knowledge that he may have put his outings with his parents at risk because of his poor behavior at the restaurant. "I'm sorry, Mom. I'm sorry, Dad. I won't do it again. I promise. Really. I didn't mean to embarrass you or hurt your feelings. Really, I didn't," Henry apologizes. The Daltons accept their son's apology.

"Henry, why don't we do this," suggests Joyce. "Why don't we keep this goal in place so that you can continue to work on controlling your behavior. We'll add an 'as needed' session on your rehabilitation program for you to come see me when you are getting stressed or upset about things. That way, we can talk about it before you get to a place where you feel like you want to act out. You can still talk to Sam or Dr. Francis about these issues too, but you can also feel free to come to me when you feel the need to." The treatment team thinks that the suggestion is a good one because Sam and Dr. Francis are not always readily available; their meetings with clients are scheduled tightly. This revision to the goal will give Henry a greater opportunity to address some of his emotions in a proactive way before any real problems occur. With that revision in the behavioral goal accounted for, Jay moves on to the rest of his residential report.

"Henry has done a great job with his personal hygiene. He is showering on a regular basis and using his roll-in shower chair with ease. He is brushing his teeth in the morning and before bed, keeps his hair nice and neat, and is wearing clothing that looks great and is appropriate for the weather. I think he has done a fantastic job with this goal."

Ellen, the direct care worker who works with Henry on his ADLs most mornings, also reports, "He is doing great with this. In the morning, if he is not sure of the weather, he will ask me what the temperature is supposed to be. This is a *big* difference compared with his first 2 weeks here, when he wanted to wear shorts and a tank top regardless of the weather. It was an argument then, and now it seems like he has really come far." Karen, the director of the day program, and Jon, the vocational specialist, nod their heads in agreement. They, too, have seen a big change in Henry's appearance compared with his first 2 weeks at PRI.

Dr. Francis comments, "Sometimes one result of a brain injury can be a lower awareness of external factors like temperature. Perhaps the medications that Henry takes have put him back in touch with his internal thermometer. What do you think, Henry?"

"I don't know about that, Doc," replied Henry, "but all of sudden I started to feel cold sometimes. And I got a bunch of new clothes right after I moved in. Ellen went with me to the mall, and we got some nice stuff for me. And I can easily get into the clothes by myself."

"Yeah, and the fact that we purchased the shower chair has no doubt made the shower more easily accessible for you, too," adds Joyce. Henry nods at this remark. "About a week after

Henry arrived at PRI, we realized that a shower chair would really help Henry become more independent with his ADLs. It sure seems like it has worked."

"Also, I think, his new friend, Judith, has something to do with Henry's consistently dapper appearance," teases Karen. Judith is another PRI client who attends the day program. The treatment team raises their eyebrows at Henry in a knowing way and Henry is embarrassed.

"Come on. Can't a guy have a girl for a friend?" asks Henry. Everyone laughs, including Henry, and the treatment team returns back to the issue of a new goal.

"So, does everyone agree that Henry has met this goal?" asks Joyce. They all nod their heads. "Well, if that's the case, I think we need a new goal to replace this one. I do think we'll continue to monitor Henry's hygiene for awhile, but I don't think we need it as a formal goal. So, do we have any suggestions?"

At this point, Henry and Jon, the vocational specialist, look knowingly at each other. Although Henry had no formal vocational goals during the last 3 months, he had been working in the woodworking program with Jon twice a week. Henry had lost function in the lower part of his body, but he certainly had full upper body mobility and excellent strength that allowed him to take part in the woodworking. "I have a suggestion," says Jon. "I think that we need to formalize a vocational goal for Henry. He has been doing a great job in the woodworking program. He is able to operate some of the more complicated tools and has been a great assistant to me with some of the other clients."

"What did you have in mind, Jon?" asks Joyce. Jon motions to Henry to explain.

"You know, I had forgotten that I used to do some carpentry in the summers when I was going to college. Do you remember, Mom and Dad?"

Henry's father slowly nods as the memory returns. "Yes, you worked with our old neighbor. I remember having to talk you out of quitting college to go into that line of work. I convinced you to stay in school because your business degree would help you to start your own building business. I had forgotten all about that!"

Henry grinned, "Yeah, I remember too. Well, I started working with Jon, and I really like it. I have made bird houses, picture frames, and I'm working on a small table for my bedroom. I sold one of my bird houses at the flea market!"

Henry's parents looked puzzled about the flea market. Jon explains, "Every Saturday morning, we rent a table at a local flea market and sell the arts & crafts, woodwork, ceramics, and jewelry that the clients make at PRI. They get to keep any profits when they sell one of their pieces. It's a great opportunity for clients to be creative, do meaningful work, and make a little extra cash. I would really like to see Henry get more involved with our woodworking program. I'd like to see him come at least twice a month to the flea market to help us sell our items. His background as a retail manager would be a fantastic asset to our program. Henry and I discussed it briefly, which is why I came to today's meeting."

"I think it is a great idea," says Sam. "But I do think that we need to consider some of Henry's behavioral issues if we are asking him to interact with people in the community and perhaps even take on a leadership position in your woodworking crew."

Dr. Francis nods in agreement with Sam. "Yes. Good point, Sam. Henry, do you understand what Sam is talking about?"

"Is this about the restaurant thing again?" asks Henry. "Because that is not going to happen again."

"Good. But why don't we build your vocational goal with some of the behavioral issues in mind," suggests Dr. Francis.

"Well," starts Karen, the day program director, "I could build some customer relations exercises into our *social interaction group*. You know, we could do some role playing of dealing with customers, even irritating ones. We could also incorporate some role playing into Henry's cognitive sessions with Sam." Sam nods in agreement.

"Okay. Jon, what is going to happen if Henry has a behavioral or verbal outburst at the flea market or, even worse, in the woodshop where potentially dangerous tools are laying around?" asks Dr. Francis.

"Yeah, I am a little concerned about that based on this meeting," says Jon. "I could put together a behavioral contract with Henry that specifies the behavioral expectations and the consequences of any violations of the contract."

"Jon, I would be glad to sit down with you and Henry and maybe Joyce?" Karen looks over at Joyce questioningly and Joyce nods, "to create the behavioral contract so that everyone at the day program, the residence, and on-site at the flea market is in agreement and understanding about it." Jon says that would be excellent, then asks Henry how he feels about the behavioral contract.

Henry says, "I would really like to do the woodworking stuff and go to the flea market, too. Do I really have to do this behavioral contract deal?"

"Henry, you don't have to do anything," reminds Joyce. "But one of the ways we get clients really on target is through the use of behavioral contracts. It's for your benefit, too. It spells out exactly what you're supposed to do and it tells you what would happen if there is a problem."

"What would happen?" asks Henry.

"What I am thinking, Henry," says Jon, "is that you would be suspended from the privilege of woodworking or the flea market for a week or two if there's a problem. Also, if you had consistent problems, maybe we would suspend your work indefinitely and work on your behavioral issues so that you would eventually be able to get back to the woodworking crew. Frankly, Henry, I don't foresee any problems unless you do. The behavioral contract is a way to make you really think about the consequences of your actions before you act. What do you say?"

"I'm willing to give it a try," replies Henry. "But I get to help put the behavioral contract together, right?" Everyone nods and mumbles affirmative answers. "And I get to sign it, right?" Again, everyone nods. "Okay, let's do it." Everyone is pleased at this outcome, especially Henry's parents. They are thrilled to see their son engage in work-related activity that takes advantage of his previous carpentry and management experience. In their minds, PRI has come through with a real match for their son's skills that can give him satisfaction and pride in his abilities. They make a mental note to stop by the flea market sometime in the next month.

"Okay. So we have covered the residential report for the most part, have modified the behavioral goal, and added the vocational goal," states Joyce. "Let's move on to the day program report."

"There were a couple of issues that we already covered," explains Karen, "so I'll just talk about things that we have not discussed so far. According to Sam, the cognitive therapy sessions with Henry are productive. They have been working on short-term memory retention strategies that seem to be helping somewhat. It is likely that if Henry would use his journal throughout each day, he would do much better in remembering the details of his daily schedule. Also, I think that the journal would also be helpful to Henry in terms of processing some of his emotions. We can barely get Henry to make one entry into it each day."

Dr. Francis furrows his brow and asks, "Why is this the case, Henry? When we built these goals three months ago, you agreed that keeping a journal would help you with your goals. The therapeutic benefits of keeping a journal are documented widely. What's the problem here?"

"I was never a writer," Henry responds. "I hated it in high school, and I hated it in college. I'm not even good at it. It makes me feel stupid and it takes a lot of time to do."

"We're not asking you to be the next major American writer here," Dr. Francis chides. "We just want you to jot down important times, dates, and happenings. This is a tool to help you become more independent. Isn't that what you want?"

"Yes. But writing all day long and carrying the journal around with me is not at all something that I want to do."

"What if we got you a Palm Pilot, Henry?" asks Sam.

"What's that?"

"It's a small, hand-held portable organizer. It's like a mini-computer with a pen, and you can store all kinds of information in it. It fits right into your pocket, too."

"How much does it cost?" Henry asks.

"Don't worry, Henry," Mrs. Dalton interjects, "Christmas is coming and we'll get that for you as one of your gifts. Your father and I were wondering what to get you anyway—so this solves part of that problem." Mr. Dalton agrees.

"I'll give it a try. Sam, will you help me figure it out?" Sam nods.

Jay also says, "I'll help you at the residence with it, too. I have one myself." Knowing that he won't be left alone to figure out this new piece of technology, Henry seems more comfortable with the idea of a Palm Pilot.

"Mr. and Mrs. Dalton, I'd be glad to look through a couple of catalogs with Henry to find one with the right kind of features for him," offers Sam. The Daltons agree that it would be a great idea. Karen moves on to the next part of her day program report.

"Henry is doing fine in all of his group therapies. He seems to especially enjoy *exercise* group. He had a couple of consultations with a physical therapist to set up a weight-lifting routine and now works on his upper body strength independently. Henry's disposition toward the other clients at the day program has been consistently positive, and he follows the direction of staff members appropriately. Overall, Henry is an active member of the day program, and many of the clients see him as a role model." Henry looks a bit surprised at the last comment, but then smiles as he thinks of himself as a role model to others. He never thought that would be the case, now that he is in a wheelchair.

"Karen, what about the transportation goal?" asks Joyce.

"I'm getting there," Karen replies. "Well, we have been working on that, and we have made some progress in that area. However, we have not completely achieved this goal. The problem goes back to Henry's lack of interest in keeping a journal. Part of his goal was to use the journal as a memory tool for the different routes that he wants to take. He decided not to use the journal no matter what strategies Sam or I used to encourage it." Sam nods in agreement. "We have not completely accomplished this goal, but Henry did find information about public transportation in the area, and Sam and he have gone through the information to identify routes of interest. The problem is that Henry needs to write his destinations down in his own words because he is easily confused by the color-coded maps of the Septa bus system. He needs to understand the maps or write down the information he needs before we commit the time of a staff member to practice with Henry. Perhaps the Palm Pilot can help here, too . . ." Karen's voice trails off.

"This goes back to the whole writing-things-down issue," states Dr. Francis. "Are you seeing how not keeping track of important details can stifle your progress and limit your independence?" Henry nods in agreement.

"Also, we thought that the behavioral concerns were enough of a problem for us to hold back in pursuing his use of public transportation," injects Joyce.

"Yes, Joyce. Good point. Do you see how all of these goals are intertwined, Henry? Your behavior affects your family relationships, roommate relationships, you vocational opportunities, and your ability to get out and about on your own. Also, it seems like the Palm Pilot will be an important tool for you. I think you need to learn to use it so that you can maximize your independence. Don't you agree?"

"Yes. I do see that," Henry replies. "And as soon as I get the Palm Pilot, I'll do my best to figure it out." The meeting ends with informal conversation between all of the stakeholders present regarding Henry's progress at PRI. Overall, everyone agrees that Henry has made excellent progress in his first few months in the program.

EPILOGUE

After 2 years of working on clearly defined goals at PRI, Henry now lives independently in a handicap-accessible housing community. Henry still attends PRI on a limited basis for cognitive therapy and woodworking. Through the monitoring of his behavior, medications, and rehabilitation program, all stakeholders contributed to Henry's progress. A participatory treatment–teach approach to rehabilitation such as this is one model of care that can be successful when stakeholders come together with a collective purpose.

RELEVANT CONCEPTS

Activities of daily living skills (ADLs): Basic skills and daily tasks that allow individuals to function independently (e.g., showering, cooking, laundry, transportation, etc.).

Community re-entry program: A rehabilitation program whose mission is to provide services that help survivors of TBI return to the community and live as independently as possible.

Direct care workers: Health care aides who primarily assist clients with their ADLs and other life skills related to their rehabilitation goals.

Participatory goal-setting: A collaborative process in which all members of the treatment team provide input to create rehabilitation goals for individual clients.

Rehabilitation goals: Specific, observable outcomes designed to increase clients' levels of independence.

Stakeholders: All individuals and organizations who have an interest in the care of a survivor of brain injury (e.g., therapists, family members, insurance company, etc.).

Treatment-team approach: A collaborative process that incorporates employees at all levels of the organization and other stakeholders in the care and treatment of survivors of TBI.

DISCUSSION QUESTIONS

1. What are the key characteristics of a treatment-team approach? How does this approach to rehabilitation differ than other health organizations? What are some of the communication issues that are necessary for this approach to be successful?
2. How effective was rehabilitative goal-setting for Henry? How did his input affect the goal-setting process?
3. Consider the various stakeholders present at the treatment-team meeting. What organizational dynamics were evident throughout the dialogue? Was there a "leader" in the group? How was leadership communicated?
4. How could the treatment approach be applied to other health care settings and organizations?
5. In this case, there are some new interpersonal challenges that Henry has to deal with as a survivor of TBI. What kinds of communication goals would you propose if you were a member of the treatment team?

ENDNOTE

[1] The content of the treatment team meeting and the dialogue between stakeholders is based on a composite of participant observations made by the author while she worked in the rehabilitation field. All names associated with the case study are fictitious.

REFERENCES/SUGGESTED READINGS

Brain Injury Association of America. (2001). *Brain Injury. An overview of brain injury, including its costs and consequences*. Retrieved February 10, 2003, from http://www.biausa.org/Pages/facts%20&%20stats.html

Centers for Disease Control. (2001). *Traumatic Brain injury in the United States: A report to Congress.*" Retrieved January 16, 2001, from, http: www.cdc.gov/ncipc/pub-res/tbicongress.htm

Fraser, R. T., & Curl, R. (2000). Choice of a placement model. In R. T. Fraser & D. C. Clemmons (Eds.), *Traumatic brain injury rehabilitation: Practical vocational, neuropsychological, and psychotherapy interventions* (pp. 185–199). Boca Raton, FL: CRC Press.

Higenbottam, J. (1998). After the brain injury: The rehabilitation team. In S. Acorn & P. Offer (Eds.), *Living with brain injury: A guide for families and caregivers*. Buffalo, NY: University of Toronto Press.

Jacobs, H. E. (1993). *Behavior analysis guidelines and brain injury rehabilitation: People, principles, and programs*. Gaithersburg, MD: Aspen Publishers.

McNeny, R. (1990). Daily living skills: The foundation of community living. In J. S. Kreutzer & P. Wehman (Eds.), *Community integration following traumatic brain injury* (pp.105–113). Baltimore, MD: Paul H. Brookes Publishers.

Osborn, C. L. (1998). *Over my head: A doctor's own story of head injury from the inside looking out*. Kansas City, MO: Andrews McMeel Publishers.

11

Communication Accommodation in Counseling

Lisa Murray-Johnson
Cat McGrew
Ohio State University

Have you ever been to see a counselor? If you have, you are not alone. Millions of people visit these helping professionals each year to feel supported in their decisions, to learn about available resources, and to make life-affirming changes. Through a process of information exchange, counselors empower their clients to believe change is possible. As communication is the mechanism through which clients' needs are identified and counseling assistance is provided, counselors must carefully craft their messages. The content of each message needs to be meaningful for clients so that clients willingly develop their skills to work toward better health and wellness. At the same time, counselors know that equal importance is given to how communication messages are delivered. That is, how counselors speak with their clients can greatly affect their receptivity to treatment and whether clients decide to continue therapy or abandon it.

The data collected for this case study were obtained from a large midwestern city that has a well-established counseling center at a battered women's shelter. The full-service facility provides both residential and nonresidential services, including legal aid, child protection, medical assistance, parenting skill support, job placement, education support, and 24-hour emergency services. Karen[1] is the Assistant Director at the shelter and a counselor with a master's degree in social work (MSW) who has been practicing for 10 years. She has been at this facility for the past 4 years, after an earlier career in county social services. This case covers her interactions with Sandra, a 22-year-old single woman with low self-esteem who is not residing at the shelter but meets Karen for weekly appointments.

THE FIRST NIGHT

It was a Thursday night when Sandra first came to the shelter. She was almost dragged inside by her friends, Donna and Cassie, after Sandra's boyfriend, Bill, decided to turn her face into a punching bag. The first 6 months they dated, it appeared to everyone that Sandra and Bill had a great relationship. They were very affectionate toward one another and eagerly made time in their schedules to go on dates. Several months later, Bill announced that he wanted to have an exclusive relationship. Sandra was thrilled! She was sure that this was the guy with whom she wanted to spend the rest of her life. Within a few weeks, however, Sandra was suffocating from Bill's attentions. Bill always wanted to know where she was, placed limits on the amount of time she spent with friends, and accused her of not loving him when she requested time away from him.

Sandra's friends became very concerned about the relationship when Bill wouldn't let them talk with her on the phone. It took 2 months for Sandra to gather the courage to end the relationship. The day she told Bill she wanted to move out and see other people, he turned violent. Karen saw the results of this violent episode as Sandra approached the shelter: a black eye, a cut lip, several cuts and bruises along her jaw, and a partially ripped earlobe, where an earring was torn out. Karen couldn't see the damage beneath Sandra's clothes, but she suspected her body was equally bruised and battered. Karen gathered the intake forms and medical supplies as her assistant helped them inside.

Karen immediately recommended a physician visit for medical treatment and documentation of injuries. When Sandra declined fervently and got up to leave, Karen began formal intake procedures. She asked about safety from the attacker, the likelihood of the attacker coming after her again, information about injuries sustained, and whether Sandra wanted to stay at the shelter. When Sandra didn't respond to a question, Donna and Cassie would take over to fill in the details. Karen continued to direct questions at Sandra, hoping to engage her in conversation. Sandra continued to look away and remain mute. Sandra only responded verbally when her friends showed their dislike for Bill and described him negatively. Her demeanor would change from outrage to shock to sadness.

When Karen had a general picture of the situation, she asked Sandra if she would be willing to discuss what happened privately, in a small office next to the large entry room. Karen didn't get a response. Karen leaned forward toward Sandra and, in a quiet voice with her elbow resting on her knees, said, "I'd like to talk with you about this. I know it's hard. You've been through a lot. I am here to help you as are the rest of the staff. We have a lot of resources and support here, but I need you to tell me more about your needs so that I can help you."

Sandra couldn't look at Karen. She was embarrassed about the abuse, humiliated that she was at a shelter, and angry at her friends for involving themselves in this situation. Sandra didn't want to talk to a stranger about a very private relationship. Sandra reasoned that Bill's violence was a shocked response to her leaving him. Even when Bill had been angry with her before, he had never hit her. Now that the relationship was over, Sandra was sure she'd never see him again. So why was everyone making such an issue out of nothing? Sandra wanted to forget it had ever happened.

Karen assumed that Sandra's lack of response was either her way of communicating her desire to avoid help or her inability to concentrate on the conversation. Karen knows that immediately after a violent event, victims tend to think about what happened and how they could have prevented it. Based on Sandra's reactions, Karen lowered her voice, speaking quietly and gently, "Sandra, your friends brought you here so that a person outside of your relationship could assess the situation. I'm here to listen, not judge you. You can tell me anything and I will be here to support you. I will not repeat what you tell me in confidence, unless I believe that you will pose harm to yourself or someone else. Since you're already here, why don't you and I talk privately so that you can tell me what has been going on in your life?" Sandra nodded. Karen took this as a positive sign, so she added, "Together, we can figure out if you really need my help or what type of resources might be of help to you." Sandra finally replied, "Okay, yeah, let's talk," and then turning to her friends said, "You guys wait for me here." Donna and Cassie smiled and helped themselves to some coffee while waiting for her.

Once seated, Karen asked Sandra to talk about her relationship with Bill. Karen asked Sandra if she could record the conversation for research purposes and, after she consented, a staff member from the shelter entered the room to take notes and record the conversation. Sandra told Karen, "He (Bill) was awesome, I mean a really cool guy. I met him through friends, and he started hanging out with us. Then, one weekend that most people were away, we went to this party and had a great time. He started calling me and we went to do stuff by ourselves."

While Sandra described the relationship's wonderful beginning, Karen listened carefully to both what Sandra said as well as what she didn't say. That is, Karen watched Sandra's body language and how her words complemented or contradicted her verbal disclosures. When Sandra described happy moments in the relationship she smiled, sat up straight, and her eyes showed excitement. At the same time, her voice got louder, she talked faster, and she was very descriptive about people, places, and events (e.g., color of clothing worn, lighting in a room).

When Sandra discussed Bill's possessiveness she said, "I just didn't get it. Before we were exclusive, he wasn't like that at all. Now, he's hammering me for going out with other friends and not calling him to tell him first. I was like, you're not my mother, and he was like, I want to be with you, too. Sometimes he'd get so pissed about it, I'd just cancel with my friends. It was like he wanted me to be with him all the time, and I was like suffocating. But I loved him, you know, and I didn't want to fight about it. I just hated when he'd yell at me."

With this disclosure, Karen observed a change in Sandra's communication style. Her non-verbal behavior showed signs of withdrawal, such as pressing her back into the sofa as if to push the pain away, rounding her shoulders and hunching, hiding her hands, and crossing her legs. When she showed anger at Bill, her voice was loud and strong, and she seemed furious with him for treating her this way. Yet, when she described her love for him, her voice became softer and more broken, as if she has accepted the relational boundaries Bill placed on her.

Karen asked Sandra to talk about her perceptions of what preceded the day's violence. Sandra's voice faded, she shuddered and then looked panicked. She says, "I called Bill to tell him I was going to take a second shift at work." Sandra interrupted her story to clarify that she is a waitress and needed to help out a friend by covering a shift for her. She continued, "He was pissed because I had already taken another shift this week and it was cutting into 'our' time. I told him I had to be there in an hour and he said he was coming over. He showed up about 10 minutes later, pounding on the door." Sandra appeared visibly agitated, as if Bill could hear what she said to Karen.

Karen reached out to Sandra with her hands, but didn't touch her, "I know how difficult this is, so just tell me what you can. Remember that I'm here to help and that you are safe here." Sandra said nothing for several minutes but rocked back and forth in the chair. She finally said in a voice of disbelief, "When I let him in, he wouldn't let me get ready to go to work. He handed me the phone, telling me to cancel or saying that he'd cancel for me. At first, I thought he was joking but he was totally serious." Sandra looked to Karen for her understanding before she continued. Then in a strangled voice, Sandra said, "I had just had enough. The relationship was getting too hard, my friends didn't like him and, although I loved him, nothing ever seemed easy. He always wanted more. So I told him it was over. That was when he lost control."

Karen stated that Bill's behavior was not a loss of control. Sandra shook her head no to say that she didn't agree. Karen clarified her statement, "Bill used violence as a means to control your actions. From what you told me, usually he'd yell at you and then you'd give in to his demands. When the yelling didn't work this time, he resorted to physical action." Sandra stared at Karen, unsure whether or not she should be believed.

As Sandra told Karen about the physical violence she encountered, Karen did not interrupt her or use words that might appear judgmental when she requested more information. Karen wanted to make sure Sandra was behaving genuinely in the encounter and not hiding anything from her. During the conversation, Karen understood how to best communicate with Sandra; that is, how to accommodate Sandra's communication style so that each conversational turn became more forthcoming and meaningful to the counseling process. Karen observed a pattern in Sandra's communication style. There was regularity in her eye contact, smiling, nodding, gestures, posture, loudness of her voice, changes in pitch, and sitting position, depending on Sandra's relationship disclosures. Karen kept careful notes of Sandra's verbal and nonverbal communication activities.

Very slowly, Karen began to integrate behaviors similar to Sandra's into her own communication repertoire. When Karen asked questions, she mirrored or paraphrased Sandra's words to reduce the potential for misunderstanding. When Karen saw Sandra become excited, Karen demonstrated greater animation by changing her posture and using more facial expression. Even when Karen wasn't talking, she responded in a manner similar to Sandra, without duplicating her behaviors. Karen was careful to only integrate those behaviors that were approximations of Sandra's when it was appropriate to do so. Karen knew that if she used the behaviors inappropriately or too often, Sandra might perceive that Karen was mimicking or mocking her. Karen did not want Sandra to have a negative impression of the counseling experience; rather, she hoped to convey through her behaviors that she was attentively listening to the disclosures and wanted to help. Moreover, Karen believed that her similarity in behavior might lead Sandra to think they were similar in other ways (*perceived homophily*) and would make it easier for Sandra to accept her support.

After 30 minutes of conversation, it became apparent that Sandra was more willing to trust Karen with information about the relationship. Even though she may not have trusted Karen completely, she responded to her questions more easily once Karen accommodated her communication style. When Sandra thought she had told Karen everything, she announced that she was done and wanted to leave. Karen asked Sandra to stay at the shelter. Sandra shook her head vigorously and said she would stay with Donna and Cassie. Karen expressed concern that Bill might find her there, hoping to apologize and patch up the relationship, or seek further retribution against her or her friends for the decision to end the relationship. At this point, Karen and Sandra joined Donna and Cassie to discuss the safest living arrangements for Sandra. Her friends indicated other people who would be happy to have Sandra stay with them who Bill didn't know, and therefore he wouldn't have access to their residences. Before they left, Karen gave Sandra resource materials and her pager number from the crisis support hotline. She asked Sandra to call tomorrow so they would know she was safe. Karen also asked her to come back in a few days, as Karen learned during the interview that Sandra had experienced abuse in prior romantic relationships. Sandra agreed to meet Karen Monday afternoon after her last class.

SIX WEEKS LATER

It was Monday again and Sandra was to arrive at the shelter in less than 20 minutes for their weekly session. Karen thought Sandra was making strides in therapy; Sandra had drawn new conclusions about her need to be in a relationship. Not only was she able to separate her own perception of self-worth from the feelings she experienced in a romantic relationship, but she was able to identify what she wanted in future relationships. Karen was looking over Sandra's file when she arrived.

"Hey, Karen, am I late?" Sandra asked, smiling and strolling into the small office. Sitting across the table from Karen she said, "It was a really good week. I made it to all my classes, and even got a B+ on my literature mid-term. I amazed myself!"

Karen was thrilled that Sandra's coursework had improved as she devoted more hours to studying each week. Yet, she was concerned about Sandra's job performance as a waitress.

Since the relationship had dissolved, Sandra found it difficult to wait on tables where romantic couples openly displayed affection for one another. She had been sent home from work one week because of her inability to provide appropriate customer service.

When Karen turned the conversation toward work, Sandra's face fell, and her answer was not very forthcoming, "I, um, I, ah, made it through the Tuesday and Thursday shifts just fine, but I, ah, Saturday was dismissed." Sandra didn't look at Karen when she disclosed this information and shifted uncomfortably in her chair. Her shoulders slumped, she began to sit on her hands, cross her legs and hunch forward; it was a demeanor reminiscent of six weeks ago. Karen assumed a more closed communication position with crossed legs, arms brought to her side, a tilted head position, and lowered voice while asking what happened.

Sandra replied, "I got mad again and angry I wasn't in a relationship." Karen asked her to clarify her answer, "What were you angry about? Being sent home or seeing two people being romantic with one another?"

Sandra understood what Karen was asking, "The second one. I wanted to be those people in that relationship."

Karen attempted to validate Sandra's feelings but altered Sandra's perception of the situation, "I know that it takes a lot of courage for you to move forward with your life. As we have talked before, it's normal to want to feel close or connected to others. It's normal to desire a healthy relationship. But there's a difference between desiring a relationship and feeling the need to be in a relationship, no matter the costs."

Sandra shifted in her chair and looked down at the table, "Yes, I realize that. I want to be in a good relationship with someone who does not need me to complete him; a person who will appreciate me and not try to change me." Looking directly at Karen, she added, "I'm worth that."

Karen and Sandra exchanged small smiles while Sandra searched Karen's face to see if she didn't believe her. Karen gave no indication of disbelief, but lifted her eyebrows as if to signal that she is waiting for Sandra to say something. Sandra recognized this nonverbal cue and said, "You're still waiting for me to address being sent home, right?" Karen nodded, and with her left arm, gestured that Sandra was still in control of the conversation.

Sandra continued her story, adding, "It was two hours before my shift ended when these two started being all lovey-dovey, swapping food and stuff. I was assigned to the table and asked my shift manager to move me to a different one. We were short-staffed as it was, so I couldn't. When they first started lip smacking, I wanted to run and then went to the bathroom to cry."

Karen responded by paraphrasing and modifying Sandra's disclosure, "So, you saw two people enjoying each other's company and became upset. At first, you wanted to run away and then you went to the bathroom. Can you clarify what you were feeling?"

Sandra replied, "I felt angry that I couldn't get rid of them as customers. I felt like they were being disrespectful to me, that they could act this way and make me feel bad about myself in my own relationships." Sandra's voice rose as she mentally recalled the incident.

Karen leaned forward placing her hands on the edge of the table, shifted in her chair and let a pregnant pause hang in the air. Karen waited for Sandra to indicate that she was emotionally ready to continue the discussion. After several minutes, Karen commented, "What you just described are separate issues. How they acted is one issue. How you interpreted their behavior is another, right?"

Sandra seemed reluctant to agree, but did. "Right," she replied.

Karen leaned back in her chair and looked at the ceiling, asking, "So which one do you want to tackle first? Which issue do you think is more important for us to talk about?" Karen's gaze met Sandra's midway through the second question.

Sandra nodded with a small chuckle because she and Karen have been through this dance before. Sandra understood that Karen wanted her to be honest with herself about her behavior. "We need to talk about how I reacted. I kind of let that situation get out of control."

"All right." Karen said, "So let's start there. We'll talk about your reaction to their behavior. What were you reacting to?"

"I, um, I got angry when they would like eat a bite and then kiss, you know?" Sandra continued, "And each time they kissed, I got more upset because I want to be in that kind of relationship. They made me feel bad that I wasn't like them. That I wasn't going home to someone like that."

Karen jumped on one of the remarks Sandra made, hoping that Sandra would change the way she discussed her feelings, "Who made you feel bad about yourself?"

Pouting and not realizing what Karen was asking, Sandra just replied, "They did. They made me feel that way." She looked at Karen tilting her head to the side.

Karen wanted Sandra to take responsibility for her own behavior and acknowledge her responsibility for personal feelings. So instead of immediately responding to the comment, Karen waited to see if Sandra alone could correct her perceptions of the situation. When Sandra didn't renew the dialogue, Karen reviewed it for her, "So far, you said you became upset because you saw two people in a relationship acting intimately, although maybe not appropriately, in a restaurant. You said that *they* made *you* feel bad about yourself."

In hearing Karen's emphasis on the words *they* and *you,* Sandra understood Karen's reaction and nodded her head. Karen looked directly at Sandra, and again both heads nodded back and forth. With a gentle voice, Karen helped Sandra to find the courage to admit her feelings about the situation, "Sandra, who really made you feel bad about yourself?"

Sandra turned her head, leaned on her right arm, closed her eyes, and with a loud sigh announced, "I did." She sighed again and then smiled, "I did it to myself again, didn't I?" Not waiting for Karen's reply she continued, "I allowed myself to think about my relationship when I should have been thinking about my job. I felt angry about a work situation that I couldn't control. It was no one's fault we were short-staffed that day. We hadn't had that busy of a night for a while. So when these two came in, I was already tired and wanted to go. I guess I was looking for an excuse . . . ."

As Sandra's voice trailed off, Karen stepped in, wanting Sandra to stay on track, "Okay, so you already felt tired by the time these two came in. What might you have done to prevent the situation from escalating, aside from not allowing yourself to think about the relationship?" Sandra looked at Karen, replying, "Well, I probably could have said something to them about their behavior. You know, that this type of behavior isn't really appropriate at our type of restaurant." Karen nodded, again allowing Sandra to keep talking. Sandra continued, "And then I could have asked the busboy to help out so that I would have less contact with them without affecting service. I should not have let the situation get out of hand. I let down the customer and my manager." Sandra was frustrated for not having anticipated this solution earlier.

Karen agreed that this solution might have been more appropriate and that she can use it in the future. Yet, Karen's focus on the solution is secondary to her desire to have Sandra focus on the process of forming the solution. She asked Sandra to think about how her behavior affected others at the restaurant. Sandra was thoughtful for a moment and then replied, "Well, I know it was an inconvenience. My manager said that I needed to work out my personal problems at home so I could focus on work at work." Karen asked if Sandra believed that to be a reasonable request, and she agreed. Karen added, "Do you think that you can focus on work at work, given the environment in which you're working?"

Sandra got out of her chair and walked around the room. Karen moved to the sofa that was parallel to the chairs, so that Sandra could command full attention of the space when standing in the middle of the room. Sandra seemed to be wrestling with the question, "You know, I don't know. I've been at this job for a while and I know everyone. The other servers are kind of like my family away from home. But I think I understand what you're asking. Because I work in a place where people come to have a good time, I'm going to always be surrounded by people. What I mean is that couples are going to come in and celebrate birthdays, anniversaries, and happy occasions. And, I'm going to have to find a way to get a grip on my feelings if I'm going to keep my job there."

Karen responded to this self-discovery, "And how do you feel about this conclusion you've just drawn?" Sandra felt unsure of herself, "I've never considered working anywhere else. I thought that I'd be there until I got a real job after college. But, now I'm thinking that I should get a job somewhere else."

Karen, concerned about how Sandra drew this conclusion, clarified her thoughts, "Sandra, I'm not telling you to get or not to get another job. That's your decision. You need to first decide whether or not you can keep a handle on your feelings no matter what job you have. Then you need to decide whether or not this current job is a job you want to continue."

Sandra interrupted her, "Yes, I know. It's just that I've only now realized the working conditions at this restaurant might be a greater challenge to me while I'm getting over this relationship. It's like being too close to fire and knowing that I've put myself in a position where it is easier to get burned." Karen gestured for Sandra to continue, while simultaneously gesturing to her to sit on the sofa. The two sat facing one another with knees supporting their elbows.

Sandra continued, "If I leave the restaurant, it might not be a bad thing. I'll still have my friends. We'll still go out together on Friday night. I can go out with them anytime." Karen asked several probing questions about Sandra's plan for a new work position, how she would terminate her current position, and her career goals for the future. Once Sandra identified possible internships in her major and contacts in her social network, Karen turn the conversation back to her current position, asking, "Before you leave this job, if you still intend to, again, that is your decision, do you think that that you might learn more about yourself by staying at the restaurant?"

Sandra looked pensive as if challenging the decision she just made, but then shook her head, "You know, if you asked me that a few weeks ago, I probably would've said yes. Although the servers are my friends, I think I need some separation from them. I think I need to figure this stuff out by myself. They watched this relationship go down the tubes and had lots of advice for me. Now that I think about it, I actually think this is part of the problem."

Karen interjected to clarify her response, "Are you saying that your friends are responsible for your relationship?"

Sandra recognized the verbal dance Karen was beginning and smiled, "No, not at all. That was a bad relationship. Although I have to remind myself how bad it was, I kept asking them for help when I should have made my own decisions. If I'm going to make better decisions for myself, I'm going to have to start making more decisions for myself."

As Sandra seemed intent on finding a new job, the next 15 minutes were spent drawing up a more formal plan for locating an internship and general job-seeking advice. At that point, Sandra looked at her watch and announced that she needed to leave. Karen and Sandra said good-bye while reaffirming the following week's appointment.

THE AFTERMATH

Karen wrote about Sandra's progress in her file. Sandra had articulated a desire for greater self-reliance in her decision making and was slowly adjusting her perceptions of romantic relationships. In addition, Sandra had demonstrated greater self-awareness of her feelings and been able to label them more appropriately. Most impressive to Karen, however, was the ease and comfort with which the two could now communicate.

Over the past several weeks, Sandra and Karen created a shared communication style. In their initial interaction, Karen focused on the meaning of each verbal or nonverbal cue as well as how these cues were tied to the content of her communication messages. That is, Karen wanted to assess Sandra's process for communication; what she said and how she delivered her messages. As Karen recognized and understood Sandra's communication style, she wanted to emulate the positive elements and help to redirect those communication cues that led to a less effective self-presentation. Thus, Karen integrated some of Sandra's behaviors into her own communication repertoire (e.g., paraphrasing language, approximating body language, and adjusting pitch, tone, and pauses), hoping to increase the self-disclosure as well as improve Sandra's receptivity to her and to the counseling process.

What began as a concerted effort by Karen to ensure that her personal communication style enhanced, rather than detracted from, the counseling sessions is no longer intentional. As Sandra's receptivity to and rapport with Karen increased, they both developed a uniquely synchronized communication style, which was slightly different from each one's individual communication style. Although Karen initially focused on Sandra's communication behaviors, it became apparent that Sandra had integrated some of Karen's communication patterns. A slight shift in facial expression from either one now speaks volumes, whether it is a raised eyebrow inviting greater discussion or a smile of shared empathy.

As their communication became a seamless dance, the atmosphere of the counseling relationship positively shifted. With increased comfort in the shared communication style, Sandra and Karen found themselves accommodating one another, even when the content of their communication messages contrasted. That is, the synchronized process of communication sustained and provided continuity to their interaction when conflict or tension arose.

As this case exemplifies, accommodation can be a useful communication technique to build rapport with others. In the beginning of the process, much time is spent watching how another person communicates and then slowly developing an understanding for the meanings behind those communicative behaviors. Yet, watching how someone else communicates brings an awareness of our own self-behaviors. This allows both individuals in an interaction to reflect on their unique communication repertoires as well as on how their communication behaviors affect others' comfort levels for that style of communication. Slowly, one or more participants in the dialogue will choose to integrate verbal and nonverbal cues that are perceived to help bridge social relations. Building a rapport with others is a process of social support and environmental and social sensitivity. Different communication styles become integrated into a more meaningful style that is adaptive to all conversational participants' needs. As a result, accommodation helps people to create messages that are both meaningful and appropriate, enabling them to focus on both *what is said* and *how the message is delivered* in a communication encounter.

RELEVANT CONCEPTS

Communication accommodation: An adaptive process by which individuals consciously or subconsciously begin to use verbal and/or nonverbal communication behaviors that are complementary and somewhat synchronized with those behaviors of the person with whom they are communicating.

Communication rapport: The level to which parties feel comfortable in their communication with one another.

Communication repertoire: The range of verbal, nonverbal, and paralinguistic behaviors that a person uses when communicating.

Communication style: The combination of the content of what is said and the manner in which a communication message is delivered, including both verbal and nonverbal actions.

Perceived homophily: The decrease of perceived similarity (e.g., behaviors, interests, background) with another.

Self-awareness: The level to which someone is able to recognize and reflect upon her/his own behavior or thoughts.

Self-disclosure: The extent to which someone voluntarily shares personal information (that is not available from some other source) about herself or himself to another person.

DISCUSSION QUESTIONS

1. Why is communication accommodation important?
2. How did Karen accommodate Sandra's communication style during these interactions? How might you accommodate someone else's communication style?
3. Would you expect it to be easier or more difficult to accommodate your family or friends' communication patterns versus an acquaintance or stranger? Why or why not?
4. Is it possible to accommodate someone's communication style while disagreeing with the content of his or her communication message? Think of a situation in which you disagreed with someone but still accommodated to his or her communication style. What did you do?
5. What other settings or context might also require communication accommodation so that interactions can be successful?
6. Is communication accommodation more important in a therapeutic setting than in other relationships? Why or why not?

ACKNOWLEDGMENTS

The authors would like to thank Gail Heller, M.S.W, and Holly Rosen, M.S.W, for their editorial comments, which strengthened this chapter.

ENDNOTE

[1] All names and identifying characteristics have been changed to protect those who participated in these therapy sessions.

REFERENCES/SUGGESTED READINGS

Ferrara, K. (1991). Accommodation in therapy. In H. Giles, J. Coupland & N. Coupland (Eds.), *Contexts of accommodation: Developments in applied sociolinguistics* (pp. 187–223). New York: Cambridge University Press.

Giles, H., Mulac, A., Bradac, J., & Johnson, P. (1986). Speech accommodation theory. In M. McLaughlin (Ed.), *Communication yearbook 10* (pp. 86–101). Newbury Park, CA: Sage.

Mearns, D., & Thorne, B. (1988). *Person-centered counseling in action.* London: Sage.

Murray-Johnson, L., & Witte, K. (November, 2002). *Using communication accommodation with counselors and clients: An evaluation of State of Michigan domestic violence shelters.* Paper presented at the annual meeting of the National Communication Association, New Orleans, LA.

12

Social Identity and Stigma Management for People Living With HIV

Lance S. Rintamaki
Midwest Center for Health Services and Policy Research

Dale E. Brashers
University of Illinois at Urbana–Champaign

The introduction of improved medications in the late 1990s dramatically increased the life span of many people infected with the human immunodeficiency virus (HIV) or who have acquired immune deficiency syndrome (AIDS). What was once treated as a terminal illness now is thought of as a chronic (or long-term) condition. Unfortunately, progress in addressing the widespread social stigma surrounding HIV has lagged behind these biomedical advances. Since the beginning of the HIV pandemic, people infected with HIV and the groups they are associated with have faced stigma and discrimination from the general populace (Herek & Capatanio, 2002). The public hysteria and lack of education surrounding HIV have led to victim-blaming of those infected and the resulting stigma since has been labeled as the most important social and psychological problem associated with the HIV illness experience.

The social stigma surrounding HIV has been well documented, including the discrimination and unsupportive encounters that people living with HIV confront. How people manage HIV stigma in their social encounters has received far less attention. People with HIV are mindful of how others feel and act toward them, and they face uncertainty in choosing whether to disclose their status and in assessing others' responses to that disclosure. Consequently, stigma impacts both how people living with HIV approach social interactions and perform during them. How they might cope with HIV stigma in general, or respond to explicit encounters in particular, is an important topic for further study. This case study highlights these dilemmas and provides examples of strategies people employ to manage HIV stigma.

The following is the story of a small support group for people living with HIV. Support groups have been very useful for people who share similar difficult circumstances to offer each other advice and comfort. Support groups exist for a number of different illnesses (including HIV or AIDS, cancer, alcoholism, diabetes, Parkinson's disease, and so on). In this particular meeting, a new member (Margaret) is brought into the group. She is struggling with a series of difficult social dilemmas and relationships with people who stigmatize her for having HIV. Members of the group console her and have a general discussion about why HIV is stigmatized in today's society, how the threat of stigma affects the way they interact with others, the types of stigmatizing encounters they've experienced, and how they respond to stigma when they are confronted by it.[1]

HIV SUPPORT GROUP INTERACTION: DISCUSSING STIGMA

Setting: Support group held at an HIV treatment clinic in a large urban hospital. Margaret is being introduced as a new member to the group.

Participants: Bobby (a White, gay male who is 32 years old), Margaret (a White, straight female who is 52 years old), George (a White, gay male who is 53 years old), Juan (a Latino, gay male who is 40 years old), Byrd (or Roberta, a Black, straight female who is 60 years old), Jack (a White gay male who is 25 years old).

Bobby: Well, it's about that time, so why don't we go ahead and get started. We have a new person here tonight, so why don't we go around and all of us can introduce ourselves to Margaret, OK? I'll start. My name is Bobby Jacobson, as you already know, and I'm something of a facilitator of this support group. I was diagnosed with HIV almost four years ago. It's been quite a trip for me since then, but right now things are great and I work to try and keep it that way. I work in Health and Human Services in the HIV division for the city and started working with the support groups about three years ago. I'm excited you're here, Margaret. I look forward to getting to know you better. I also hope you get a lot out of coming to our group tonight. OK, who's next?

Juan: I'll go. My name's Juan Martinez. I've been HIV positive for six and a half years now. I've recently gone back to work after coming off of disability and I think that's gone really well. I do a lot of outreach work now in HIV care and I love it. I've been coming to these meetings for a while now, and I'm glad to see Margaret is joining us. This group is something of an extended family for me. I hope it becomes like that for you too. How's that for starters?

Jack: My turn? OK, my name's Jack Chase. I'm a Taurus, my favorite food is Thai, and I like long, romantic strolls along the beach.

Byrd: Boy, don't make me smack you upside your head!

Jack: Hey! I bruise easily! I'm very delicate, you know. OK, my name is Jack and I've been positive for about five years, since I was 20. My life is good, though, and I haven't had too many serious problems with my health. In fact, I just opened my own gallery in Up Town which I'm very excited about! You should all come and I'll give you the grand tour. I even have senior discounts, Byrd.

Byrd: Hey! I don't look a day over 60 and don't you forget it. Margaret, honey, you pay this child no mind. If he gets out of hand you have to just smack him around until he shapes up. I'm Roberta Jackson, but everyone just calls me Byrd. I'm happy you decided to join us tonight, honey. It'll be nice to have another woman in the group—not that I mind spending time with all you handsome men!

Jack: You know you love us Byrd.

Byrd: Even if you don't deserve it, you little trouble-maker.

George: I'll take my turn. I'm George Gunthry and I've been living with HIV for what seems like just about forever. I guess it's been, let's see, I was diagnosed in 1986, so how long does that make it?

Bobby: A long time! You're a veteran George.

George: Yeah, I'm a bit of an old timer. It's good to meet you Margaret.

Margaret: Thank you George. I guess I'm the only one left, so here goes. My name is Margaret Hawthorne. I found out I was HIV positive almost a year ago. It's been hell. The doctors had been misdiagnosing me for years now. I've had an assortment of ailments over the past six or seven years that I just couldn't shake. Half the time I think the doctors thought I was making stuff up or they thought it was "just menopause." I guess I didn't fit their profile for someone who might have HIV, so they didn't even think to check that out. Finally, a friend of mine who's a nurse told me I should have my immune system checked out. That's when they finally diagnosed me with HIV. Only, it's really far along and I have full-blown AIDS. It's bad enough that my body is falling apart, but I was engaged to be married and when my diagnosis came back positive my fiancée broke it off. The rest of my family has pulled away from me. Even my own kids. I have two grown children from my first marriage and my son won't even let me hold my grandchild. I see Bobby a lot when I go in for check-ups. Both Bobby and Juan were nice enough to come visit with me when I had to stay in the hospital for pneumonia, and they're the ones that convinced me to come to the group tonight. I thought maybe I could ask you about how you cope with people when they treat you badly.

Bobby: Well, I think this is a really important issue and its well worth talking about tonight. Even though there are a lot of improvements in how society approaches the disease, there haven't been as many positive changes in how society accepts people with the disease.

Juan: I agree. It's not even so much anymore the disease of death, it's the disease of stigma.

Jack: Right, right.

George: There's still definite stereotypes being made about people with the disease.

Byrd: People like to put labels on others. If you have AIDS you're either gay, a prostitute, or promiscuous in your early life, or whatever. Or a drug user.

Juan: I think they're also specific to different groups. Such as, if you're a White man you're probably gay. If you're a woman you're probably a slut. If you're a Black man you probably shot drugs. Just negative stereotypes that people use to rationalize why "it'll never happen to me."

Bobby: When people find out that I have HIV they often say, you know, "I always wanted to ask you if you're gay or not." I look them square in the eyes and say "Well, I think the only reason you'd ask me is if you want to have sex with me."

Jack: That's a good one! I'm gonna have to use that. "Are you trying to have sex with me? A relationship?"

Margaret: "How'd you get it?" That's what everybody wants to know.

Bobby: Right. When I go out to speak publicly to kids and to adults, the first question that always comes up is, "How'd you get it?" I mean, that's the first question, and if you say you got it through a transfusion or something that's no fault of your own, then you're an innocent victim. But, if you got it through sex or IV drug use, then you get the, you know, "Well, that's too bad but you kind of got what you deserved" attitude.

Byrd: I hear a lot about it in my church. A lot of the ways HIV is transmitted are "sins" and our pastor has even referred to AIDS as punishment for those sins.

Margaret: And I know a lot of older people who have been like, "Alright, you've got the plague, stay away!"

Jack: Well, even though the new medications have really extended the lives of people who are infected, in the eyes of a lot of people we're still walking corpses.

George: Well, we're all going to die. I think the fact that we make them think of death and dying makes a lot of people uncomfortable.

Bobby: There's still just a lot of ignorance out there about HIV. There's this guy who keeps calling the radio station I listen to. He keeps calling in and warning people to stay out of Up Town "cause there's all those homos and queers, and the mosquitoes are so bad that you better just stay out of Up Town."

Byrd: It seems like it always ends up having straights against gays. I've been in conversations where it's turned into kind of a verbal bashing. "This is a gay disease" or "This is a straight disease" or "This is a no disease" or "You brought it on yourself." So, you kind of get that tug of war about whose disease it is. I think you have to look at this as something that happens, big deal how it happens, cause someone with HIV is still a person.

Margaret: With all the stigma out there about HIV, how does that affect you? Does it affect you?

Bobby: No matter how long you've had this disease, I think there's still always a fear of how someone's going to react when you tell them. I know it still makes me leery around other people and I'm always looking for signs of how someone might react if I were to tell them. Do I think they'll be supportive or are they going to run screaming from the room?

Margaret: I know I worry about that. I worry about all the stereotypes out there about people with HIV and how this is going to affect my reputation.

Byrd: I think that is something that bothers a lot of people, honey. I think it's a big problem for straight men, in particular. We've talked about this before, that we know several straight men with HIV who won't come to these support groups or even go to get treatment because they're afraid people are going to see them, put two and two together, figure out they have HIV and then think they're gay. They're more afraid about people thinking they're gay than that they have HIV! I think that's just so sad.

Jack: I love you Byrd.

Byrd: I love you too, honey. As a Black woman, I think I've seen this to be especially true in my community. You know, "African American men are not homosexual!"

George: Gay African Americans don't exist.

Byrd: No, they "don't exist." You know, my nephew is gay and there was an article about him in the paper where he talked about it. I couldn't believe how so many people turned to me and were all, "Damn, I can't believe he said it!" I think homosexuality gets viewed and treated differently across different ethnic communities. In some you might face worse discrimination than in others.

Margaret: I guess my big thing is over how I can tell other people. How do you guys deal with that and the possibility of people stigmatizing you?

Jack: I've learned to think about it a real long time. Like, I haven't told anybody in my family. When I was diagnosed, I said, "You know, I really do think there's a need there, but Jack, you had better wait and think about this for, oh let's say, two years." Because when I told them I was gay, I kind of decided in the afternoon and told them in the evening. And it was very, very ugly. So I thought, I'm not going to have an ugly scene like that again, so I kind of have done that with everyone.

Bobby: I think there is a lot of uncertainty about whether or not you'll be accepted. I think I'm a little like Jack, where it's similar to coming out to people about me being gay. I mean, it's kind of like going through the same thing twice.

Jack: My group of friends, uh, you never know how they're going to react, so I thought about it a while and there are some people that I've told and there wasn't a real bad reaction, but I know not to mention it again. I don't talk about what studies I'm in or what medication I'm taking or how I'm feeling. They know about the HIV and that's all they want to know. You know? But, because of the uncertainty on a lot of things, treatments, relationships, telling people, jobs, I think about it a long time. That doesn't mean you always make the right decision, but you do the best you can.

George: Yeah, but you have to balance that. There's a time and a place where it's to your personal benefit for people not to know you're HIV positive. I'm always advising people, I mean if you're working or whatever, "Hey, if you feel like you have to lie about it, you know, there comes a point where you've got to protect yourself." We're talking about protection. I mean, people can make you suffer a great deal.

Byrd: I went from one extreme to the other. I went from complete denial to saying "Hell, I'm just going to tell everybody!" After having gone through the pain of being rejected by some people and feeling bad about myself for having HIV, I've turned that around and now I find a lot of validation in myself. I'm intentionally open about it because that steals the power people have over me when it's a secret. I feel like I have less to lose because I'm so open about it. No one can out me, no one can tell other people about me behind my back.

Juan: I used to work in construction, which is a very macho sort of work, and a lot of my friends were straight. I mean good friends, not just anybody, but friends. For a long time I basically dealt on a need to know basis. I was like, "If I'm not sleeping with you, it's none of your business." But now I'm a lot like Byrd. I'm open about it because after hiding it for so long it's very cathartic to be open about it. Also, talking about it is a large part of my work.

Margaret: Something that's really bothered me is people gossiping about me behind my back. I'm always worried about who's telling people without my consent, you know?

Bobby: Sometimes friends or family find out from other people. It's not always necessarily in a positive way that they find out, so you kind of have a mess to clean up afterwards. Or just knowing how certain people are going to react—you know—if they write you off they're just going to write you off, so . . . .

Byrd: If I were to give any newly infected person a piece of advice it would be to not isolate themselves. That's why I'm glad you're here tonight, Margaret. Keeping your HIV status from people for strategic reasons is one thing, but to hide it is quite another, and dammit, that's more damaging than the virus. Get out into the world and especially seek out other people with HIV, especially when you're newly infected. That sense of community will help you survive.

George: Right, and I think it's important to teach people to advocate for themselves. Teach people they don't have to take it from other people who give them a hard time about their HIV. We don't have time for that sort of thing.

Bobby: A lot of what I do is going out and educating others about HIV and what it is. That's how I tackle the stigma that's out there. I'm proactive. When I go out and do presentations I never reveal my status until I'm midway through or at the end. Then I'll say, "Hey, I don't have any t-cells, and I have AIDS, and blah blah blah" and they go, "You! No, wait a minute!" Especially with the young kids, because they have this picture of what AIDS is and it's important to challenge that. I think that changes the stigma that's associated with you. That's one way of tackling the social stigma out there, by going out and talking with people, letting them know what HIV and AIDS are, and putting a face to the disease.

Margaret: What are the sorts of things you've dealt with from other people?

Juan: When I was diagnosed I associated with several people from work and I socialized a lot with them. You know, these were reasonably intelligent people. Some were socialites and some were egg heads, but nonetheless, they were all pretty intelligent people and you know, went to college and all that. There was this one guy, a good friend of mine at this office, who didn't know I was positive. One day he said to me, "The way I set my life up, you know, I'm never going to meet somebody who has been infected with AIDS. It just won't enter my life because of the way I've structured my life." And I just looked at him. Then I went nuts and said, "You are completely wrong!" I was amazed that there are a hell of a lot of people in this world who don't think that their lives will be in some way, shape, or form touched by HIV. You know, I never did tell him about me. I wish I had.

George: At first, I didn't share with my sister that I was HIV positive, but I stayed with her for a short while one summer after I was diagnosed. I just didn't know how to talk about it back then. Then, she comes home one evening and says, "Don't you have something you need to tell me?" I was like, "No." "Don't you have something you need to tell me?" Well, I knew what she was driving at so when I finally told her, she said, "You put me and my child at risk." And I'm like "Huh?" Here's someone who has a Master's degree and wants to work on a Ph.D. I said, "You can't get this externally and there's nothing I've done or would even dream of doing that could put you at any risk of infection." But I noticed that when she would cook dinner and ask me if I was ready to eat, if I said "Naw, I can get something later," she would say, "No, I've already cooked." Then I noticed I kept getting the same plate, the same utensils, the same glass. And that hurts coming from a member of your own family, you know?

Bobby: I think what bothers me the most is when people keep their distance from you. I even see it within the gay community. For example, Friday night used to be a bowling league. There was like maybe five or six that were positive and like five or six that weren't positive and there was definitely a line as to who associated with whom. I mean, it was cordial, but the ones that weren't positive weren't inviting the ones that were positive to parties, out to dinner, and so forth and so on, cause they didn't want to be associated with it other than in the bowling league.

Jack: I know what you mean. I go out every now and then and I've had a great time when I've gone out. But it makes a big difference once people find out that I'm positive. You're kind of like labeled, you know? And most people are like "stay away, stay away, stay away."

Juan: That pisses me off. I know this guy that is super friendly, the salt of the earth. He's financially independent, too, which isn't necessarily a bad thing. He told me he once mentioned to a close friend about his HIV and the next time he went to the bar his friend had gone around and told a lot of other people, and as a result, people wouldn't even talk to him. He said he doesn't go to that bar anymore because people still shy away from him.

George: And if anyone does talk to you they probably do it on a one on one basis because they don't want to be affiliated with you in public. "Guilt by association."

Jack: I think when family and friends do that sort of thing it hurts the most. A friend of mine, when he passed away, his mother stood at the casket and as everybody came up she said, "My poor son died of leukemia." I was just appalled that she was so embarrassed to say that her son had AIDS and he died and that he was a wonderful person. I can't seem to believe me having AIDS makes me any less of a person. And I won't accept or tolerate anybody assuming I'm less of a person because I have HIV.

Margaret: Sometimes it's kind of ambiguous, you know? Other times, it's a lot more in your face. My family acts like that—they say I have cirrhosis of the liver and lung cancer. My children pretty much stay away and have nothing to do with me. My ex-husband managed to tell all these people without asking me if that was OK. I hadn't even told anybody that I had AIDS but he managed to tell all his sex partners, you know, that his ex-wife had AIDS and that they better get HIV tested. I hadn't even told anybody before he went out and told them.

Bobby: Has anyone had weird experiences with their doctors?

Byrd: I had my dentist tell me, he says, "I think that you should find someone who deals more with your kind of people." I was like, "What do you mean, my kind of people?"

Margaret: An ophthalmologist turned me down. Can you believe that? My ophthalmologist I had been seeing for years and years and years. I called him just to find out what they would do and they said, "We think you should go see an AIDS ophthalmologist who deals in that."

Jack: I have a friend whose dentist told him that he could continue to come to him but it was going to be a lot more work for him, the dentist. It's like, well what? Does that mean you're going to have to start sterilizing your instruments or what? I've had doctors who didn't want to touch me. There was this neurologist who would be all the way across the room examining me. I was like, "girl, you have to come over here." Or I see a nurse drawing blood from somebody else without gloves but when they come to me they put on a gown, gloves, and a face mask. You know? I was like, " I can pop my own line for you. Just let me do my blood draws if you're that afraid to touch me."

George: When I first came to town I registered at City Hospital clinic and they gave me this whole intake thing for an hour and a half. Although they don't say it directly, the definite inference was that if you're HIV positive you have essentially given up the privilege of having sex and you shouldn't be sexually active. They're also very quick to point out if you have sex in this state with someone and don't tell them that you're HIV positive, you'll be subject to felony prosecution. But the thing that got me was the definite inference that it's your fault that you're HIV positive so now you've given up the privilege of being sexually active.

Byrd: I never went through that, but I did get turned down by my beautician who refused to cut my hair.

Margaret: Do you have tissues? You guys gotta realize I get emotional. Sorry for the tears guys.

Jack: Oh, no, it's OK.

Margaret: It's just menopause, it's old age.

Bobby: There we go, there's a whole box of them.

Juan: I have a friend who's told me several times that he has a tremendous support system. He's always been very up front about it with people and his family has always been right there for him. His parents were with him the first time he went to the doctor, the whole nine yards. He's never really had any negative experiences. No one has denied him housing or medical treatment or dental treatment or anything. I guess it's important to recognize that not everyone feels stigmatized or has bad experiences. Although, he is the first to admit that he knows there aren't very many people who have had all the same positive experiences he has.

Margaret: There was this time where my son and his wife became pregnant with their first child and they didn't want me to be around them. They were so fearful. Now I look at it as, "what am I going to tell this grandchild?" How is she going to look at me?

Byrd: You just tell her the truth. There's no use in hiding it. You're her grandmother, you have HIV, and you love her.

Margaret: Now I'm thinking about children with HIV. My heart really goes out to them. They didn't ask for it.

Juan: Nobody *asks* for it, Margaret.

Byrd: That's true. None of us.

Margaret: But they were innocently born with this disease. Do they live very long? I've not seen that. That they don't live very long, even on medication. They might live to fifteen, sixteen, seventeen, or eighteen, but. . . .

George: There's a few of them that are living up into their 20s.

Margaret: They're the ones that are feeling really alienated. That's just a few kids that I've talked to. I don't mean to offend you Juan.

Juan: No, I just don't react very well to that whole children thing.

Margaret: Why?

Juan: Because I don't think *you* asked for it, I don't think *I* asked for it, but that's the way that many people justify bigotry against people like you and I. That's what your comments trigger in me. It's not you caring for the kids, because obviously we all care about children.

Margaret: But the kids have this wrong impression about being HIV positive.

Juan: I'm sure it's very difficult.

Margaret: They need a community just like I need a community.

Juan: Sure.

Byrd: Honey, you've still got that stigma in you. You didn't go out asking for this, right? Don't think you're not a good person because you have HIV. That stigma inside of you will eat you alive if you let it.

Margaret: Have any of you ever wanted to die? I've had those thoughts. I feel worthless. I used to be superwoman, now I'm nothing. I feel like a piece of crap.

George: You have to shake that. You're with us now. We'll see this through together.

Byrd: That's right. And this is a place to deal with some of that bad energy.

Margaret: OK.

Bobby: Maybe what would be useful is talking more about how we deal with stigma when we encounter it. That would probably be helpful for all of us and we might all learn something.

George: I've noticed in a few support groups how once people get outside the group they act differently towards you. They get out of the group and they hide from everybody when they see somebody from the group outside in the general neighborhood. They shy away from them, as if they don't want to be seen with them. I think that's internalized stigma. Just don't do that Margaret, OK?

Margaret: I won't. I promise.

Bobby: The truth is, when you're first coming to terms with all of this it can be really hard to deal with other people when they discriminate against you.

Jack: I wouldn't say that it's necessarily something that becomes easy, though.

Juan: No, but I think I see where Bobby is going. I think all of us probably used to just take it when we were first diagnosed. You haven't built up any defenses to that and I think you're really sensitive to being rejected and ostracized by people. You know? When people do or say something to you, maybe you'll just take it. Maybe you'll slink away. But you have to see their ignorance for what it is. You need to become resistant to that, shrug it off when people treat you badly.

Jack: I have a friend whose motto is "if you don't pay me, feed me, or sleep with me, I don't care what you think." Maybe you and I can both work on thinking like that Margaret.

George: When people become HIV or AIDS, or I think with any kind of terminal illness, their tolerance level for the mundane is very, very low. And we don't take shit from nobody cause we don't have time to take shit.

Bobby: I get pissed off. I've grown away from my parents. I still have a relationship with them, but it's a different kind of relationship than what it used to be. We're civil to one another. We speak to one another. But the closeness isn't there. I don't think the respect is there. I also realize that they're not going to come over to my side and I'm sure as hell not going to go over to their side. So this is the way it's going to be. And, like I said, I draw my support from the friends in my life. And I don't need to deal with that. I don't have to deal with my mom's stuff.

Juan: When I see people stigmatize others with HIV it makes me want to go out and march. I want to go out into the schools and the businesses and the hospitals and educate others. That's how I try to respond to it. It's the most constructive way to handle it, I think. It also makes me want to go out there and get everyone else who is living with HIV and get us together. I want to teach people to be self-advocates. I want them to stand up for themselves. And I want them to become activists and stand up for their community.

Margaret: What about when they're your doctors and nurses? How do you deal with that? They've got all the power.

Juan: You know, when I went back for my master's degree I was a sheep. I just followed the herd. I did whatever my doctors told me to and never said anything when I got the nurses who put the ten pairs of latex gloves on before they'd get within fifty feet of me.

George: I think a lot of us are like that after we're first diagnosed.

Jack: I know I was.

Juan: But once I became empowered about my illness and I did a lot of research, I realized the doctor is my employee and I want both high quality of life and high quality of care. I don't let them tell me what to do anymore. In fact, I find that a lot of times I'm more knowledgeable about the current treatments than they are. I make them listen to me and take me seriously. If they don't, I get a new doctor. The same holds true if I get any sense of discomfort from them. Right now, I have a good doctor and our relationship is a pretty good one, I think.

George: When people stigmatize me I usually confront it directly. Remember the nurse I was telling you about who basically told me that people with HIV weren't allowed to be sexual beings anymore? Well, I let her have it on that stuff. I said, "That's bullshit." I said, "What makes you think that anybody with any disease, as long as they take precautions and engage in safe sex practices, can't have sex? Can't have an orgasm for heaven's sake? Or have a loving relationship with somebody else?" I said, "That's the most asinine thing I've ever heard." I said, "You need to go to New York and talk to some physicians and social workers out there. You are really behind the times here. You don't say that to cancer patients, so why would you say that to somebody like me?"

Juan: Sometimes I'm in a better state of mind for handling this sort of stuff than others. Sometimes I can be constructive and address the stigma directly and try to educate someone. Other times I don't have the patience and I want to get in a fight.

George: Sometimes, too, I might use their stigma and fear against them. "Do you know I have AIDS? You might just want to move along." I've done that a few times and they have left me alone pretty quick.

Byrd: Haaa! I can hardly imagine it.

Jack: I'll bet it really freaks them out.

The support group interaction continued for several more minutes, sharing more stories of how they've managed interactions with others who stigmatize them and then the group started their customary social time, enjoying soft drinks, brownies that George had baked, and casual conversation. They've found over time that ending their support group meetings with uplifting social time helped further reduce their stress of living with HIV.

RELEVANT CONCEPTS

Activism: Persuasive efforts of a group that are in the interest of both members of the group and others.

AIDS: A disease in which a person is infected with HIV and also has had a serious decline in the function of his or her immune system and/or a corresponding opportunistic infection or malignancy.

Chronic illness: Illness that lasts for an indefinite amount of time (that is, it is not considered to be curable).

HIV illness: Illness that occurs as a result of infection with the human immunodeficiency virus, which negatively affects the infected person's immune system.

Self-advocacy: Persuasive efforts of an individual that are in the individual's interest.

Self-disclosure: Intentionally revealing personal information about oneself.

Social identity: The part of people's identity that is attributable to their group memberships (Tajfel, 1978).

Social support: One's social network of family and friends; the assistance, advice, or comfort that others give; or the perception that others are available to give assistance, advice, or support if needed.

Stigma: Characteristic of a person that invokes negative stereotypes; "an attribute that is deeply discrediting" (Goffman, 1963, p. 3).

Stigma management: Communication strategies that stigmatized people use when they encounter discrimination (such as either confronting or avoiding the stigmatizer) or actions they take to preempt social stigma directed towards them (such as concealing the stigmatized attribute if possible).

DISCUSSION QUESTIONS

1. What characteristics of HIV illness have led to stigma? What are some of the ways that others communicated or expressed stigma to the members of the HIV support group?

2. What are some approaches that people in the group took to disclose their HIV status to others? Why did they feel the need to be cautious revealing that information? Are there advantages or benefits to disclosing one's HIV infection to others?
3. How did different members of the group respond to stigmatizing behaviors of others? Identify those that you might consider "self-advocacy behaviors."
4. What recommendations would you give Margaret for dealing with the reactions that others have to her illness? How do you think you would cope with the stigma associated with HIV if you were in her place?
5. What other illnesses are stigmatized? How is the stigma associated with those other illnesses similar or different from the stigma associated with HIV illness?
6. Some people argue that it is better when members of a support group are very similar to each other. Do you think diversity in this group was an advantage or disadvantage? Do you think having groups for targeted segments (for example, straight men) might be helpful in some circumstances? Why or why not?

ENDNOTE

[1] Although this support group interaction was fictionalized for the purpose of this case study, the dialogue was constructed from the actual narratives of real people living with HIV. The authors collected these narratives from individual and group interviews of over 120 men and women living with HIV, in research funded by the National Institutes of Health (grant number 1R29NR04376). Those men and women described to us their experiences and feelings associated with their HIV infection. We are grateful to them for sharing their stories with us. They told us that HIV illness creates a lot of uncertainty about how long they will live and how others will treat them, but that it also creates opportunity for personal growth and the development of new, important relationships, like those that Margaret may have found in her new support group.

REFERENCES/SUGGESTED READINGS

Adelman, M., & Frey, L. R. (1997). *The fragile community: Living together with AIDS.* Mahwah, NJ: Lawrence Erlbaum Associates.

Alonzo, A. A., & Reynolds, N. R. (1995). Stigma, HIV, and AIDS: An exploration and elaboration of a stigma trajectory. *Social Science and Medicine, 3,* 303–315.

Brashers, D. E., Neidig, J. L., Haas, S. M., Dobbs, L. K., Cardillo, L. W., & Russell, J. A. (2000). Communication in the management of uncertainty: The case of persons living with HIV or AIDS. *Communication Monographs, 67,* 63–84.

Crocker, J. (1999). Social stigma and self-esteem: Situational construction of self-worth. *Journal of Experimental Social Psychology, 35,* 89–107.

Crocker, J., Major, B., & Steele, C. (1998). Social stigma. In D. Gilbert, S. Fiske, & G. Lindzey (Eds.), *Handbook of social psychology* (Vol. 2, 4th ed., pp. 504–553). New York: McGraw-Hill.

Goffman, E. (1963). *Stigma: Notes on the management of spoiled identity.* New York: Simon & Schuster.

Herek, G. M., Capitanio, J. P., & Widaman, K.F. (2002). HIV-related stigma and knowledge in the United States: Prevalence and trends, 1991–1999. *American Journal of Public Health, 92,* 371–377.

Rintamaki, L. S. (2003). *HIV identity trajectories and social interaction.* Unpublished doctoral dissertation, University of Illinois, Urbana-Champaign.

Tajfel, H. (1978). *Differentiation between social groups: Studies in the social psychology of intergroup relations.* New York: Academic Press.

Additional Resources

An excellent video that focuses on people living in an HIV group home is *The Pilgrim Must Embark: Living in Community* (produced by Mara Adelman & Peter Schultz, available from Lawrence Erlbaum Associates, Inc., on the Internet at www.erlbaum.com).

The Northwestern University Medical School's patient narrative video series (available on the Internet at www.pcm. northwestern.edu) offers several enlightening videos that address the patient's perspective on illness, including how they face stigma (for examples, see *Sara: A Woman with Diabetes*, *Gwen: A Woman Living with Chronic Pain*, and *Ann-Jeanette: A Woman with Parkinson's Disease*).

Pandemic: Facing AIDS, an educational program designed to help people understand the global pandemic of AIDS that includes videos and student workbooks, is available on the Internet at www.pandemicfacingaids.org.

13

"Every Breast Cancer Is Different": Illness Narratives and the Management of Identity in Breast Cancer

Leigh Arden Ford
Brigitte Cobbs Christmon
Western Michigan University

Each year in the United States, approximately 267,000 new cases of breast cancer in women will be diagnosed. Based on current life expectancy for women in the United States, one woman out of nine will develop breast cancer in her lifetime—a risk that was one out of 14 in 1960. Breast cancer is the second leading cause of cancer death for all women and the leading cause of cancer death in women between the ages of 20 and 59. This year, 39,800 women are expected to die of breast cancer—one woman every 13 minutes. Given these statistics, it is not surprising that breast cancer is the most feared of diseases among women.

A diagnosis of breast cancer evokes a complex set of physical, psychological, and social conditions, circumstances that threaten a woman's sense of self and of her place in the world. She lives within a psychosocial context that may include stress, body disfigurement and/or body failure, loss of productive functioning, stigma, and threat to previous selves. Faced with challenges to valued identities, she works to make sense of her illness by reflecting on her experiences and renegotiating her identities with children, spouse, friends, coworkers, medical providers, other women with breast cancer, any and all with whom she has relationships.

This process of redefinition and transformation of identity is a distinctly communicative act in which narrative is the central process and product. Each woman's breast cancer story becomes a mechanism for "explaining" the experience of breast cancer to herself and to others. The breast cancer narrative may recount events and/or may account for events by explaining or justifying actions taken or feelings expressed in the story. Through constructing and presenting her narrative she creates and recreates her self and her life and redefines its meaning.

Breast cancer narratives, then, reflect the struggle to manage identity in the face of a life-threatening chronic illness, but there is not one true breast cancer story. Each breast cancer narrative reflects a different version of a different story rooted in a specific political and cultural context. As every breast cancer is different, every breast cancer story is different, deeply personal and true to the person living it.

In this chapter, we present the breast cancer narratives of four women. These women come from diverse backgrounds and experiences, and each has a different diagnosis and prognosis.

Each represents a struggle for identity. Through the juxtapositioning of these narratives, we hope that the meaning of these lives can be found in each story and "in the spaces between."[1]

BETTER THAN *THE BRADY BUNCH*: HELEN'S STORY

I first met Leo Grady about six months after my first husband had been killed in a car accident. I had three young children under seven years old to raise and had gone back to teaching to try to support us. Leo also had lost his wife about six months previously. He was trying to run his fledgling business and raise a son on his own. Some friends of mine at my school set us up on a blind date and, frankly, that first meeting didn't go all that well. Nonetheless, we did go out again and sort of fell into dating. At the time, I think we both just needed someone to talk to who was experiencing the same things we were experiencing. I needed someone to do the occasional household repair and he needed someone to prepare the occasional home-cooked meal that consisted of more than things that could be nuked in a microwave or grilled on a barbeque. For about a year, ours was a rather casual relationship, but one where we increasingly spent time together with and without our kids. For some very practical reasons, we decided it just made sense to get married. I remember telling friends that I fell in "like" with Leo and that liking each other was more than a lot of people had who had been married for many years.

After our marriage, Leo continued to work hard building his business, I continued to teach, and our two families began the difficult challenges of merging together. I won't say that this time was easy, but we did survive this difficult transition and eventually we adopted each other's children, becoming one family legally as well as emotionally. Three years into our marriage, Leo's business took off, and I left my teaching job and began to work with him in the office a few mornings a week. Oh, and somewhere along this journey, we actually did fall in love.

I don't remember who first called us the Grady Bunch, but the name quickly stuck. In fact, our kids made up their own words to the Brady Bunch song to fit our family story. They serenaded us with their version at our 15th wedding anniversary party held at our cottage on the lake. That was a great day, a special day—you know the kind of day where all the elements of your life seem to be in harmony—everyone is well, everyone is happy, your financial future is secure, you are content in your emotional and spiritual life, and the weather is great!

I know this is supposed to be my breast cancer story, but you can't understand my story unless you know where Leo and I and our family had come from, how great everything was, how great my life was. Two weeks after our anniversary party I was in the hospital. I had a diagnosis of breast cancer and a prognosis that said I likely had less than two months to live.

After my initial shock, I told my doctors that they were wrong. I told them I had no intention of dying any time soon and that I thought their prognosis was flat out wrong. So I had a mastectomy and began chemotherapy, determined to prove that they were wrong. I was certain that I could beat this thing, but Leo and I decided that it would be prudent to address all the legalities, like our will and ownership of the business, as a precaution. So we went to a lawyer as soon as I felt up to it and moved everything we owned from joint ownership to sole ownership in his name.

The next few months were difficult. I was undergoing chemotherapy, losing my hair, gaining weight, and living—and maybe dying—in a house full of young people home from college for the summer. It all seemed so normal—and yet it was all so abnormal. I could feel the dynamics of the family shifting around me and I could do little about it. I no longer was the center of stability in the family. I just was never sure how much energy I would have on any given day. I had to give up so much to concentrate on fighting my cancer and the nausea and exhaustion of its treatment. I watched as the tasks I took pride in—planting and nurturing a lovely vegetable garden, cooking good meals, having friends and family gather at our home—either disappeared from our family's routines or, what was worse somehow, they would appear but in greatly altered form and without me as their prime mover.

My daughter suffered the most during this time, I think. She was living at home while going to college, so she was in the middle of everything. Emily both tried to be me and resisted being me. How could she take on her mother's role when her mother was just up the stairs lying on her bed trying not to be sick? For Em, a mother who occasionally felt well enough to be the mother and then would strongly reassert herself in that role must have been more difficult than having a ghost mother that lives in the shadows but doesn't interfere as you struggle to emulate her actions and to hold your family together, as you try to keep everyone's fear, especially your own, at bay.

I think my boys were affected during this time, but they found ways to escape. They, of course, had summer jobs and participated on various sport teams, and then two of the three went off to college again in the fall. It's not that my sons were not concerned, but I think they didn't want to confront my cancer directly.

I thought a lot about my children during this time because they were home for the first few months of my treatment. I was glad that they were older and nearly on their own. If I was going to die, I felt like I had at least given them a good foundation for their lives. I also thought I had to teach them something by the way I approached my disease and the way I lived my life right then. My lesson in cancer turned out to be especially true for my middle son. During his first year of medical school, he found out that he had testicular cancer. The dean of the medical school told him that he would have to drop out because he could never keep up with his studies while undergoing treatment. My son said, "Well, my mother did it. She went everywhere and she did everything and I'm just going to do it unless I am kicked out." And he did. I could hardly stand that one; watching him go through his cancer experience was much harder than my own.

Some women worry about their husband's reaction to breast cancer. Some men have even divorced their wives. During my cancer, my Leo was a rock. When I had my breast removed, my husband could not have cared less. During those first weeks and months, I would lie awake at night and think I am certainly not attractive—I am bald, one-breasted, and 15 pounds overweight. But I think my husband absolutely adored me. He didn't care; he just wanted me to stay alive so we could grow old together.

His plan to keep me alive required me to follow the doctor's advice, to stay home in bed, to save my strength. My philosophy was that the outcome was so unpredictable, caution was a waste of time. I was pretty sick, but I did not want to spend any more time in bed and away from my family, friends, and activities than I had to. He was really angry with me at first, but I insisted. I told him, "I will probably throw up wherever I go, but I am going to go!"

My breast cancer altered our lives, of course, but nothing could have prepared us for what came next. I had completed about six months of chemotherapy when my beloved husband had a massive heart attack while playing a pick-up game of basketball. He died before emergency help could get there. He was 49 years old, had been in excellent health, and now he was gone from us. The shock of that was nearly more than I could bear. He was my emotional center and so important to my ability to get through this cancer every day. Even though I believed with all my being that I was going to survive, I also depended on the idea that he would be there to carry on if I did not. Now there I was, alone, not yet fully recovered. I still had children to raise. I now also had a business to run alone, to take over quickly, a business that was not even in my name and legal control because we thought I was the one at risk for dying.

At times, I was very angry with Leo for leaving me with all that work and the worries and no money. Fortunately, many people stepped in to help. Friends and family were supportive, of course, and even vendors and customers of our business worked with me, and the lawyers were understanding and helpful. It took time, but eventually the legal mess and business mess worked out. The children were just amazing. They had to work through this unexpected loss, stave off their fears of losing me as well, and contribute in every way possible to help save the business.

It was a terrible time for us, but when I look back at it now, I feel nothing but pride in our resilience as a family and in the love that allowed us to make this work. As for my cancer during this time, I tell my friends I just didn't have time for it. I don't mean to be flippant because cancer is very serious but I just didn't have the time to think beyond when I needed to go to a treatment or an appointment. My life was consumed with securing a future for my children.

My first diagnosis of breast cancer was a little over 10 years ago now. So I did prove the doctors wrong, and I made it past the critical 5-year mark. Then I had a recurrence of breast cancer 2 years ago, had another mastectomy, and went through another round of chemo. It was tougher the second time around without my Leo's support. On the other hand, I knew much more what to expect, so that made it easier to handle the surgery and the treatment. Now the docs keep a pretty close eye on me and, so far, things seem to be going well.

I have been close to death a few times during this breast cancer experience, but I have survived much longer than the predicted two months. Some might call me lucky or healed by faith or saved by a positive attitude or by excellent medical care. I know that there is no simple explanation for why I survived when someone else with the exact same prognosis as mine might not have. The why of it all remains a mystery to me. I do know one thing for certain: nothing in life is certain. So I try to live just this day, sometimes I try to live just this moment. I spend time with my children and grandchildren, I continue to run the family business with one of my sons, I go out with my friends, and I visit with other cancer patients. I want to spend whatever time I have left well. I want to remember it all so I can tell Leo everything when I see him again.

I AM A CREATION OF GOD: SHAWNA'S PRAYER

About a year ago, in February, I found a lump in my breast quite by accident. I didn't do regular monthly breast self-exams nor, for that matter, did I think that I should. I didn't see myself as a candidate for breast cancer. I am a 29-year-old, African American female, and most of my understandings of breast cancer at that point had come from the media—women on talk shows or in movies-of-the-week. The women in these stories were always White, upper middle class, and in possession of a great health insurance plan and a supportive husband and family. I had known personally only one woman who had breast cancer, a woman from my church who was diagnosed with late-stage cancer in her 60s and died within a few months. I did not see myself in these breast cancer stories, so I decided that the lump was probably temporary and that finding it was simply an accident. I told myself I had likely had such lumps before but never noticed them, as they disappeared before I could become aware of them.

I ignored the lump for a week or so. It didn't hurt, and I was too busy to think about it, much less do anything about it. I was taking the last of my classes and was just a few months away from graduating in June with a master's degree. I also was in the midst of planning my wedding. But the lump didn't go away, and I finally had to have it checked out. I saw a doctor and then had a mammogram. When I went to hear the results, the doctor informed me that the mammogram showed a dark mass, and he recommended a needle biopsy so the lump could be checked for cancer. I heard the word *cancer*, and then I doubt I heard another thing. I think I was on autopilot for the rest of the appointment, trying to process the doctor's words as he explained this test to me. While I was still trying to focus on the possible meaning of this turn of events in my life, I heard the swoosh of the door as he left the room.

In the next few minutes, I relied on the one certain thing in my life: I gave this up to God. It is my belief that the power of life and death is in His tongue, and He can speak things into existence. I am His creation and He is my foundation. So I prayed and asked for God's guidance and peace in this moment and His steadfastness to help me see this journey through no matter its conclusion.

For the next day or so, I kept the news to myself that I had this lump that needed further examination. I didn't tell anyone—not friends, not family, not even John, my fiancé. I love my family very much, and we are close, but we are also complicated. My mother is African American, and my father is European American. They are no longer together and haven't really been together since I was a young child. My mom lives several states away, but my extended African American family lives in this community and I am close to them, especially my grandmother. My dad has remarried and he lives nearby with his wife and children.

I wanted to tell my mom, but I knew she would tell my grandmother, who is elderly and not in the best of health. She's also the family telegraph. No doubt, this news would be passed to other family members and outsiders as well. The family support network then would be activated, and that would make me feel worse if they came to my rescue while ignoring their responsibilities. I also didn't want them to pity me. I am a strong Black woman, and I have always been independent. I was the first girl in my family to earn a bachelor's degree. That was not easy. It took nine years of working in a factory to support myself and studying when and where I could and resisting the temptation to quit when the journey seemed long and the goal so far off. I have always managed my own life.

Although I definitely was not ready to tell any family member, I knew I had to tell John. I had met John in July, in December we had gotten engaged, and we were planning to be married on the same day as my commencement for my master's degree. I knew that nothing would ever change my love for him, but this lump carried in it the potential to change all of our hopes. This frightened me. I put my trust in God that He would take care of the illness, but I was so afraid that this could change our relationship. I didn't think that John would leave me, but could I ask him to take this on, if the lump proved to be cancerous? I also didn't want the quality of our relationship, the ease of our day-to-day conversations, to be overshadowed by this potential.

At that time, John and I had a long-distance relationship. He lives and works in a city about 400 miles away. We met at a church-related conference, where we spent some time together talking, but the first few weeks of our relationship were actually carried out on the phone and through email. Email became the link we used to keep daily contact, and so I decided that I could use this form of communication more easily to let John know my status and my concerns. In my email, first I asked him to pray for me and then I told him about the lump. I also included some information and breast cancer web site addresses I had found to try to help him understand the situation. While I was typing the message, I was crying. I knew that when I clicked "send," our relationship would be forever changed, and we would not be able to go back. This situation was forcing our relationship to another level at a time when we should be picking out china patterns.

John got the message while he was at work and called me within minutes. He prayed with me over the phone in the middle of his workday while he was in his office. Then we talked. He was all things wonderful to me at that moment: a strong Christian, a friend, a protector, the man whose commitment to me would not waver.

John's reaction gave me the courage to tell my dad. Because of our complicated family history, I am just getting to truly know and love my dad and to have a father–daughter relationship. My dad loves me in his own way, but until recently, he often spoke to me in sarcastic or humorous ways. I think he does that as a way to ease the tensions we both feel at times, but during this phone conversation, he just listened to me. I appreciated that and, for that time,

I felt like his daughter and not just his African American child. After telling my dad and John, I felt empowered, and I began to disclose to others as my experience unfolded.

As the week progressed toward my scheduled needle biopsy, the pressures of school and life were starting to wear me down. I felt like I was too busy for even the thought of breast cancer. I simply could not fit this into my already overbooked schedule. It also seemed to me that the people around me were complaining about the most insignificant things. Why couldn't people look at me and recognize that I could be sick? This, of course, was foolishness. If I wanted release from my concerns, I could go to God, but I also could go to my friends and family. I needed to let go of my independence and image as the caregiver and seek the care that I needed in that time.

Getting support from others created some contradictions for me. When I told my church family, they said things like, "Oh, you have the faith, you will be all right," or "God knows what you can bear!" Even though these were things I had said to myself and had said to others facing other concerns, I was somehow dissatisfied. I knew what they were saying was scriptural, but I wanted more. Faith is not perfect. During these days, at times, I let my fear about the unknown overwhelm my trust in God. My older female friends said things like, "Oh, a biopsy is nothing. I have had them, and they always come back negative," or "You know that 9 out of 10 of them are benign." I wanted someone to take this seriously. I wanted to shout, "If it is not a big deal, then why do so many women die from it?"

I think these momentary doubts occurred because I had been back and forth to the doctor so many times before the biopsy, it increased my anxiety. I just wanted to have the procedure and find out whether the "suspicious lump" was cancerous. On the day of the procedure, I was quite calm. They put a fine needle into your breast where the lump is located and then extract some cells for diagnosis. I went in with my mind focused on my faith. I just repeated to myself over and over again, "I am a creature of God's creation. I am a beloved child of my Heavenly Father." The biopsy was negative.

I felt as though a heavy burden had been lifted from my shoulders just in time for me to prepare for finals. I was sleeping better, and I felt like I had more energy. My planned wedding and graduation could go forward. John and I could start our new lives without this added challenge. But then, about two weeks later, I unexpectedly received a call from the doctor's office that I needed to come in ASAP; that we needed to discuss something. I asked the nurse if anything was wrong, but she would not tell me over the phone.

I went to the doctor's office almost immediately after that phone call. You can imagine my fear. I prayed all the way over there that I would be given the strength to hear whatever I would be told and the courage to bear the news with grace. When I arrived, the doctor said that they had found another dark area, and they wanted to do a regular biopsy this time to make sure that what they were seeing was not malignant. Of course I agreed to the procedure, an outpatient surgery, requiring anesthesia.

To me, this procedure upped the chances I might actually have breast cancer. Once again, I turned to my faith, but this time I also prayed for all those around me, that they might have courage. On the day of the scheduled biopsy, I awoke with a feeling of peace. I was ready for whatever the outcome. I opted for a two-stage procedure. They would first do the biopsy, and then if the mass was cancerous, they would immediately remove the lump. This time, I had everyone holding positive thoughts for me—my family, my friends, my church family, and, of course, John. He was with me. We held hands and talked and then prayed. When I awoke from the anesthetic, I learned that cancer had been present in the mass, and the physician performed a lumpectomy.

I don't put myself in the same category as other breast cancer survivors that they make the movies about. I didn't require radiation treatments or chemotherapy. I got to go ahead and finish my degree and marry the man I love in front of all my family, and friends. I didn't have to fight to stay alive like those women in the movies or the women whose stories become books and inspiration to other women. My story is simple. I had breast cancer. Now it is gone. My God, my family, and my friends sustained me during those weeks of uncertainty. I know they sustain me still.

CAN'T ANYONE SEE THE GENDER POLITICS IN ALL THIS?: ELLEN'S LAMENT

I am a 54-year-old divorced woman with one adult child. I make my living by writing and teaching. I have followed the rules for good health for most of my life. I eat a low-fat diet, I exercise regularly, don't smoke, and think positively. After a youth and young adulthood of loving the sun and shore, I now enjoy the shore while slathered in sunscreen and shaded by a rather unfortunate-looking straw-brimmed hat. I do have two vices, I suppose. I drink a glass of Merlot each evening and frequently find my blood pressure raised as I engage with friends in spirited political debate. I am a committed feminist, and I have been active in the Women's Health Movement since the 1970s.

Today, I also am a woman who has breast cancer. I claim that part of my identity, but I resist with all my words and actions the culture's efforts to define that identity as a breast cancer survivor. I see the mythologizing of breast cancer survivors in the media and through the larger social structures of our society as oppressive and hegemonic. I guess it's not very surprising that I am not well loved in breast cancer circles. In this culture, if you refuse to enact the role of the noble survivor, you are invisible and marginalized, not just by mainstream society but also by most other women who have experienced this disease.

A year and a half ago, I had a mammogram as part of my annual physical and a "mass of some concern" was found in my right breast. About two weeks later, I had a surgical biopsy. Still groggy from the anesthetic, I awoke to the news delivered in lugubrious tone by the surgeon, "I regret to inform you that there is cancer." With those words, I fell down the rabbit hole into a whole new world, a world where the language spoken and the cultural customs observed created a sense of disorientation as I tried to negotiate my way through this sojourn.

My trip to this other world actually began with that mammogram. At the time, I barely noted the décor of the small room where I undressed. My mind was on an article I was writing that was due for submission in a week. I dismissed the room's ambiance as the usual sort of thing a decorator thinks of as appealing and comforting to women, a little island of pink femininity in the otherwise sterile medical environment. The room was so pink, five or six different shades of pink. How many pinks can there possibly be? I was suffocating in pink, right down to the pink-flowered gown they gave me to wear as I prepared to bare my chest.

The walls in this little room were decorated with cartoons and poems and those items other women send you via email. These jokes supposedly celebrate womanhood, but I find often they just make me realize that the jokes we make about men have a kind of maternal know-it-allness about them that mimics the condescension that men have used on us for years. Most of all, I am struck by the upbeat aphorisms on the posters that decorate this space. At that time, I dismissed them for their sentimentality. I realize now that little pink un-dressing room, with its kitsch posters and decorations, was my introduction to the tension between the trivialization and the valorization of women with breast cancer.

In the weeks following my surgeon's announcement, I did not do what many women in my place have done. I did not engage in days and weeks of study of the disease and its possible treatments, reviewing the options, and interviewing doctors. In truth, after just a few hours of reading, it seemed to me that the breast cancer path is fairly straightforward. The choices are not that wide-ranging—lumpectomy followed by weeks of radiation or mastectomy. In either case, chemotherapy follows if your lymph nodes have been invaded by cancer cells. With chemo treatments come all the side effects that are so vivid in the public mind—nausea, mouth sores, baldness, immunosuppression, weight loss for some, weight gain for others. I considered alternative therapies briefly. I even considered doing nothing—relying on the power of the mind to heal the body. But the exhortations of my loved ones and the pressure from my doctors, and if I am honest, my own faith in science, led me to the knife followed by better living with chemistry—a little gallows humor rarely appreciated in my support group.

Yes, I did join a breast cancer support group. Self-help, mutual support, and networking with other women for health information were all strongly advocated by the Women's Heath Movement and reflect my ideology. Today, most people forget that when postmastectomy women proposed forming support groups in the mid-70s, the American Cancer Society responded with a firmly patriarchal, but loving, no. It's hard to believe that support groups were seen as revolutionary activities then. Today's support groups have been given the blessing of the medical establishment. In fact, participation in such a group is strongly encouraged, if not exactly prescribed as part of one's treatment.

Because I appreciate and value my women friends who have supported me throughout my life, I looked forward to interacting with the women in my breast cancer support group. I looked forward to the solidarity brought about by our common experience, but after several meetings, I found I was an alien in this sisterhood. I always hesitate when I tell this part of my story. I don't want to sound strident or self-righteous. I believe that each woman must find her way to cope with the great indignities, fear, and uncertainties of this disease. Indeed, this is an oft-repeated premise of my support group, "every breast cancer is different and each woman copes in her own way," but I found very quickly that this was not the case at all. In truth, there is a great mythic breast cancer story that has predictable themes, standard rhythms and turning points, and restricted identities for the women with breast cancer who are the central characters of these stories. The plot follows the woman's progress from lump to mammogram to treatment to coping to surviving, with an emphasis on the words of hope and encouragement for fellow sufferers. This is not the story I want to focus on—at least not every week.

I want to talk about the causes of this disease and the promising research that focuses on environmental carcinogens, such as plastics, pesticides, and industrial runoff in ground water. No direct causation between these factors and breast cancer in humans has been found—in fact, most causal factors for breast cancer have not been clearly delineated—but these environmental factors have been found to cause the disease in mice, a significant result. I also am convinced that the rate of increase in breast cancer since the 1950s surely can find its explanation in ecological factors. At the least these factors deserve more attention than they are currently given.

I want to talk about the treatments as the source of the pain and illness, not the disease itself. Why are the options for experimental treatments offered only for advanced, metastasized cases? Even if a woman would elect to try one of these treatments, they would not be available. I want to talk about the limitations that cost places on a woman's choices, from the availability of mammograms to the doctors she can see to the treatment she can pursue. The inherent unfairness in our health care system is writ large in the breast cancer story.

I want to talk about the corporatization of breast cancer. I am deeply grateful for the courage and visibility of women like Betty Ford and Betty Rollins and Rose Kushner, who broke the silence surrounding breast cancer. But I am deeply troubled by the popularization of this disease as a cause. Corporate America has signed on to breast cancer in a big way. Corporate sponsorship of runs, walks, bikes, hikes, and climbs for the cure are ubiquitous. Support for breast cancer research is now linked with the purchase of particular products (buy $\times$ product, we'll donate $\times$ sum of money). When I ask my support group members if they are troubled by this, their response is dismay at my dismay. I point out that we probably could make more money for breast cancer research if all participants simply wrote a larger check. They tell me these events are really about awareness. I wonder if we are aware. Does corporate sponsorship mean that we don't say the things we ought, that we don't express our anger in fear of losing that sponsorship? These events also feature breast cancer paraphernalia. Breast cancer is now part of the market economy. We have pink ribbon pins and scarves and bears and T-shirts and coffee mugs and wind chimes and breast cancer candles and tchotchkes galore. There is something offensive about this. Most of these items advertise that "part of the proceeds go to breast cancer research." I wonder how much—and to what end? I prefer a straight business transaction—at least the motives and agenda are clear.

I want to talk about the women who die from breast cancer. Over a million women in the United States have died from this disease since 1970, but the focus is always on survivors. I am not against survivorship. I, like all women who have experienced this disease, hope that I shall live for many more years and I celebrate with those who live. What I want to talk about is the determined effort to marginalize those who have not survived this disease. At most breast cancer events, the dead are given scant attention. Sometimes, there's a brief memorial ceremony, sometimes a moment of silence, sometimes someone carries a sign remembering a loved one lost. When we consign the dead to the margins, we diminish the urgency of this disease. We need to be reminded that since the 1930s the death rate from breast cancer has changed very little. We need a breast cancer equivalent of the AIDS quilt, a visual reminder of lives lost before their time. We need to mourn and remember and build our action on our anger that the death toll has changed but little in 70 years' time.

I want to talk about the tyranny of relentless cheerfulness and the exhortations to a positive attitude that are part and parcel of the survivor identity. The eternally optimistic breast cancer culture goes largely unquestioned. Doubts and fears and anger must be suppressed in light of claims that thinking positively makes all the difference. I think about the woman who dies. Is she doubly victimized—by the disease and by her inability to think positively enough? I don't want to wallow, but surely space should be made for honest emotions. I also have been told often about the transforming power of breast cancer. Women in my support group regularly testify to how their lives are so much better now, their purpose is much clearer, they live more fully each day, and so on. I have even had women tell me that chemo can be seen as sort of an intense beauty treatment—chemo softens the skin, helps you lose weight, and when your hair grows back, it's usually curlier and may be a different color. What are we saying? The sainted, and potentially lovely, survivor awaits, if we just are patient and positive.

I want to talk about this tension inherent between femininity and feminist in the total breast cancer experience. I want to discuss the challenges to cultural definitions and expectations of womanhood and beauty that arise from breast cancer. I don't want to spend time on cosmetics and ways to look better—meaning more feminine—during treatment. I want to talk about challenging the whole notion of beauty and breasts. I want to talk about the contradiction in pink ribbons and the language of war. Cancer is always described as a battle and a fight. Surely we can find a metaphor less patriarchical and more feminist, and hence more empowering, a metaphor that creates a space for all the experiences of breast cancer.

I do believe that every breast cancer is different, and I expect that there should be space for each story. I don't expect that women who are scared and in the midst of a medical crisis can turn around and become activists—to take to the streets or to the halls of government in protest. But I do expect that we won't just accept a unifying definition of self—one more palatable to corporations, media coverage, and the patriarchy. If women cannot be free to frame their own experience in this uniquely womanist context, I despair.

But in my breast cancer support group, there is no space for dissent. So I no longer attend. I have found some kindred spirits through online support groups. We dissidents have formed our own group, where we discuss the strategies we might use as activists for change. One way we've decided to resist is through the creation of a web site. We will talk, we will organize, we will act. We won't be selling any T-shirts.

HOPE IS A FRAGILE THING: DIANNA'S TALE

For about a year and half now, I have been fighting a recurrence of breast cancer. I am 43 years old and I have two young daughters, 6 and 8 years old. I am doing everything I can to stay alive for them. My children are my number one priority, and I will do anything to keep their world safe and secure. My own mother died when I was 14, and I still feel that loss today. I will do everything I can so that my daughters will not have to face that.

I was 33 when I met my husband, Jack. I was a middle-school English teacher working on my master's degree in counseling. I was busy with my career and had reached the point where I thought I might never marry. I had even decided that if I didn't marry, I would adopt a child as a single parent. I love kids, and I could not imagine my life without experiencing parenthood. Then I met Jack. I was at the airport to pick up a friend, and he was waiting for his mom. The plane was delayed and, while we waited, we struck up a conversation. We married three months after our first date.

Jack had been married before but did not have any children in that marriage. We both wanted kids, so we decided to start trying for a family right away. It took us a year to get pregnant, but we were finally successful, and nine months later our Jenny was born. Two years later, we were pregnant again, but in my fourth month of pregnancy, I discovered a lump in my breast. Faced with a hormonally induced breast cancer, we had to choose among very difficult options. First, I could terminate the pregnancy and proceed with the approved medical protocol with the best odds to treat my cancer. My other option was to stick with the pregnancy and proceed with the medical protocol and perhaps risk damage to my baby. The normal process with my type of breast cancer would have been lumpectomy and removal of some lymph glands followed by radiation therapy. Radiation was not possible while pregnant, so that left surgery followed by chemotherapy. Jack wanted me to terminate the pregnancy and focus on the breast cancer, but I just could not do that. Even though the research on the effects of chemotherapy on the fetus is limited and focused on a small number of cases, the results of those few cases were positive. That is, it seemed from this research that there were no short-term effects if chemo was administered after the first trimester. I wanted this baby very much. I just believed so strongly that both the baby and I would be fine, so despite Jack's reluctance, I decided to proceed with the pregnancy and to have a mastectomy followed by chemotherapy. The doctors watched my progress and the baby's development in utero very carefully over the next months. Our Amy was born about a month early, and she was perfect. Of course, we watched her carefully the first year or so, but she came through with flying colors. All of her development thus far has been normal.

After that very difficult pregnancy, the next few years we felt so blessed. My cancer treatment was over, and we were going on with our lives as any family would. I had fairly regular checkups every three months to watch for recurrence of the cancer, and things were fine each time. I had stopped working after Jenny's birth, but I went back to teaching part time when Amy turned three. I job-shared in a sixth grade class and enjoyed getting back into my career. Don't get me wrong, I loved being home with my girls, but I also missed the challenges of my chosen profession. My mother-in-law helped out with child care, and we were able to save some money.

Two years ago, we bought a new larger home with a big yard for the kids. After we moved, I did most of the landscaping, working pretty hard for a week. I had quite a bit of pain each night. I thought—I am 42 years old, and I am feeling all this pain because I am not used to this physical activity. And that's why I put off going to the doctor. This happened to fall into the gap between my cancer checkup visits. I finally went to the doctor and learned that my cancer had metastasized to the bone. The cancer came on very quickly this time, and when it was finally discovered, it was like cancer emergency therapy mode. The prognosis was grim. They said that if I didn't respond to chemo, I was short term.

The recurrence was very devastating. To be told that one is "short term" is chilling. I had asked the doctor to be honest and I am rather blunt myself, but those words froze my soul. I tried to maintain my positive attitude, but in the dark of night, I felt like a failure. I could not understand why this was happening to me, to my husband, and to my girls. We had already been through so much.

So I began chemotherapy. The type I was on required the administration of a megadose once a month. I did seven months of that form of chemo, and it was uphill climbing. I was in a lot of pain, so they gave me morphine—heavy duty, and it had some obnoxious side effects. I actually had a hospital bed in my living room at one point because I was too ill to get upstairs. It also was easier for people to help out with my care with my bed downstairs. I especially appreciated this time because I did not feel so cut off from my girls and the activity of the house. I wasn't in the "sick room" away from the life of my family.

Then I ran into a wall. Apparently, I developed a resistance to that chemo and so I had to change to another type of chemo coupled with radiation treatments. This turned out to be a blessing in disguise. The chemo I am on now is so much better. I don't feel sick all the time. Rather than a megadose once a month, I take a lesser dose once a week. I still have pain, especially if I sit for any period of time, so I take about 10 pain pills a day, and they are helpful while still allowing me to function. As to my cancer, I have multiple tumors from my hips to the top of my head, but it appears that this battle between the cancer and me has reached a kind of stalemate.

Besides the physical and medical aspects of breast cancer, this recurrence has also caused some significant challenges to the relationship between my husband and me. We haven't been together at all to fight this.

Jack has become very distant emotionally, just when I need him the most. He would never leave me physically, but I can't seem to get him to understand that his emotional abandonment is nearly as devastating to me as if he had packed his bags and moved out. Jack finally told me that he thinks I made the wrong decision when I went ahead with my second pregnancy, that I would be okay today if I had gotten the best treatment then. This was difficult to hear. I know he loves Amy, and I know he loves me. I think this outburst was just a way to express his fears of losing me forever. I know all these things intellectually, but the words have done their psychic and relational damage.

Jack and I live in the same house and carry on. I have only about two or three hours a day where I feel strong enough to engage in my life. I don't have the strength to do the typical motherly duties and rely on friends and family to carry out daily chores. I no longer attend my breast cancer support group. I try to spend my good time with my daughters. Yesterday, we made cookies; today, we will work on our embroidery project. Some days we just sit together and read.

Some people in my support group would talk about how they believed that they had breast cancer for a reason and that they needed to learn something about living from having cancer. At first, I dismissed this notion out of hand because this was a lesson I did not need or want. Now, I think about that idea differently. I have learned something. I have learned that hope is a fragile and fierce thing. It is made up of gossamer threads, able to support the human spirit in order to bear the most terrible of burdens. And so I live in hope. I hope that my husband will find the courage to join me again in the promises we made to each other when we married. I hope my children will remember and treasure these hours we spend together and that someday we will tell this story together to my grandchildren. I hope my treatment continues to keep the cancer at bay. I hear about different women who have had what I have. The longest running is 13 years, so I figure I have at least 13 years—think of all the advances in cancer research and treatment that can be made in 13 years. Most of all, I hope that I am an example of the power of hope.

CONCLUSION

The breast cancer narratives presented here are just a small sample of the thousands of stories that are told everyday by women with breast cancer. A chronic and life-threatening illness, breast cancer affects every aspect of a woman's life. It threatens physical functions, valued social roles, and important personal activities. It challenges marriages and families, friendships, and work relations. It creates opportunities for self-examination and reevaluation of belief systems, values, and ideologies. With each challenge, threat, or opportunity, the woman with breast cancer works to define and redefine her identity through telling her story. For us as readers or listeners, each breast cancer narrative offers an opportunity to understand the meaning of this complex illness experience and to observe the deeply human process of managing identity dilemmas in the search for the authentic self.

RELEVANT CONCEPTS

Contradiction: The dynamic tension of oppositional forces; conceptualized as a continuum, these opposites are experienced as "both–and" rather than as "either–or."

Identity management: The presentation and negotiation of self in interaction with others.

Illness narrative: The telling of the story of one's illness experience; the storytelling process becomes a means for making sense of the experience for self and for others.

Lumpectomy: A surgical procedure to remove the cancerous tumor and a small margin of surrounding tissue.

Mastectomy: A surgical procedure to remove all or part of the breast; may include the removal of auxillary lymph nodes.

Social role conflict: An experience of tension among the various socially defined obligations and expected behaviors that arise in the performance of more than one role in interaction.

Social support: Verbal and nonverbal communication between providers and recipients that manages the uncertainty about the situation, self, the other, and/or the relationship.

Sociopolitical and cultural context: The larger social, political, economic, and cultural institutions, ideologies, and norms within which our interpersonal interactions are embedded.

DISCUSSION QUESTIONS

1. Compare and contrast these breast cancer narratives. Which did you feel most comfortable reading? Which did you feel least comfortable reading? Why?
2. Narratives provide the reader/listener with a word picture of an experience and allow us to make attributions about the persons involved in the story. As you read each narrative, did you develop a portrait of the storyteller and her family? How would you describe the narrator of the story to another person? How would you re-tell her story?
3. What did you learn about breast cancer from reading these narratives? What are the strengths of the narrative form for learning about breast cancer? What are the weaknesses?
4. Examine one of the breast cancer narratives. Suggest three identity dilemmas faced by this woman. Are these dilemmas resolvable?
5. Within these narratives, how do the women describe their communication experiences with friends, family, spouses, support group members, health care providers? What did you learn about communication during chronic illness from reading these narratives?
6. These are written narratives. How would your experience of the narrative change if someone told you her story? Select one of the narratives and try reading part of the narrative aloud.

Does your experience of the story change? Do your perceptions of the persons in the story change?

ENDNOTE

[1] Three of these narratives are based on interviews with breast cancer survivors. These interviews were conducted as part of a larger research project conducted by the first author. Ellen's Lament is a composite narrative based on two research interviews, a published account of breast cancer by Barbara Eihenreich entitled "Welcome to Cancerland," that appeared in *Harper's Magazine*, and various commentaries and articles from the newsletters of the Women's Community Cancer Project, Cambridge, MA.

REFERENCES/SUGGESTED READINGS

Anderson, J., & Geist-Martin, P. (2003). Narratives and healing: Exploring one family's stories of cancer survivorship. *Health Communication, 15*(2), 133–143.

Bochner, A. (1997). It's about time: Narrative and the divided self. *Qualitative Inquiry, 3*, 418–438.

Charmaz, K. (1994). Identity dilemmas of chronically ill men. *Sociological Quarterly, 35*, 269–288.

Eihenreich, B. (2001, November). Welcome to cancerland. *Harper's Magazine*, 43–53.

Karp, D. A. (1999). Illness and identity. In K. Charmaz & D. A. Paterniti (Eds.), *Health, illness, and healing* (pp. 83–94). Los Angeles: Roxbury.

Kleinman, A. (1988). *The illness narratives: Suffering, healing, and the human condition*. New York: Basic Books.

Mathieson, C. M., & Stam, H. J. (1995). Renegotiating identity: Cancer narratives. *Sociology of Health and Illness, 17*, 283–306.

Additional Resources

Web sites offering information about breast cancer abound on the Internet. For example, popular and reader-friendly sites are supported by The Susan G. Komen Breast Cancer Foundation (http://www.koman.org/) and the Y-ME National Breast Cancer Organization (http://www.y-me.org/). A Web site devoted to political activism and grass roots organizing around breast cancer issues is supported by the National Breast Cancer Coalition (http://www.natlbcc.org/).

14

"They Make Us Miserable in the Name of Helping Us": Communication of Persons With Visible and Invisible Disabilities

Dawn O. Braithwaite
Phyllis Japp
University of Nebraska–Lincoln

MARGARET'S STORY

Running a bit late, as usual, Margaret left the house in a near panic, hoping there would still be an open handicapped parking space near her office building by the time she arrived on campus. However much she planned ahead and tried to organize her life, there were always unexpected and uncontrollable problems. This morning, for instance, she woke up with a violent headache and vision problems that slowed down her morning routine. Her teenage daughter, Stacy, not a cheerful morning person in the best of times, stumbled into the kitchen while Margaret was trying to get herself together for the day. "Mom," she whined, "you promised to help me with the homework assignment that is due today and you didn't! And I need a note for gym and some money for lunch." Usually Margaret would have dealt with these details the evening before, but she had come home from the office with such extreme fatigue that she'd gone straight to bed. "Single motherhood would be hard in the best of circumstances," she thought, "and these aren't the best of circumstances." Her health problems had eventually taken their toll on a marriage that was not particularly strong to begin with, and she had been coping alone for the last two years. She knew Stacy was frustrated with her inability to do things other mothers could do and probably blamed her for the divorce.

In fact, until recently, Margaret had been able to handle most of the demands of her career and family. She came from a large and active extended family used to constant activity. Family gatherings revolved around boating, swimming, mountain climbing, skiing and other outdoor sports. Sibling rivalries were often settled on the tennis courts in the park down the street from the family home. Those who didn't participate were designated as wimps or couch potatoes. Brad, her ex-husband, had grown up next door, playing with Margaret and her siblings. In high school, she and Brad fell in love, at least in part because they had so much in common and enjoyed the same activities. Her energy level had been such that she was able to handle marriage, motherhood, a full-time teaching job, and work on her PhD, often going without meals and sleep to do everything that needed doing. Brad had been supportive of her work as

171

long as she continued to participate in his beloved sporting activities and didn't expect him to do much around the house.

But several years ago, Margaret found herself dealing with chronic fatigue, muscle pain, digestive upsets, and other symptoms that gradually became too much to ignore. After seeing a number of doctors and trying both traditional and alternative treatments, she finally was given the diagnosis: she had a chronic autoimmune disease. There was no cure, she was told, but with care she could manage her disease. Unless it progressed rapidly, she should be able to live a relatively "normal" life. But what, she wondered, was normal about dragging through a day so tired that she could hardly sit up? "OK, enough!" she scolded herself as she pulled into the parking lot. "Stop feeling sorry for yourself. You can see, you can walk, you can hear. So you can't do everything you used to. So Brad decided he couldn't spend the rest of his life with someone who couldn't go skiing and climbing, someone who was usually in bed by 9:00 p.m. You have a job, a tenured teaching position. You have Stacy. You have at least one understanding sibling who doesn't tell you to 'get up and get moving and you'll feel better.'"

Arriving on campus, Margaret spied a handicapped parking spot and pulled her car into it. She waved at Joanne, who was parked next to her, unloading her wheelchair from the back of her car. Joanne, who appeared to be in her mid-20s, supervised the mathematics tutoring center on campus. Margaret watched as a history professor reached into the car, grabbed Joanne's chair, and set it on the pavement. "He actually looked sort of proud of himself," Margaret thought to herself. Joanne responded with a rather curt "Thanks!" and rolled her eyes at Margaret. "Well that answers my question," Margaret thought, "Joanne doesn't appreciate the unsolicited help." As Joanne rolled toward the building, Margaret unloaded her book bag and noticed several people staring at her. One young man yelled loudly at Margaret, "Aren't you ashamed of yourself, taking a handicapped spot when you're obviously not handicapped?" Much like the history professor, this man looked rather proud of himself, too. For Margaret, the comment cut deep; in fact, she often did feel ashamed. She knew she looked perfectly healthy and, on good days, was able to walk without a limp or any visible symptoms of her disease. In fact, on the best of days, she could walk several blocks without experiencing distress. On bad days, however, even the few feet from the car to the door were exhausting and painful. She had started to use a wheeled book bag rather than try to carry her overloaded briefcase. And some of her colleagues made fun of her for looking like an "old lady." Even though they probably would have said they were just teasing, the comment hurt.

Until recently, Margaret had kept her health problems to herself. She did not want to be pitied. And, given the initial reaction of her family, she was afraid people would think she was exaggerating her symptoms or using her illness to avoid extra work. The few colleagues she had told of her problems were stunned and responded, "But you look so healthy!" She could tell that her disability didn't really register on their radar. After all, she didn't look disabled. She had no visible signs of illness. "Looking healthy is great," she thought, "but it means that people tend to forget that I'm not completely healthy."

As she entered the building, Margaret heard a wheelchair coming and held the elevator door open for Joanne. Although they often met coming and going from the building or in the parking lot, Margaret and Joanne had seldom talked of anything besides the weather. Margaret had never told Joanne why she had a handicapped sticker and now, after hearing the man yell at her in the parking lot, Margaret wondered if Joanne thought she was taking a slot from someone who needed it. But today, as they rode up together, Joanne unexpectedly turned to Margaret and asked if she would be interested in joining a support group for disabled women that met weekly and was, in fact, meeting at 4:00 that afternoon. "I've gone to several meetings," Joanne said enthusiastically, "and I think you'd find it very helpful." "I'll think about it," Margaret told Joanne, "and maybe I'll see you there."

Margaret was torn, trying to understand why she was reluctant to attend the meeting. She realized she had a hard time thinking of herself as disabled, although she knew that was the case, or at least was becoming the case. Did she fit with this group of women? Disabilities were supposed to be visible, something everyone could see without having to explain it, right? In fact, in this one respect, she even envied someone like Joanne because her disability was open and obvious. People probably didn't tell her to "just try to stand up and walk," or "you're exaggerating your problems." No one yelled at Joanne when she parked in the handicapped space. At the same time, Margaret realized she felt fortunate that in most situations she wasn't automatically identified or stigmatized as disabled. She did not have to cope with the embarrassment nondisabled people often felt around those who were not physically "normal." For Margaret, attending the disability support group would be more than a decision about how to spend her afternoon. She realized that, by attending, she would be crossing an invisible boundary, publicly identifying herself as disabled.

Deep in thought, Margaret entered the corridor outside her office, pulling her book bag. She realized she was once again a bit late for her office hours; several students were already standing impatiently by her door. She knew they were hoping she had finished grading last week's exams; she'd certainly taken them home with that goal in mind. But she'd been unable to put in several more hours of work last evening after having taught her classes, attending two long and somewhat frustrating meetings, and answering a number of emails from colleagues and students. "Sorry guys," she explained, "the exams aren't done. But you know I didn't promise them until Monday." After listening to a bit of good-natured grumbling and answering a few questions on next week's assignment, Margaret headed for the monthly staff meeting.

After a few preliminary announcements, the department chair, Dr. Long, brought up an emergency report that was due to the Dean in 1 week. The department chairperson expressed her regrets for piling the extra work on everyone, but enthused, "I know you'll all be willing to do your share. If we all will 'burn some midnight oil,' I think we can get it done on time." As everyone else around the table nodded in agreement, Margaret froze in anxiety. She wanted to do her share; certainly her colleagues deserved her best effort. However, she well knew that a week of too much stress and too little sleep could propel her into a serious relapse that would take weeks to work out of. She had learned to cope with her illness by meticulously organizing her time so that she could apportion out her energy and reduce the stress of deadlines, always allowing for health-related interruptions. "Well," she thought, "I'll just have to try and hope for the best. I can't ask for special favors. After all, what I don't do will fall on someone else's shoulders. And they wouldn't understand. I'm afraid they'd think I was using my disability as an excuse."

As she left the meeting, Margaret again grappled with her confusion about if, when, and how to bring up her physical limitations. She had decided to remain silent in the meeting. She was uncomfortable asking for favors and not sure what accommodations she was entitled to. Yet, just two weeks ago, she'd had to tell Dr. Long that she had chronic health problems and ask her to reschedule her classes next fall so that the times and locations would be easier for her to manage. Although Dr. Long agreed to the changes, Margaret had sensed her discomfort. "The communication problems are almost as difficult to deal with as the physical problems," she mused.

After teaching her last class of the day, Margaret decided to attend the support group. Just going into that room felt like a big step. As she entered the room, Joanne wheeled toward her with a smile, "Let me introduce you around." A number of women in the room had obvious disabilities, but there were several who, like Margaret, looked perfectly healthy. As the women introduced themselves, Margaret was both reassured and disturbed. One the one hand, she realized how much she needed confirmation and support for the many problems she faced; on the other, she was reminded of what she might have to face in the future as she looked at others whose diseases had progressively limited their mobility. Today, the leader suggested they discuss their experiences in the workplace. Some, Margaret discovered, were still struggling to hold down a full-time job and experiencing the same stress that she so often felt. Others who could no longer manage full workdays were on partial disability status and finding they felt isolated and no longer accepted by their colleagues, almost like half a day meant half a person.

When it was her turn to contribute to the discussion, Margaret decided to bring up her problems communicating about her invisible disability, although she felt ashamed to even admit to problems around those she felt were experiencing even greater challenges and limitations. As she talked about her experiences with family, friends, and colleagues, they all agreed that problems in communication were a major part of their daily lives. Some offered experiences that paralleled Margaret's, but others had almost the reverse problem. Katie, sitting next to Margaret in her wheelchair, captured it best, "People look at me and label me 'disabled' and forget that I have many skills and abilities intact. People look at you and label you 'healthy' and forget that there are skills and abilities you may have lost. I have to continually remind people of what I *can* do; you have to continually remind them of what you *cannot* do." Joanne added, "Like this morning in the parking lot. That guy from the history department reached over and tried to help me because my disability is obvious; but you were treated with hostility because yours is not. Katie has been on both sides of this dilemma, as her disability has progressed from being invisible to being obvious. So she can relate to what you are going through."

As Margaret drove home, she replayed the conversation in her mind. One thing she realized was how conflicted she had been about her health status. Her uncertainty, she realized, affected not only how she defined herself but how she presented herself to others. The lack of understanding she was picking up from others might well be the result of the mixed messages she was constantly sending. Whereas on a good health day her message might read "treat me as healthy," on a bad health day it could be "treat me as disabled." She acknowledged that she wanted her family to pretend she was the same old Margaret, yet became frustrated when they forgot that she wasn't able to do everything she once had. Margaret realized how important it was to understand how this disability fit into her own sense of self—her identity—and she hoped that she would grow to be more comfortable with who she was becoming. Margaret also vowed to be more clear and consistent in her communication with others and more direct and unequivocal about setting boundaries and dealing with others' expectations.

Arriving at home, Margaret decided to put her goals into action immediately. Extricating Stacy from her headphones, she asked for some help preparing dinner. As they worked, she reminded Stacy that their mornings had become very stressful. "So," Margaret said firmly, "I need to know as soon as I get home any tasks that you need done by the next day. Then I can do them before bedtime, and we can both start the day without being stressed and angry. If you forget to tell me at night, you'll have to go without my help in the morning." Stacy pouted a bit but agreed to try and be more organized. Margaret was sure this would take some time, and she made a mental note to be consistent and also to express her appreciation when Stacy remembered on her own.

After dinner, Margaret called her sister Ann, the high-energy but chronically disorganized sibling who was planning the family reunion next summer. Margaret volunteered for tasks she could do ahead of time, such as preparing mailings or menu planning. She reminded Ann that her health situation meant that she would not be able to do last-minute shopping or cooking. Surprisingly, Ann agreed and thanked Margaret for her willingness to help. "Now," she thought, "if I can just figure out how to be as confident and assertive at work!"

Finally, thinking how grateful she was to Joanne, Margaret gave her a quick call to thank her for the invitation to the support group. Joanne was delighted and suggested they have lunch the following week. "You know," she informed Margaret, "before you go much further in talking to your colleagues, you need to consult the disability office on campus. They can help you determine what accommodations you have a right to and give you some advice about how to bring up the topic with your supervisor, colleagues, and students. And I'll be happy to share some of my experiences and strategies with you over a sandwich."

JOANNE'S STORY

As Joanne brushed her hair, she glanced at the clock and saw that she was actually running a bit early for work. That was a good thing, as the freeway was likely to be jammed on a Friday. She thought about what her schedule held today—run by the store, go to work, the disability support group at the university, and then that party at Juan and Maria's tonight. For each large step or task, she planned ahead, making sure that she had her "ducks in a row," as she called it.

Ever since her accident five years ago, Joanne found that she needed to plan out her day more than she ever had. Because she now used a wheelchair, she planned ahead to make sure that she would be able to obtain any assistance she needed to do her daily tasks. Although she could get her wheelchair out of her car by herself, she did need assistance getting the chair back into the car. Joanne thought through her to-do list, "Let's see, at the grocery store I might need some help getting any items off tall shelves. The dairy case I can handle myself. If I just get juice and donuts, I can carry the purchases in my lap." She remembered the party tonight. "Oh, shoot, I should bring a bottle of wine for the party tonight. Yes, I think I can carry all that. That would be good, and I would not need to ask for help from anybody." Once she arrived at the university, things would go smoothly. The university was very accessible, and usually she needed very little help to get through the day. Not that help would be a problem, she mused; actually, it was the opposite, as she usually received many more offers of help than she needed or wanted. I wonder how many times today I'll have to say, "No thank you."

Because she was running early, Joanne had time for a cup of coffee and a chance to read the newspaper. Friday was the day that the personal ads ran in the paper. Joanne read these ads without fail, trying to picture what kind of men would write advertisements to find dates. Although she sometimes thought about answering one of these ads, she never did. What would she say? "Woman, 28 years old, math whiz, attractive, red hair, green eyes, likes movies, jazz, loves to cook, uses a wheelchair to get around." No, she just could not picture it.

Sometimes, she really missed Jeff. They started dating her sophomore year in college. They met on the running track at the university and hit it off immediately. Part of what they had in common was competition—running, working out in the weight room, and comparing scores on their mid-terms. Joanne was an excellent student, especially in mathematics, whereas Jeff barely pulled "Cs." He could have done the work, but Jeff was not good at sticking to things, except for sports. "And he wasn't very good about sticking to relationships, either," Joanne said to herself. After her accident, she was in the hospital and then rehabilitation for six months. At first, Jeff was with her around the clock, cheering her on, telling her she would walk again someday. But as the weeks turned to months and it was clear that she would not walk and that her life had changed, Jeff started visiting less often and soon hardly at all. When he did come, he would give her a quick peck on the cheek and not stay for long, treating her more like a friend than a girlfriend. In fact, although Joanne had lots of male friends, that was how most men seemed to treat her since her accident. "Good old Joanne," she imagined men thought about her.

Joanne finished her coffee and put the dishes in the sink. She fed her cat and was out the door. As she pulled into the parking lot at the grocery store, she drove to the front of the store, looking for a handicapped parking space. There was none to be found. She was even more irritated when she noticed that two of the cars did not display handicapped parking placards.

Joanne was angry. "Do these people have any idea how much extra time and energy it takes just to go to the store, get the wheelchair in and out of the car, and maneuver around a busy parking lot? If these yahoos had to spend one day in a chair, they would be singing a different tune," she said under her breath.

As Joanne got into the store, she decided to buy fresh donuts from the bakery counter. She wheeled up to the tall counter at the bakery and looked for someone to wait on her. She could see the employees in back, but was not sure if they saw her, as she was fairly hidden behind the counter. There was a bell but she could not reach it. Joanne finally called out and one of the employees approached the counter. Peering down at Joanne, the woman looked surprised, "Uh, um, um-what-can-I-help-you-with?" the woman said very loudly and incredibly slowly. Joanne had heard this before—why did they think that because her legs did not work that her ears and brain did not work? Joanne, answered, "I need two dozen donuts, go ahead and mix them." The woman answered, again loudly and slowly, "OK! Let-me-get-these-for-you. I'll-take-them-to-the-cashier-for-you." "No need, I can get them just fine," Joanne replied, sighing to herself.

Earlier in her experience as a person with a disability, Joanne might have reacted differently. In fact, she had to admit that she would have probably gotten angry and told the clerk, or anyone else talking down to her, that she had a brain and could do things for herself. However, as the years wore on, Joanne had figured out ways to handle these kinds of situations. Although it still made her angry at times, she also came to realize that many nondisabled people were trying to help and they were simply very inexperienced with folks who were disabled. What made it worse was that so many nondisabled people also seemed so uncomfortable around people with disabilities. Those two things together added up to interactions that were often unpleasant for Joanne and, she imagined, for the other person as well. Although it all made her crazy at times, most days she could pass it off. But if she could tell nondisabled people anything to make this situation better, she would say, "It is best to help me when I ask for help . . . and when I do ask, please listen carefully, as I know what kind of help I need."

As Joanne arrived at work, she was glad to see several handicapped parking spaces available for her to use. As she pulled in, she saw him. "Oh no, not that guy from history," she said aloud to herself. Dr. Phillip Gray had been at the university for 38 years. Although Joanne appreciated that he wanted to be helpful, whenever he saw her pull in or come up to her car, he always approached her, and would say quite loudly "Here, allow me to do that for you." Worse, he would never listen to her when she would tell him, "No thanks," or when she would explain how best to get her chair into the car. She sighed to herself, "We are supposed to be forever grateful to all the wonderful nondisabled people in the world who make our lives miserable in the name of helping us!"

Although there were days when she would drive around the parking lot if she spied Dr. Gray and he had not yet seen her, today she needed to get to her office, as she had an appointment scheduled. So she gritted her teeth, "Let's just get it over with," and endured the unpleasant interaction. Just as Joanne was settled into her chair, she noticed a blue car pull into the handicapped spot next to her. It was Margaret Crane. Although Joanne did not know Margaret well, she had seen her on campus for several years, and the two of them had a passing acquaintance. She had heard rumors that something was "wrong" with Margaret and had heard everything from arthritis, to multiple sclerosis, to even one wild story that Margaret had a drinking problem. Joanne had heard one university employee exclaim, "Have you seen that poor woman walk? She must have had one too many martinis at lunch!"

Joanne had witnessed a steady decline in Margaret's health, too. Sometimes she seemed to be doing very well and, at other times, clearly the woman was in serious pain. It was hard to see her struggle by on campus, trying to walk to the library clear across the quad. Joanne wanted to invite Margaret to the disability support group. This was very delicate, though. She did not know for sure that Margaret had a disability and, even if she was sure, she did not know how Margaret would feel about being identified as disabled and invited to this meeting. Once Margaret started using the handicapped parking spots on campus, though, Joanne thought perhaps it would be safe to invite her.

Just as Joanne finished with the ever-helpful Dr. Gray, Margaret was getting out of her car. Joanne rolled her eyes and Margaret smiled. Within seconds, this jerk yelled at the poor woman for using the handicapped parking space. Margaret looked humiliated and froze for a couple of seconds. Joanne started to say something, and then stopped, telling herself, "Slow down, Jo, you do not know this woman well. Let Margaret handle her own business." She did shoot Margaret a sympathetic glance and rolled her eyes. As their eyes met, Joanne decided to ask Margaret to the disability support group that afternoon.

As Joanne came to the door of the building, Margaret opened it for her. That was fine with Joanne. She sensed that Margaret did this out of kindness, and that she would open the door for anyone approaching. This was so different from how people like the history professor would have done it. Even though there was a button and she could open the door herself, Joanne entered, smiled, and said, "Thanks." As they rode up in the elevator, she screwed up her courage, figuring "the worst she can say is 'no,'" and asked Margaret to the support group meeting. Margaret did look a bit taken aback. She hesitated, as if really thinking about it, and then she said she would think about it. "Whew," Joanne thought, "I'm glad that went OK. I really do love these meetings. I think there could be some good information and friendship there for Margaret, too."

As she finished up her work that afternoon, Joanne thought about Margaret. Joanne remembered how hard it was after her accident. Like she did with everything in life, she pushed herself hard at the rehabilitation center. There she learned how to take care of her physical needs and got some counseling in adjusting to her disability. She mostly kept to herself; she just did not feel like she had much in common with the others there. She worked hard and got herself home and back to college more quickly than anyone else who had been in the center with her. But the thing was that she did not feel disabled. She did not have any people with disabilities in her life. She thought that everything would be the same—just from the vantage point of a chair.

However, things were not the same. When Jeff moved out of their apartment, her parents had her belongings moved home. Although she appreciated their help, she hated needing to live with her parents, even if it made the most sense. Joanne worked hard in school, arriving home exhausted each night, and then spent each weekend lonely for companionship. In addition to Jeff, she had lost most of her friends. They came by now and then, but their visits were short, and it felt like she did not have anything in common with them anymore. Her classes were a struggle, too. Whereas school had always come easy, each trip to the library or copy center wore her out. Everything took so much longer to do! Even trying to find the elevator in an unfamiliar building was a major undertaking. And though the physical adjustments were big, sometimes it felt like the emotional adjustments were huge. She just did not know who she was anymore or what she wanted, or could expect, out of life. She was lonely. She was tired of people staring at her and being so uncomfortable around her. Sometimes, she just wanted to shout, "What's your problem? Haven't you ever seen a person in a wheelchair before?"

On a particularly rotten day when she was very close to quitting school, Joanne ran into Guy, who had been in the rehab center with her. Guy, who was now a senior, invited her to a support group on campus for people with disabilities. Joanne was not sure she wanted to go, but Guy invited her to lunch and talked to her about how helpful this had been for him. "Joanne, I have been there, and this group has been a lifesaver for me."

Going to that first meeting was truly scary for Joanne. It was like admitting that she was "one of them." Not only did Joanne find the support group helpful, some of the members also introduced her to online support groups for people with disabilities. Joanne started visiting these chat rooms at night after she finished studying. Her favorite was called "On a Roll." It was much easier for her to be open with people online. She could talk about her fears and concerns, and it helped to see that she was not alone. Joanne even started writing poetry about her experiences and posting it on the Web site, something brand new for this math major.

As Joanne thought about it, her situation and Margaret's situation were both similar and different. Both had to cope with becoming a person with a disability. It ranges from thinking you will get better, to thinking life will not change much, to actually accepting and learning to live as a person with a disability. "Kind of like adjusting to living in a different country or culture," she thought. Both she and Margaret came to the new culture in different ways. Joanne had to cope with becoming disabled very quickly—literally waking up disabled after her accident. Yet, it took time to actually feel like a person with a disability. On the other hand, Margaret had to adjust to becoming disabled over time. Because Joanne's disability was visible to others, she had to cope regularly with the stares and too much help. People like Margaret, whose disability was not usually visible to others, faced the opposite challenge of not knowing what to say to help people understand her disability and limitations she might have.

Joanne cleaned up her desk and got ready for the women's support group. She readied all her materials for the morning and checked the tutoring schedule. Mid-terms were coming, and she knew the math tutoring center would be swamped for the next two weeks. Joanne checked her email one last time and laughed out loud at some of the jokes on the "On a Roll" Web site. Grabbing the donuts and juice she bought that morning, Joanne headed out to the meeting. She loved these meetings and appreciated how understanding the women in the group were and how much they laughed together. She would have to tell them the latest exploits of Dr. Gray. As she approached the door to the meeting room, she hoped she would see Margaret there.

RELEVANT CONCEPTS

Disability communication: Communication of a person who has experienced physical or social limitations affecting one or more key life functions: self-care, mobility, employment, communication, or socialization.

Identity: An identity is a relatively consistent and enduring set of qualities and characteristics that define who a person is, both to oneself and to others.

Invisible disability: A disability or limitation that is not immediately observable by others, giving the disabled person a choice of whether to disclose or to keep the limitation hidden from others.

Social support: Behaviors or messages that demonstrate that we are cared for, valued, and part of a network of mutual obligation; information support, tangible assistance, esteem support, network support, and emotional support.

Stigma: Attributes that are deeply discrediting; being different in ways that are unexpected to those with whom we interact.

Uncertainty: Discomfort that occurs when we interact with people, groups, or cultures that are unfamiliar and we perceive we are unable to predict what the other person will say or do or what we should say or do.

DISCUSSION QUESTIONS

1. From the situations discussed in this case, what communication challenges do people with invisible disabilities like Margaret face? What communication challenges do people with visible disabilities like Joanne face?

2. An invisible disability is defined as "one that is hidden so as not to be immediately noticed by an observer except under unusual circumstances or by disclosure from the disabled person or other outside source" (Matthews & Harrington, 2000, p. 1). What sorts of health problems would be included in this category? What do you think about using the term "invisible"?

3. For Joanne and Margaret, how is the process of becoming disabled similar and different for each of them? How can they let others know when they desire help and when they do not? How is becoming disabled like becoming part of a new culture?

4. What benefits are there for support groups for people with disabilities, both face-to-face groups and online groups?

5. What issues concerning communication with people who are disabled are you unsure or uncomfortable about?

REFERENCES/SUGGESTED READINGS

Braithwaite, D. O., & Braithwaite, C. A. (2003). "Which is my good leg?": Cultural communication of people with disabilities. In L. A. Samovar & R. Porter (Eds.), *Intercultural communication: A reader* (10th ed., pp. 165–176). Belmont, CA: Wadsworth.

Braithwaite, D. O., & Eckstein, N. (2003). Reconceptualizing supportive interactions: How persons with disabilities communicatively manage assistance. *Journal of Applied Communication Research, 31,* 1–26.

Braithwaite, D. O., & Harter, L. (2000). Communication and the management of dialectical tensions in the personal relationships of people with disabilities. In D. O. Braithwaite & T. L. Thompson (Eds.), *Handbook of communication and people with disabilities: Research and application* (pp. 17–36). Mahwah, NJ: Lawrence Erlbaum Associates.

Krigher, S. M., & Jurkowski, E. T. (2001). Life after a national nightmare: Coping with invisible illness and disability. *Health and Social Work, 26,* 211–216.

Lyons, R. F., Sullivan, M. J. L., Ritvo, P. G., & Coyne, J. C. (1995). *Relationships in chronic illness and disability.* Thousand Oaks, CA: Sage.

Matthews, C., & Harrington, N. G. (2000). Invisible disability. In D. O. Braithwaite & T. L. Thompson (Eds.), *Handbook of communication and people with disabilities: Research and application* (pp. 405–421). Mahwah, NJ: Lawrence Erlbaum Associates.

IV

Issues in Family Dynamics

15

Communicating About Family History in an Age of Genomic Health Care: Expanding the Role of Genetic Counseling

Roxanne L. Parrott
Judith Weiner
Pennsylvania State University

No one is likely to be prepared for a telephone call regarding the unexpected hospitalization of a family member. Still, when Susan received the call about her sister, Lynn, she was particularly shocked. Lynn was only 18 years old and in her first semester of college. Eight years older than Lynn, Susan had recently talked with her sister about the decision to seek birth control pills from the student health center on campus. The last thing either of them had considered was that after beginning use of the oral contraceptive, Lynn would develop a life-threatening blood clot in her leg and have to be hospitalized.

"You knew she was taking the pill?" Susan's mother hissed into the telephone. "And you didn't tell us?"

Both statements were expressed as questions, but the mother expected no answer, and there was none that Susan cared to go into with her parent. At least, not right now. Although a large and close-knit family, nonetheless, there were topics that just simply were not discussed in their household, and sex was one of them. That was not unusual or surprising, given the taboo nature of talk about sex within the United States (Parrott, 1995). In this case, such a conversation would likely have made little difference, as the problem had to do with family health history associated with blood clots. Susan doubted that *any* conversation about this specific issue, or their family health history in general, might have taken place regarding the use of birth control pills. She predicted that a conversation about the use of oral contraception would have turned to a discussion about morals and family values, with her parents implicitly linking the use of birth control and premarital sex to inappropriate behavior falling outside the boundaries of their religious background and upbringing.

"How's Lynn doing? Are you sure you don't want me to come home? I could catch a flight later today," Susan offered, sidestepping an argument about failing to disclose information about her sister's decision to take the pill and Susan's advice in that regard.

"You don't need to do that. Your father and I will handle it."

"Have any of her friends been visiting?" Susan asked.

"I doubt that they know about it," the mother responded. "She hasn't exactly been in a position to call anyone. I certainly am not going to call them. And we haven't told any of our friends or anyone outside the family either. What would we say?"

Susan felt flushed as she filled in the unfinished statement about her parents' embarrassment over their daughter's behavior. She also made a mental decision to call the office and take the rest of the week off so she could go to visit Lynn in the hospital. She had an uneasy feeling about the nature of her parents' visits with her sister in the hospital.

"OK, Mom. I'll talk to you later. I need to get to work."

As she drove to her office, Susan developed a mental checklist of what needed to be done to take the rest of the week off. Luckily, the project she was lead on was ahead of the release schedule date. She worked with an outstanding team who collaborated well, so she was not too worried about being able to take the time off. Still, she needed to organize what should be accomplished in her absence.

"Good morning," Pam called brightly as Susan entered her suite of offices.

"Hi, Pam. Would you have a few minutes to join me in my office?"

The two women walked into Susan's office and took seats at the small round conference table. "My sister has been hospitalized with a blood clot in her leg," Susan said, and Pam raised her eyebrows. "I want to go spend some time with her. Probably just over the weekend, but let's plan the next week's schedule and put it out. Then call a meeting for the group early this afternoon. Also, if you could make my flight reservations, that would be a tremendous help."

"I'm on it. Want me to do that while you pull stuff together to outline the week's project aims?"

"That sounds good."

Pam rose and walked out of the office, while Susan rose and went to her desk. An hour later, the women had completed a summary of project tasks for the coming week. Pam went to print it out and make copies, while Susan sorted through her mail, selected folders that she would take with her to work on in her absence, and prepared a list of calls to make before leaving.

It was after nine that evening when Susan stood in line at the airport rental car counter to pick up the car that Pam had reserved for her. One of the factors in her decision to accept her current position was her ability to catch a direct flight that was just two hours from where her parents lived. As she drove toward her parents' home, she considered whether to stop by the hospital on the way and decided against it because she was uncertain about the schedule for visiting hours and her parents were not expecting her. She pulled into the driveway and grabbed her suitcase from the back seat. Getting out of the car, she headed toward the front door. Her parents had seen the headlights and turned on a porch light as she walked up the sidewalk. Her father opened the front door and, upon seeing her, called out to her mother, "Jean, it's Susan!"

Her mother rushed from the kitchen and threw open the screen door. "Oh, Susan! I'm so glad you've come," she said and then began to cry as she embraced her eldest child. Susan was shocked and immediately concerned, as neither of her parents was given to emotional displays.

"What's wrong? Has something happened to Lynn?" Susan realized that a blood clot like Lynn had could cause a stroke to occur.

"No, no," her father quickly reassured her. "But some blood tests have been done that I don't understand." Susan felt a moment of panic, as her mind leaped ahead to the possibility of a positive HIV test. "Lynn may have the Factor V Leiden mutation," her father said.

"What?" Susan had never heard of such a thing and raised her eyebrows as she looked to her dad for further explanation.

"We will meet with the doctor in the morning. All I know is that it has something to do with risk for blood clots. We'll learn more tomorrow."

The three went to the kitchen for a cup of tea and talked about other matters unrelated to Lynn. Dad had gotten the garden planted just this past weekend. Mom was still working on her flowerbeds. "So many bulbs need to be pulled up this year. They're really thick along the border of the house near the garage." As the teacups emptied, Susan began to yawn. Her mother said, "Your room is just the way you left it the last time. Of course, I washed the linens, so they're fresh. Want any help getting the rest of your stuff out of the car?" They walked together to her car, got out her briefcase and laptop, and strolled back to the house. Both parents kissed her good night, and Susan went into the bedroom that she had shared with Beth, the middle sister. Beth was married and had a two-year-old, so she could not easily travel home on short notice. Beth had been one of the people on her list to call earlier today and was relieved to learn that Susan was going to go home and would be able to relay "what was really going on."

All three slept well but awoke early the next morning, rising to have breakfast together and then prepare to visit the hospital. It was nearly a 40-minute drive across town to the location where Lynn was being treated. The hospital was the one nearest campus, so Lynn had been taken there by ambulance when she woke up with pain in her right calf, swelling, tenderness, and discoloration. Her roommate had been insistent that Lynn go to the university's Student Health Center right away. There, a doctor ordered the ambulance that transported her to the hospital.

"Dr. Fredericks, this is my daughter, Susan," her mother said as they entered Lynn's room at the hospital, and the physician turned toward them.

"Susan!" Lynn smiled, and her older sister looked past the physician to the bed where her younger sibling looked pale and small in the oversized bed. She crossed over to the bedside and the two sisters embraced. Then Susan turned and extended a warm greeting to the physician.

"Dr. Fredericks," she nodded.

"I'm glad you're all here," he said. "I was just beginning to explain to Lynn what we may learn from her blood work." He looked like a nice man, Susan thought; probably mid- to late 40s. He was maybe 6 feet tall and average build, a bit of graying at the temples. "We have a couple of pretty good ideas of what is going on when someone so young develops a clot and has recently begun using oral contraceptives. With the work that has been done in the area of human genetics research, some factors relating to the increased risk for DVT—deep venous thrombosis—or blood clots, have been identified. Lynn's blood work may reveal that she has one of these factors." The doctor paused.

"Well, I have a sister that had problems with blood clots," Susan's mother said. "It happened when she was much older. Lynn probably got it from me."

"Perhaps," Dr. Fredericks nodded. "But it will take a few days for the results to come back. If we find something, we will want all of you in Lynn's immediate family to be tested. That's the best way to prevent any problems in any future surgeries that you might have. Oral contraceptives and hormone replacement therapy are not usually appropriate for individuals who have these factors. But we'll talk about that later."

Susan looked at her father and could tell that he was uncomfortable with this discussion. She suspected that he had a number of questions but wasn't asking them because the doctor had not asked if they had any questions. She also knew that her father was a very private man and her sister was in a semi-private room, so the conversation could be overheard by the patient behind the curtained screen and anyone who might be visiting that patient. It really wasn't very private. Still, this seemed to be the time if not the place to ask her questions, so she said, "I guess I have a couple of questions if you have the time."

"Sure," Dr. Fredericks responded.

"Well, first, I don't really understand what it means to say that someone has a mutation that showed up in their blood work. A mutation of what—the blood itself?"

"It is a genetic mutation," Dr. Fredericks said. "You've probably heard about the work that has been done to map the human genome and efforts to use this work to be able to improve human health. Well, so far, we are finding that many common diseases, such as diabetes, heart disease, and cancer, have many genetic links. Unlike the more traditional work of genetic disease, in which there were single gene disorders such as cystic fibrosis or sickle cell disease, we now know that heart disease, for example, is linked to a wide array of genetic disorders. And we know that this mutation that Lynn has inherited greatly increases the risk of thrombosis, or a blood clot that blocks an artery or vein and stops the blood flow."

"Yes, I have read and heard about the breast cancer gene," Susan's mother said nodding.

"That's right," Dr. Fredericks nodded. "The two primary methods of communicating about human genetic research to the public are consultations with physicians or genetic counselors, and through the media. Most patients still have no specific reason to have a genetic consult, so what most know depends on their exposure to media. Unfortunately, the media tends to take shortcuts, using shorthand phrases and terms, such as 'the breast cancer gene,' which may lead to misunderstanding. Breast cancer risk is increased for women who have been found to have any of the genetic mutations linked to the disease. However, a very small percentage of women who get breast cancer have any of the genetic mutations linked to breast cancer. So, one challenge is to continue to keep women interested in having screening tests to detect the disease early when they do not think they have the gene that predisposes them to risk.

"The Factor V Leiden mutation, for example, is a bit different in that regard. It is the most common inherited cause of blood clots. Having the mutation is a sign of increased risk for blood clotting, and many people who get blood clots do indeed have this mutation." The doctor paused and looked at each of them. "Lynn tells me that there are also other siblings—another sister and a brother. They would need to be tested, too, because each child has a chance of having the mutation just like Lynn. Since each of you inherited one gene in each gene pair from each parent, and each of your parents inherited one gene in each gene pair from their parents, you have to know what the parents' DNA is like to predict your own DNA. The DNA of reproductive cells will carry hereditary mutations like the Factor V Leiden Mutation. Then, cells containing the mutations will combine and be present in all of the offspring's body cells."

Susan looked at her father, whose jaws were clenched. It was too technical and too much. "Thank you, Doctor," he said. "We'll wait for the results and then see what you recommend."

Dr. Fredericks nodded. "I left some information with Lynn that you might want to read. She's receiving a drug intravenously to thin her blood. She will have to limit her activities for the next half-dozen weeks even after she leaves the hospital, which should be in a few days. She'll continue to take a blood-thinning medication, probably for the next 6 months, so Lynn will be at higher risk for bruising and internal bleeding. I've ordered a Medic Alert bracelet for her to wear while she's taking the medication. If you have any other questions, let me know, or tell Lynn to ask me. You folks take care now." And the doctor left the room.

Susan and her parents then visited with Lynn for awhile, talking about the weather, Susan's work, and most everything except the reason Lynn was in the hospital. "We should go run some errands," their dad finally said. "But you girls go ahead and visit. We'll stop back and pick Susan up after lunch if that's OK with you two." The sisters nodded and waved as their parents headed out the door and Susan walked over to the window to watch them leave from the parking lot. Then she turned back to her younger sister.

"So, how are you doing—really?" she asked.

Lynn looked at Susan. "I'm fine. I'm just worried about all the classes I'm missing."

"Well, I can talk to your department and make sure they let the university know, so you can get excused absences."

Lynn's lower lip suddenly began to quiver.

"What?" Susan demanded.

"I'm just so embarrassed," Lynn said. "Dad told me that me that they couldn't even put my name on the prayer list at church because then everyone would want to know what happened, and they couldn't tell them. He said that nobody will ever look at me the same way again if they find out what I did. Do you think that's true, Susan?"

"Of course not!" Susan felt herself growing hot with irritation and anger at her parents for upsetting Lynn more. Their father's comment served to compound Lynn's fears and anxieties over her present condition with guilt regarding her decision to be a responsible sexual adult. "You know that, when we talked, I told you I have been using the same pill for the past several years. I just must not have the same blood condition that you have. And I'm not sure that I would've thought about Aunt Mona even if I had been asked whether we had a family history of blood clotting. I can barely remember her, and I don't know if Mom ever told us that she had blood clots. If she did, it didn't really mean anything to me. Did you remember that? Did anyone ask you about a history of blood clots when you went to get the pill?"

"I think it was on the history form, but I didn't know Aunt Mona had that history. I think the things that I knew about were related to heart disease. That's all I checked on the form, and no one asked me any further questions."

"Well, I'll take care of school and you don't need to give it another thought. If there are any friends you want me to contact, I'll do that too. What about your roommate? Hasn't she even been up to visit you?"

"She came to see me the first couple of days, but Mom and Dad were so quiet around her, I think it made her nervous. So she told me to call if I needed her."

"OK, well if you want me to get in touch with any of your friends, just let me know. In the meantime, is there anything I can get you? That lunch didn't look too good. How about if I go to the library this afternoon and see what I can learn about this Factor V thing, and then I'll come back and bring us both some dinner. How's that?"

Lynn smiled, and the two sisters continued to catch up until the phone rang, and it was their Dad telling them that they were waiting just outside the hospital's front entrance. Susan bent over to give her sister a hug before heading out the door. She took the brochure that the doctor had given Lynn so she could go to the library and see what she might find out about all this on the Internet.

"I'm going to go back out after we get home," Susan informed her parents. "I promised Lynn I would go to the library and see what I could find out about all this." Her parents nodded, seemingly not surprised. Susan had been a debator and on the high school newspaper. Her parents often referred to her as the "reporter" in the household, even though her career in technical writing for a large computer company had taken her in a different direction. She got out of her parents' car and walked toward the rental, waving as she headed for the library.

It took some time to get past all the greetings with familiar faces at the local library. Susan wasn't ready to disclose to anyone what information she was seeking. So it was a bit challenging to dodge the questions and raised eyebrows, because everyone knew it wasn't the usual time of year for her to be visiting. Finally, she found her way to an isolated computer monitor and sat down to do a search. She had her laptop and could have done it from home. But her parents didn't have any broadband connection, so it would have been very slow navigating the Web through the local phone lines. Besides, this was easier because she didn't have her parents peering over her shoulder into the monitor trying to decipher what information she retrieved.

Susan quickly realized that the problem would be too much information rather than too little. She started with the search term "genetic conditions" on Google.com and got pages and pages of hits. She decided to narrow her search to the Factor V Leiden mutation test. Most of the information she found was technical and not very helpful in extending her knowledge. Next, she decided to do a little background research on genetics. It had been awhile since her last biology class in college, and at the time, the Human Genome project loomed against a backdrop of speculation. What she was most interested in at the moment was genetic mutations. She quickly found information about research relating to mutations as changes in genetic information and some discussion about mutations that are automatically repaired. She made notes to explain some of what she was finding to her parents. She started with the statement that a gene is made of DNA and that a genome is an entire set of genes. Genes come in different forms, called alleles, and if two alleles are the same, they are called homozygous. When the two forms are different they are called heterozygous. "Hmm," Susan thought to herself. "If both parents had the same version of a gene, the children would have been homozygous rather than heterozygous."

Susan found so much information that she lost track of time. When she next looked at the clock, it was after four in the afternoon. No time to go home before going back to the hospital with some dinner, as she had promised Lynn. She looked around the library and found a pay phone near the front entrance. She went to call her parents. "Where have you been all day?" her mother asked with both anxiety and irritation apparent in her voice.

"Sorry. I found so much information at the library that I lost track of time. I promised Lynn I would come back with dinner, so I'm on my way there now. Are you coming back this evening, or do you want to take a night off since I'm here?" There was a long pause. "Mom?"

"I'm here. I was just wondering what Lynn would think if your father and I 'took a night off,' as you put it."

"I'm sure she would be fine with it. In fact, I'll tell her that I suggested it so that we could do some more catching up. OK?" There was a sigh into the phone, and Susan couldn't tell what her mother was thinking, so this time the daughter waited for her mother to speak.

"All right then. But if Lynn seems upset or wants us to come, give me a call."

"I will." Hanging up, Susan considered briefly where to get dinner for her and Lynn. She headed to the nearby A & W, ordered chili dogs, onion rings, and large root beers. The aroma brought smiles to Lynn's face as she entered her hospital room and began to arrange a spot for the two of them to eat.

"So, what have you been up to?" Lynn asked between bites of hot dog. "Mom called here twice this afternoon."

"I'll show you when we're done. I collected a bunch of information from the library off the Internet. So, now that Mom and Dad aren't around, want to tell me some more about what happened?" Susan talked quietly so that the other patient in the room would not hear her. She moved her chair nearer to Lynn's bed, so she could respond in a near whisper.

"It was awful!" Lynn whispered with emotion. "Dad looked at me like he didn't know me. Mom cried. And not about me being in the hospital but about what I had done to put myself here—to use her words."

Susan shook her head. "I'm sorry you had to go through that. Revealing that private information because you had to must have been really tough. When I was at the library looking up information about genetics, one of the things I kept coming across was about how families develop patterns for disclosing information about health. One researcher named Sandra Petronio talked about how if family members don't freely reveal personal information, it protects privacy but can pose risk for health-related matters. One article said that family members should remember that no single family member 'owns' genetic information, because every member could share certain genetic traits, links, or diseases. It's natural to feel like we own private information and try to control who has access to it. Issues of ownership may become really intense with genetic health information because the notion of genetic inheritance is brought into the forefront." Lynn was looking at Susan blankly. "Sorry. I know that was a lot of mumble jumble. But I just thought it was interesting to realize that we aren't the only family to keep secrets and worry all the time about what other people are thinking about us."

"Well, how many times when we were growing up did we hear that what goes on in the family is the family's business and no one else's?" Lynn said. "If we hadn't learned that rule of behavior before this, we surely would learn it now. Mom and Dad are going to have to be pushed to get tested, couldn't you just see that in their faces this morning? I don't know how we'll convince them—or, I should say, how you will convince them to do it." The sisters shook their heads and resolved to give the matter some thought and talk about it the next day. For the rest of the evening, Susan caught up with Lynn's college activities, so she would be able to go to campus in the morning and take care of her absences. Her parents were already in bed when she got home, so she quietly went to bed after locking the front door and putting the kitchen and porch lights out.

It was a surprise when, the next morning before anyone got out the door, Lynn called to say that the doctor had just left and the results were back on her blood work. She was diagnosed with Factor V Leiden mutation, heterozygous. So, that meant that she had inherited this risk from one of her parents, but not both. Susan's parents called the family doctor, and he placed an order at the lab for the blood work required to determine which other family members had the Factor V Leiden mutation. "We made an appointment for you, too, Susan," her mother announced. "We read the brochures that Dr. Fredericks gave us when we got home, and we need to know this information before any of us have any future surgeries, including dental work. Aren't you supposed to be getting your wisdom teeth out next month?"

Susan covered her surprise by turning toward the coffeepot to pour a cup. "That's right. But the results won't be back before I leave on Sunday. It took this whole week to get Lynn's results and that was with a rush on the tests to be completed. But I guess the report can be forwarded to my doctors if need be. What about Beth and Allan?" Susan asked referring to the other siblings in their family that needed to be informed and tested. Allan, the third child in the family, was on assignment with his National Guard unit, taking leave from his position at an area home improvement store.

"We called him last night after we finished reading the brochures," her father said. "He was coming down to visit with Lynn and see you tomorrow anyway, so he's coming to town this afternoon and will go with us. The lab is open until five, and the order is there so we can go anytime." Susan nodded and reached for the phone to call Beth, who agreed to take care of it with her own doctor.

"I told your brother that I am probably the one to blame in this situation," her mother said. "This is one of those times when 'blood ties' linking us is not such a good thing. But better to know than not know. They put Lynn on that blood thinner, you know. Her treatment is being closely monitored in the hospital, but this event may still impact her ability to get pregnant or carry a child to term."

"What do you mean? I went to the library yesterday and read quite a bit, but I didn't see anything like that in the information. Do you mean that you think she might decide not to have children because of this? My understanding is that when an obstetrician is informed of any genetic risks prior to pregnancy, she just needs to be more carefully supervised. So it won't be like taking birth control pills—which she can't do now."

"Well, it's something to think about, that's for sure. We don't have any control over the risks we inherit."

"But we do have some control over whether any serious or life-threatening effects will occur. Even when it relates to our inherited genes. So I'm really glad we are all going to be tested. I think it's better to know. People usually take family history into account figuring out their risk for diabetes, cancer, and heart attacks. This test will help us make better decisions about our own behaviors around blood clotting risks."

Before going to visit Lynn that morning, Susan went by the university, where she ran into more familiar faces. She had been an undergraduate in the same college as Lynn, and both sisters had used work-study positions in various departments to help pay their way through college. Susan found her way to the office administrator in the English Department and briefly filled her in. Rita agreed to take care of the rest. "Tell Lynn not to worry, and when she gets back, we'll figure out how to catch up then." Susan nodded and headed to the hospital. It was almost noon, so she went through a drive-through window and picked up some tacos, just enough for Lynn, who loved them. Susan lost her appreciation for them after her exchange program experience in Mexico City. The American version just wasn't very authentic.

"No Mom and Dad?" Susan said as she entered Lynn's room.

"You just missed them. They brought the morning paper and coffee, and told me about the appointments at the lab. Dad even said, 'It's just a simple blood test.'"

"I know. Do you think he realizes the implications for discrimination both at work and buying health insurance?" Susan saw Lynn's shocked expression and attempted to back off from her statement. "I mean, federal and state levels are trying to address that, so I don't think you'll have to worry about it. But Dad—he's older and it might impact him more, you know with the cost of having Mom covered if she has it. Anyway, let's not worry about it right now. We're doing what we need to do, and that's all we can do. Eat your tacos before they get any colder." Susan pulled out a deck of cards and the two played for awhile before Susan left to go join her parents and brother at their home.

"Hey, Sis," Allan greeted Susan as she walked in the family home's front door. "How ya doin'?" The pair embraced and then let their parents guide them out to the family car. The four talked about everything but the upcoming blood test. At the lab, Susan's mother checked them in and was told that they should have a seat and would be called shortly. Forty-five minutes later, Susan walked up to the desk to inquire why it was taking so long.

"I apologize, but the tests your doctor ordered are not ones that our techs usually do, so we are having to do some special preparation. They're almost ready."

Susan noticed that people were looking with curiosity as she turned to rejoin her family, having overheard what the receptionist had told her. "It's just about time," she said to her mother. "They're setting up to do us all." And then they were called and streamed together to take seats at stations where each rolled up a sleeve. Susan noticed her Dad's clenched jaw and her Mom's forced smile. At least this part was almost over.

"OK, well the results will be back next week," the tech said as he released the band around her arm and pressed the spot, then applied gauze and a band-aid. "Well, mostly. Two of these tests take a couple of weeks. The reports will go to your doctor." Susan nodded. No point in going into her request to have the report forwarded. She would let her local family doctor take care of assisting with that when the results got in. Susan nodded, rolling down the sleeve of her blouse and then rejoined her family in the waiting room.

The rest of the weekend went by quickly. Lynn was doing well and would be released in the coming week. Susan felt that she could return to work with no worries. As she prepared to leave on Sunday afternoon, her father came into the bedroom and said, "I read in one of those brochures that you shouldn't sit for long periods of time in the same position, like in an airplane seat or a car traveling somewhere if you have this thing. So, be sure to get up and walk around in the plane every hour, OK?" Susan nodded.

The next two weeks went by quickly. Susan called Lynn each day. She was doing well and got back to school at the end of the first week that Susan was back. The sisters talked about alternative birth control methods, recognizing that the main one—condoms—depended on cooperation with a partner. Maybe Lynn learned a thing or two about how to navigate the disclosure of sensitive information and to negotiate issues concerning her health. Susan was at work when she got the call from her dad. "Hello."

"Susan," her dad sounded tentative.

"Dad? What's wrong?"

"Well, we got the results back. The results from the blood tests. Remember that you told them they could give us your results? Anyway, Susan, it's you and me. You and I have the Factor V thing. Mom and Allan don't."

Susan didn't respond immediately. She was stunned. "But how could that be?" she asked. "I mean, you don't have any family history at all. Do you think that maybe they made a mistake? Should we get a second opinion?"

Now it was her dad's turn to pause before responding. Finally, he said, "Well, we could do that. But I talked to Uncle Rick last night," he referred to his brother. "Remember when he had the bypass surgery last year. Well, as part of the preparation for that, they did some blood tests. He has it, too. They put him on blood thinner during the surgery and for awhile after. I remember when I visited him, he said something about it all, but it didn't make any sense to me. I guess I was more worried about how he was doing and didn't think much more about it. Rick says that when Janie got pregnant, they tested her, too. She has it, and they're doing some precautionary things with her. So, I guess it seems pretty clear that it's in my family. And I guess I passed it on to you kids. Sorry about that."

"Wow," Susan said. "That's a lot to take in. So, Janie's pregnant? She's doing OK?" She wasn't really listening. She was thinking about her own use of oral contraceptions, her upcoming dental work, and future children to whom she might pass on this condition. Genetic testing was a "simple blood test," but the information clearly had implications for the rest of her life. She suddenly felt sad and angry all at the same time. She remembered Lynn telling her about similar emotions and felt embarrassed that she had dismissed them so lightly. And she wondered if her insurance company, because they had paid for the test, would be entitled to know the results and even use them to deny future claims.

"Susan," her father intruded into her thoughts. "I know it's a lot to take in. You might want to schedule an appointment with a genetic counselor to discuss the results. I think Dr. Fredericks said he could help with that. But he also said that it is different talking about this sort of risk issue with a counselor compared with more traditional genetic disorders. Anyway, I love you. Try not to let this ruin your day, and we'll call back tomorrow to see how you're doing." And he hung up.

Susan hung up as well, looking at the phone and thinking about how seldom her parents ever verbally expressed how they felt to their children. It would be interesting to see how her family handled issues relating to this genetic health history in the coming months, issues such as who to tell and when, and how to keep each other informed about their experiences. She shook her head realizing what a short amount of time had passed since she received that first phone call about her sister's hospitalization. She sighed, realizing that she now needed to inform her doctors about the results from the *not*-so-simple blood test and that it would likely mean changes in her health care. Still, she decided it was better to know than not know because she really did have some control in the situation. Starting with now, as she picked up the phone to call her dentist, telling the receptionist, "Hello. This is Susan Simmons. I have an appointment to get my wisdom teeth removed late next week, and I need to discuss some recent blood test results with Dr. Benjamin. If you would have him give me a call at his convenience, I would appreciate it. Thanks."

RELEVANT CONCEPTS

Boundary management theory: Asserts that individuals decide *who*, *what*, *where*, and *when* to share information with others and have metaphoric boundaries around private information. For example, a daughter may choose to have very open (fluid) boundaries when it comes to sharing information about her friends with her mother, and yet, she may have very closed (restricted) boundaries when it comes to discussing her romantic relationship with her mother.

Family boundaries: Family members have a complex set of boundary linkages (i.e., parameters) in terms of the different kinds of private information they individually, as well as collectively, own. In addition, how information is shared within the family may be similar or differ from how information is shared with individuals outside of the family.

Family health history: Also known as medical genealogy; involves obtaining and recording your own, as well as your family members', health records. In essence, you create a sort of family tree with respect to medical issues. This includes major illnesses, allergies, emotional or behavioral problems, health routines, etc., for your family members. It also includes interpreting patterns of health, illness, and genetic traits for you and your descendants.

Genetic inheritance: The genetic material (i.e., DNA, genes) an individual receives from her or his biological parents. In other words, children have traits transmitted to them from their parents.

Genomic health care: Medical care that is based on knowledge about genes and health generated from the Human Genome Project. It is based on the reality that many common diseases (e.g., heart disease) have numerous genetic components that predict a person's susceptibility and severity to health threats. For example, health care will be changed and tailored by knowledge of individual genetic predispositions.

Insurance discrimination: When individuals are denied insurance based on race/ethnicity, sexual orientation, socioeconomic status, age, and/or a medical condition. For example, individuals with chronic health conditions (i.e., heart problems) may be denied insurance coverage because their condition is "costly."

Privacy and confidentiality issues: When individuals share personal health information with physicians, there are often legal, as well as familial (i.e., interpersonal), concerns. For example, once a young female college student reaches the age of adulthood as defined by the law (i.e., 18) and she goes to her physician to request birth control pills, the physician must legally protect information regarding her use of birth control pills; prior to that age, a physician may be legally required to provide that information and get parental consent to prescribe contraception.

Religiosity: The role of religious faith as a social and personal resource. More specifically, extrinsic religiosity functions as a social resource that provides information and/or assistance through direct communication or vicarious observation. Intrinsic religiosity functions as a personal resource associated with cognitive and emotional functioning and may thus provide a coping mechanism in association with information about genes and health.

DISCUSSION QUESTIONS

1. To whom should one talk to learn about one's family health history?
2. What is the role of religiosity in health beliefs and behaviors, including discussions about both?
3. How does the discovery/disclosure of an inherited health condition affect family dynamics?
4. How do individual family members negotiate the balance between dialectical tensions, such as privacy versus public information?
5. How will the organization and delivery of health care be affected by genomics? Why will more than genetic counselors be involved in discussing genetic testing with patients?
6. Why is the Internet an important source of genetic-related information (GRI)? What advantages and disadvantages are associated with use of the Internet for GRI?

REFERENCES/SUGGESTED READINGS

Parrott, R. (1995). Topic-centered and person-centered "sensitive subjects": Managing barriers to disclosure about health. In L. K. Fuller & L. M. Shilling (Eds.), *Communicating about communicable diseases* (pp. 177–190). Amherst, MA: Human Resource Development Press.

Parrott, R., Silk, K., & Condit, C. (2003). Diversity in lay perceptions of the sources of human traits: Genes, environments, and personal behaviors. *Social Science & Medicine, 56,* 1099–1109.

Petronio, S. (1991). Communication boundary management: A theoretical model of managing disclosure of private information between marital couples. *Communication Theory, 1,* 311–335.

Taylor, M., Alman, A., & Manchester, D. K. (2001). Use of the Internet by patients and their families to obtain genetics-related information. *Mayo Clinic Proceedings, 76,* 772.

Additional Resource

Popular Video: *Gattaca*.

16

Catching Up With Down Syndrome: Parents' Experiences in Dealing With the Medical and Therapeutic Communities

Carol Bishop Mills

University of Alabama—Birmingham

No child is "perfectly" whole in mind, body, spirit, and ability... nor can any child meet all of a parent's hopes and expectations. Yet there is a wholeness of each and every child, a wholeness that is unique and brings with it a set of possibilities and limitations, a unique set of opportunities for fulfillment.

—Fred Rogers (1994, p. 6)

Most mornings, I wake up to a beautiful voice calling, "Dad, Dad, Dad," and if my husband, Jon, rolls over and tries to ignore the voice calling from the other room so that he can sneak in five minutes more sleep, the voice continues, "Dad, Daddy! Daddy! Up, Daddy up! Eat!" If he continues to ignore the voice from the other room, I will finally be called into action with a somewhat disgusted and deflated voice saying, "Mom, up."

Though the voice from the other room might see me as the last resort for her morning wake-up calls, I delight at the rare opportunity to rescue her from her mini-jail cell that we properly call the crib. You see, my daughter is simply a daddy's girl and because she is my second child, I know that her current affections are a phase.

When I walk into the room, my 20-month-old daughter's face lights up. Her calls have been answered, and she giggles with anticipation of being picked up. She'll grab her doll, throw her from the crib, and hoist her own arms straight up. Even though I am currently her second choice, she'll smother me with kisses and hugs for a few moments before she finally announces "eat," and downstairs we will go for her morning breakfast. As she and her four-year-old brother eat, they take turns initiating games such as pound the cup until mom says stop, or feed each other, or trade food. The adore each other, and eating often takes far too long because it is more of a play session than a nourishment activity.

Our days vary considerably from day to day. Most days, my four-year-old son has pre-K; my four-month-old son still does not conform to much of a sleep schedule and may sleep until 11 a.m. or be up hours before my daughter. Some days, I go to work, and my husband runs our son to school; other days, I do the running. And sometimes, we might have grocery shopping on the agenda; yet, other days, I might need to be at work early for meetings. Then, as if our lives are not hectic enough, a few days of the week, my daughter might have visitors stopping by to play.

195

In most ways, we are a fairly typical and loving family with a hectic schedule. But for outsiders looking in, my family may not seem so typical. The visitors coming to play are not just any visitors; they are part of the therapy team assigned to us by Early Intervention and include a speech therapist, a physical therapist, a developmental therapist, and a music therapist. In fact, my gorgeous little girl, Maren Flannery, was born with an extra 21st chromosome in each cell of her body. The official name for my daughter's diagnosis is trisomy 21 (T21), but most people know it as Down syndrome. In our family, it is simply a gift we were given that we would have never known to ask for and probably would have never understood before our Little Miss Magic captivated our hearts.

As you may have guessed, my husband and I do not see Down syndrome as a negative part of our lives. T21 is simply a small part of who our daughter is. Her extra chromosome is never a problem. Sadly, any negative feelings we have about our daughter's diagnosis come from the world around us—outside of our family's control—and often stem from some members of the medical and therapy communities that are supposed to make her life, our lives, better and easier.

In this case, I explore some of the major medical and therapy provider interactions my husband and I have experienced as the parents of a child with trisomy 21, as well as discuss the experiences of several of the friends that I have made along this journey.[1] Some are joyous experiences, others are infuriating, and still others are heartbreaking for the parents. Each is presented so that you might better understand the life of a parent of a child with special needs and the importance and power that interactions with the medical and therapeutic communities have on us.

BACKGROUND INFORMATION

According to the National Down Syndrome Society, one in every 800 to 1,000 live births is a child with trisomy 21, and over 350,000 families in the United States are affected by Down syndrome, which is the presence of 47 chromosomes rather than 46.

So, what causes Down syndrome? We do not know precisely what causes it. In approximately 98–99% of the cases, the extra chromosome is a "fluke." T21 is an equal opportunity chromosomal anomaly: Children born with Down syndrome are from all races, religions, ethnic backgrounds, and socioeconomic statuses. Advancing maternal age increases the possibility of having a child with an extra 21st chromosome; but the majority of children with Down syndrome are born to mothers under the age of 35 (Stray-Gundersen, 1995).

Though we do not know the "cause," we do know about the processes resulting in T21. The majority of the cases are explained as a nontypical division of the cells at conception that results in an embryo with three number 21 chromosomes instead of the typical two. According to researchers, as the embryo develops, the extra chromosome is replicated in every cell of the body. This type of cell division occurs in 95% of the cases classified as Down syndrome. In a few other cases, called mosaicism, the cells divide properly at conception, and in later cell divisions, the chromosomes split unevenly; thus, some cells have 46 chromosomes, whereas others have 47. In the final type, Translocation, a piece of one chromosome breaks off and attaches to another, typically the 21st. It is only in the final type that the extra chromosome is hereditary, and the estimates for hereditary Translocation account for less than 1% of all cases of the diagnosis.

GETTING THE DIAGNOSIS

Jon, Carol, and Maren

On May 15, after a fairly difficult pregnancy that was at week 36 and bed rest orders that I had trouble following, my nurse midwife, Kim, strapped me to a non-stress test machine. My baby was not moving much. Kim did not want to alarm me, but said I needed yet another ultrasound. The technician seemed alarmed during the exam and sent me back to Kim's office. Kim summoned the doctor in the practice.

Dr. Jackson began slowly, "Carol, there are some indications that your baby is not continuing to thrive in utero, and I have called a top-notch neonatalogist at the Chicago Hospital. He thinks you should go there right away for induction." A bit stunned, I asked, "Can you please tell me specifically what you are seeing that has you so concerned?

"Well," he continued, "it appears that there is an enlargement of your baby's heart and a significant amount of fluid in the kidneys. Further, the baby's head appears to be flattening."

"What are you trying to tell me?" I asked.

"I do not want to alarm you, but there are indications that this baby may not be thriving," Dr. Jackson responded.

"Are you telling me you think this baby may not make it?"

After a long pause, he said, "All I can say at this point is that there may be some complications, and you should be at a hospital with specialists."

I was terrified and, despite his relatively calm demeanor, just hearing, "I don't want to alarm you," was reason enough for alarm. I was sick and scared when my husband arrived to take me to the hospital that was about 40 minutes away. I begged him to stop at the house, where I proceeded to clean my living room, pack food for my son to take to the neighbors, call my family, and make the beds. Finally, my husband's patience had been tested, and we left.

The entire drive to the hospital, I kept hoping a wreck in front of us would slow us down, that construction would keep us from reaching our destination, that we'd get there and the doctor would be gone and they would send us home. All I knew was that if my baby was going to be stillborn, I wanted to keep his or her heart beating inside of me as long as possible. I wanted to stay his or her mommy, and I could not escape the ominous feeling that this baby would not be born alive. I was terrified by the thought of telling my son, $2\frac{1}{2}$ years old at the time, that he was not going to have a baby brother or sister after all.

When we finally made it to the hospital, the doctor was clearly a bit agitated. Dr. Cassidy began our initial interaction by asking, "What took you so long? I've been waiting three hours." In an effort to shield me, my husband Jon responded, "We hit horrible traffic."

"Okay, let's just get started," Dr. Cassidy replied. He immediately hooked me up to an ultrasound machine and, after a few minutes of calmly looking at the baby, he spoke, "Um, this does not look bad at all. The heart looks just fine to me. Kidneys are a bit enlarged. And they shouldn't have even made a comment about the head because the baby is already so low."

He did some measurements on the baby and was the second doctor during my pregnancy to comment on the baby's "small for dates" proportions. He then said, "Since you are here, though, given the kidneys, we ought to induce. Get some sleep and we'll start a oxytocin drip in a few hours to induce labor. Looks like you are already having some mild contractions anyway."

Dr. Cassidy was calm and did not use any words that caused alarm. By the time he left, my fears were quelled. My husband and I had known for a while that something "wasn't quite right" with this pregnancy and even discussed the possibilities of having a child born with medical and developmental issues. What we wanted was a live baby to love and hold. Because the doctor showed no signs of urgency or panic, and because we knew he was one of the best doctors in the area, we were confident that everything was going to be all right.

Thirteen hours later, my labor room was filled with at least 12 people. Dr. Cassidy, two of his partners, three residents of the teaching hospital, two neonatal intensive care unit (NICU) doctors, and several nurses, all there waiting for the entrance of the baby and ready to spring into action if anything was wrong. The baby was born.

We were told we had a girl, and immediately she was whisked away from us to the prep table. I heard lots of whispers and chatting, but I also heard a beautiful cry. She was alive!

Dr. Jacobs, the NICU doctor, approached my bed about 15 minutes later and handed me a gorgeous baby girl. He was very pleasant and smiled when he told us all about her. "Mr. and Mrs. Mills, your daughter is quite healthy. She seems to have a strong heart, and her kidneys will be fine. There was some fluid pooled, but it will eliminate itself naturally. Her APGAR scores[2] were 8 and 9. She's a beautiful little girl. There are some preliminary indicators in her features that she might have trisomy 21, Down syndrome, but we need to run some blood work to confirm that."

I have replayed his words in my head many times, and perhaps with each replay they get altered, but the biggest thing I remember is that he was so upbeat about her health and so matter of fact about her diagnosis.

He did not apologize as if there was something to be "sorry" for. He did not say, "I hate to give you this news," as if he was preparing me for something awful. He did not look upset, disappointed, or disgusted. He simply told us about an aspect of our daughter that would be forever part of her existence, and he did so in the same manner that he told us about her APGAR.

He treated her diagnosis as "normal" rather than "abnormal." He then looked at us for our reactions, I think searching for denial, anger, and refusal. He offered to send counselors, geneticists, and support parents to see us, but reminded us that only karyotype testing could confirm the diagnosis.

My husband and I simply looked at our daughter and said, "Thank you. We do not need to wait for the results; we kind of had a feeling about this." I'm sure this was not the reaction he expected, and I have learned over the past 21 months that I was fortunate to have his reaction, as well. His tone, his choice of words, his professional manner set us on a path for our own acceptance of our daughter's diagnosis.

A few hours later, we were later greeted by a wonderful geneticist who gave us information about Down syndrome and told us all of the wonderful things that children and adults with Down syndrome do. At that time, we were even given a poem called "Welcome to Holland," by Emily Perl Kingsley that we know now is the credo of parents of children with Down syndrome. In this poem, Kingsley, an Emmy-Award winning writer for *Sesame Street* and a mom to a son with T21, likens becoming the parent of a child with special needs to a trip that is detoured to an unexpected destination. We were then given the contact numbers for a support group in the area and asked if we would like to initiate contact or if they could have permission to call us.

In every way, our experience of the diagnosis of our daughter could not have been more positive, and I am sharing our own story with you so you can see how well things can be done, and are done, by many professionals. The truth, however, is that many people are not told in such a positive way and, in fact, those early encounters are quite traumatic for some and can leave lasting emotional scars.

Kate, Chris, and Joshua

I was 40 years old when I finally got pregnant for the third time. Chris and I had been trying for two years to conceive, but two earlier pregnancies had ended in miscarriages by nine weeks. Early ultrasounds and alpha-fetoprotein results indicated no markers for T21 or any other birth defect, so when offered an amniocentesis based on maternal age, I refused.

I couldn't see taking the risk of a miscarried pregnancy, which can happen following the invasive procedure, and besides that, Chris and I would not consider termination after all we had been through to get this baby. In retrospect, there was also some arrogance of thinking, "I am a professional. My husband and I have degrees from wonderful colleges, and we are healthy. People like us do not have babies that aren't perfect."

In the labor room, we anxiously waited to greet our son. We heard a cry, we saw our boy, and then heard the following from Dr. Lee, "I am so sorry to tell you this. This baby looks like a Down's. I'm so sorry." The doctor fumbled for words for a few moments as he looked over Josh. He then said, "In 20 years, I've never delivered a Down's. Didn't you have tests?"

I remember these words as knives piercing my hearts. I quickly informed the doctor that ultrasounds *he* had performed indicated no reason to look for Down syndrome in an amnio, and that, in fact, he prided himself on seeing markers in the tests.

"Well, at 40 you should have done the amnio. Older mothers should always do one, but I can't force you to watch out for yourselves. This looks like a Down's baby to me. I'm sure it's a Down's. I am so, so sorry" he repeated. He was visibly upset.

Chris grabbed my hand and told me not to forget we had a wonderful son that needed us, but I was obsessed by the doctor's admonishment, "Didn't you have tests?" In my heart, I knew the Down syndrome was my fault, and it was clear that the doctor was angry that there was a Down's baby in his practice now. I didn't have a boy, in my mind, I had an "it," a Down's, one of those short, funny, retarded kids that work at grocery stores. My mind flooded with thoughts of drooling, retardation, the little yellow buses, the teasing, and the problems.

I thought to myself, "Was Dr. Lee right? Why didn't I test? If I had—if only I had, then I would not be to blame for this defective child. It was easy to say I wouldn't test when I thought my baby was perfect!" I kept thinking, "I do not want this—him—it—a Down's. I want a normal baby like everyone else gets to have! Why me? What have I done to bring this curse on me and my family?"

I was terrified of voicing these thoughts to Chris for fear he would think I was a terrible human being, especially while he was acting so strong as the thought of his son playing professional baseball and becoming a corporate CEO must be slipping away from him too. I knew how much he wanted a son, and I felt like I had let him down. Dr. Lee said he "couldn't force us to look out for ourselves," and I knew he thought Josh was going to be a serious burden.

To make matters worse, the baby's pediatrician was called, and when informed that Josh had an extra chromosome, the pediatrician refused to come, telling the hospital that she didn't deal with "that kind of baby." We were stunned, and Chris yelled at the nurse who delivered the news, "What kind of baby? A wonderful baby? A human baby? A baby that needs love? A baby that is going to go home to a room that is decorated with a teddy bear theme?"

Chris was ready to accept his son's extra chromosome almost instantly; he had worked with lots of individuals with Down syndrome and had some wonderful interactions with them. In addition, given our ages, he always accepted the possibility that our child might have challenges.

Now, when talking with friends about that day that was one of his happiest and yet saddest, Chris tells people, "Sure I was disappointed. I could feel many of my dreams slipping away from me, but I was so very angry at the reactions of the 'so-called' professionals and the need to fight for my son's rights that I didn't have a chance to feel sorry for myself. Somehow, they were treating my son as a pariah and he was a gorgeous kid with a full head of hair and a sweet little face. And, seeing Kate look so sad, I knew she was feeling guilty and hurt. I just had to focus on the baby to get me through this."

A few hours later, an on-call pediatrician did stop in and check the baby, Joshua, out. After a brief examination, he asked, "Did anyone tell you anything about Down's?" "No," replied Chris as he held my hand tightly, "but I've had some experience with great people. . . . " Quite abruptly, the pediatrician cut him off and began rambling.

He said, "Well, the people you met are probably the exceptions. In truth, your child will be retarded. You just can't expect that he'll ever be normal. He will have a hard time learning how to walk and talk, and he'll probably never read or have a normal life. You need to prepare yourself. They say the Down's kids are the sweetest, but beware, there are lots of problems. The best you can do is to love him and to understand that he will be a huge drain on your life.

These kids have a ton of health problems. You'll need to get an echocardiogram immediately. They always have lots of heart problems."

I thought he'd stop, but he didn't. He just kept piling it on, "You have to be willing to make a serious commitment to be able to take care of one of these types of kids. You need to be aware that lots of marriages end in divorce over things like this. There are people who will take him if you can't handle this."

Chris and I now openly talk about the horror of those early hours, how the doctor was clearly not accepting of people with Down syndrome, how utterly uninformed and wrong he was, how the pediatrician shared those views and outdated stereotypes. Most of all, I look back and cry when I remember how painful those first days were: how I kept thinking about how awful and terrible my life was going to be with Joshua.

Today, as I watch our son stack blocks and bee-bop to his favorite kids' music, or clap wildly with his father when their favorite basketball team makes a three-point shot, I know that things will be okay. That doctor was simply clueless about the real life of people and families with Down syndrome in their lives!

Looking back, I wish those doctors would have shown me the artwork done by adults with Down syndrome, let me read about the adults with Down syndrome who graduate from community colleges with associate of arts degrees, or given me the web address for Karen Gaffney, a young woman with T21 who swam in an English Channel relay and travels the country speaking as a self-advocate. I wish they would have given me some of the poems and books written by adults with Down syndrome, or let me watch videos of their national organization's annual talent shows to see that some people with Down syndrome play multiple instruments, sing beautifully, or have an amazing talent for dancing. I wish they would have told me that teens with Down syndrome are frequently not classified as "mentally retarded," but only as "learning disabled," and that many have IQ scores in the mid-80s, some even higher.

I guess what I really wish is that they would have told me about some of the things our son might do, rather than telling us what they thought he never would do. I admit that I would have never been happy when I received the news that my son had Down syndrome, but I know that the way I was told made things worse, much worse.

One week after his birth, Joshua's karyotype confirmed the doctor's suspicions; he does have T21. Quite honestly, I spent five months on antidepressants and had a hard time coming to terms with our son's diagnosis, and without Chris's love and support, I'm not sure I would have made it through all the sadness. Today, I actively work with new parents who have received diagnoses of T21 and try to help them get more updated information about Down syndrome. I try to help them deal with the roller coaster of emotions they will face. I know because I've been there.

Comparing Our Experiences

You might be guessing that Kate's experiences and mine were years apart. Wrong. Her son is one month younger than my daughter. You might be guessing that it happened in an entirely different area of the country then. Wrong. We live less than 10 miles apart.

The difference? The doctors that delivered my child were at a teaching hospital that also happens to have one of the country's best clinics for children and adults with Down syndrome, and the doctors were well trained and prepared for all types of birth experiences. They were familiar with the most recent information on Down syndrome, but more importantly, they were cognizant of their language choices and the impact of their interpersonal interactions. Had my daughter, Maren, not shown signs of distress, she would have been born in the same hospital as Josh.

By now, most people have heard about people-first language, but many may not fully understand how important it is to a parent of a child with special needs to talk first about the child and only second about the diagnosis. Children with Down syndrome are first and foremost children. Talking about them as "Down's children" only focuses on one aspect of their identity and obscures their individuality. Individuals with Down syndrome should be talked about as babies, children, teens, and adults with Down syndrome or with T21.

Further, medical professionals who reject the child as a diagnosis, rather than a child, as happened in Joshua's case, cause significant emotional harm for the entire family unit. Kate says she would love to talk to the doctor who delivered Josh and the pediatrician who first talked to them about T21 and let them know about the harm they caused with their language and judgments, but she's still too angry and afraid. She thinks she will only be effective when she can rationally discuss their behavior with them.

GETTING A PRENATAL DIAGNOSIS

As you were reading Kate, Chris, and Joshua's story, you may have been thinking, that could not have happened, but in fact, it did, and it does. Sadly, though, the communication of the diagnosis and the provider interactions after the birth of a child with T21 are frequently problematic and poorly managed; believe it or not, however, they are thought by many to be much better than those diagnoses that occur prenatally. At least in many post-birth diagnoses, the caregivers recognize that the child is here to stay and work to help the parents adjust to the news. However, in a prenatal diagnosis of T21, a doctor's words can be even more powerful and painful. According to medical studies, 9 of 10 who receive a prenatal diagnosis of Down syndrome through amniocentesis will choose to abort (Hook, Mutton, Ide, Alberman, & Bobrow, 1998; Smith-Bindman et al., 2001).

Many parents of kids with T21 argue that the reasons that many couples choose to terminate reside, at least in part, with the negativity of the doctors presenting the information. Several of those parents readily admit that they, too, considered termination after they left the doctors' offices because the information that the caregivers provided was so negative. Down syndrome is often framed as a life-shattering experience, as was the case with Joshua. One mom, who has a 12-year-old with T21, says:

> I will never judge a parent for choosing termination. Each parent has the right to choose whether or not they can handle the responsibility of a child with special needs. However, I will judge doctors who paint unnecessarily negative pictures of what life with a child with Down syndrome is like. I believe in my heart that most people who chose to terminate because they can't handle having a child with special needs do not have accurate information about Down syndrome. If they did, they would see that it's really not that big of a deal. Most days, we forget Nate even has Down syndrome. No joke.

For this mom, how doctors talk about T21 has a dramatic impact on the families receiving the diagnosis and can often result in unnecessary fear and worry. In fact, doctors' negative interactions with parents of prenatally diagnosed fetuses are one of the most commonly addressed topics on support boards.

In response to his own experience with a prenatal diagnosis of T21 with his own son, one father, Bob Lincoln,[3] wrote the following piece to help doctors think about the implication of the way they frame Down syndrome.

> "Warning: this post is intended to make a serious point in an interesting way. It is not meant to offend anyone, except possibly doctors."

NORMAL SYNDROME

How to give parents a prenatal diagnosis:

I'm very sorry, I have the results of the genetic tests and they have confirmed our suspicions that your fetus is what we call... Normal. Some people prefer the terms "Ordinarily Challenged" or "Normal Syndrome." The syndrome can be easily identified by a complete lack of any interesting genetic characteristics. I know this will come as a shock to you, but you should be aware of what this is likely to mean.

If your fetus manages to survive the rest of the pregnancy and the birth, which is becoming more common these days, he or she will face some daunting challenges. Children who suffer from normalcy are prone to health and psychological problems. It is almost certain that the growing child will suffer a seemingly endless stream of viruses. They will frequently damage themselves, and sometimes others, from their excessive energy.

Their relentless demands will put a strain on your existing family and, of course, your relationship with your partner will suffer, and possibly end in a painful and acrimonious separation. Any children you already have, even if they also suffer from normalcy, will be jealous of the newcomer and all their extra attention. Many siblings are liable to be psychologically scarred by the new arrival.

I need hardly mention the financial consequences, although disastrous, will be nothing compared to the emotional turmoil your life will suffer.

After a while, you may be lucky and find they can be kind and loving young children. They may find some temporary happiness in things such as music, dancing, food, or playing with toys.

But if they survive early childhood, a Normal child is almost certain to grow into a Normal adolescent. Your years of sacrifice will be thrown back in your face as they become disobedient, wild, and reckless. Unable to find happiness and contentment, they will treat you with contempt until they manage to leave home. Even then, the suffering will continue as they will often return to try and extract money. They will blame you for their own faults and leave you bitter and twisted.

They may well become criminals. Over a quarter of Normals will have trouble with the law, many will spend time in jail. Many will have problems with alcohol or drug abuse. Normal marriages are often unhappy and short, and over half end in divorce.

Even if they become successful, this is likely to be because of the often-observed tendency of Normals towards excessive greed. The chances of them sharing their success with you are remote, and they will tend to see you as an embarrassment.

Finally, Normal people are likely to die before their time. Twenty-three percent will die of cancer, 33% of heart disease. Hundreds every year in this country alone are so distressed by their condition that they take their own life. I'm sorry to say that many will have had a lonely, painful and pointless existence.

I am afraid that Normal Syndrome is a genetic condition that affects every cell of the body, and so is impossible to cure.

Termination is an option. Shall I book an appointment?

—From a parent who received a diagnosis rather like this

This piece clearly highlights the ways that parents are frequently told about their child's diagnosis and offers a perspective on the importance of framing an issue like T21 for parents. It also shows the power of the medical professional for shaping the ways in which T21 is understood.

Parents discussing this piece in online chat rooms and electronic bulletin boards repeatedly said things like, "Wow, this captured thoughts I've had but have never been able to put into words," and "This perfectly captures my experience of getting Jess's amnio results. I can remember the doctor rattling off all the things my child would never, ever do. I went home and cried for days, pitying myself and was ready to schedule the termination. Finally, a friend said to me, "'Lisa, there are no guarantees with any child, and even a child born normal could develop problems later. At least, with this child, you'll know to get a jumpstart on her learning and education. You'll know her challenges and be able to get her all the help in the world.'" Jess's mom continued, "If every doctor would read this, they [sic] might think twice about being so negative. It's a fabulous spin on the words we have all heard. Thank you!"

Ultimately, the doctors involved in the diagnosis and care of fetuses and infants with an extra chromosome have tremendous power to shape and alter the way parents feel about Down syndrome. The language they use, the scenarios they present, and the nonverbal cues they display have tremendous impact on the parents' ability to understand and accept Down syndrome.

When most parents find out that we are pregnant, we often say that all we want is "a healthy baby with ten fingers and ten toes." Truthfully, what most of us also want is a gorgeous child who will make strangers stop and gawk, who will be the smartest kid in the play group and will have the most friends. We want a child who is a superstar in dance or football, who will star in the school play, who will get a full scholarship to Harvard. And, in our truly selfish moments, perhaps preposterous pondering, we even wonder if it is too much to wish for dimples.

Hearing a diagnosis of Down syndrome, either after birth or prenatally, may seem like all of those dreams shattering in an instant. Clearly, when a child is conceived, parents do not hope for a child with an extra chromosome, and that news can be devastating, even when presented well. Doctors need to think about the implications of the ways in which they present the news and the language they use. Though they cannot remove the extra genetic material, they can help lessen the pain, even pave the way for acceptance, by presenting the information in nonthreatening and nonjudgmental ways.

UNCERTAINTY AND TENSIONS SURROUNDING A CHILD'S DEVELOPMENT

Though the interactions with medical professionals during the diagnosis period are formative, interactions with medical and therapy providers will continue throughout the child's life. Professionals need to be cognizant of their power in these later interactions as well.

Kara and Mitchell

A few months after Mitchell's birth and diagnosis, my biggest question was, "Well, is it severe? He doesn't look that much like he has it." The doctor started to explain everything to me, and I just started to cry. He began, "First, we cannot tell you how functioning your child is going to be on the basis of his diagnosis. Just as with any child, by looking at the cells in his body, we cannot determine how smart he will be. You will find that out in time, like you would with any kid."

I continued, "But he doesn't look like he has it. Doesn't that mean anything?" I remember reaching and grasping for any straw. I needed a glimmer of hope that he would be okay. "No, I'm sorry;" said the doctor. "There is no relationship between his outward appearance and his developmental level."

Somehow, I didn't believe him. I didn't want to believe him. Every parent should be able to look forward to the mysteries of a child unfolding, wondering what the next day will bring, how smart, how funny, how athletic the child will be. Most parents look forward to the child becoming his or her own person, but I didn't want that. I wanted to know what Mitchell was going to be like. If he was going to be smart, I could sit back and enjoy him and help work to make him smarter, but if he was going to be severely retarded, I needed time to adjust, to start making plans for him.

Now, Mitchell is 4 years old, and I cringe if people ask if he's retarded or if he is high functioning or low functioning. I can't believe they do not see that he is just Mitchell and that the beauty of him isn't contingent on his functioning! Each day, he grows and learns and loves. Had I known from the outset he would be high functioning, I might have pushed him so hard that he'd hate to learn. And, if I had been told he would be low functioning, I might have given up and never exposed him to this beautiful world. It may have been a self-fulfilling prophecy.

Funny thing, Mitchell is like every other kid; he has strengths in some areas and weaknesses in others. He walked at 16 months and has great motor skills now. His talking is still delayed, and we rely on lots of sign language. But I know one thing for certain; part of being his mom is learning that there are no certainties with children.

A few weeks ago, we had Mitchell's checkup at a clinic for kids with Down syndrome, and the doctor started to tell me where Mitchell was at developmentally with his peers. I stopped her. She said, "Don't you want to know how he's doing?" "Not by your standards," I told her. "I know what he is doing everyday. He's learning to read. He knows his colors. He counts to 12. He loves watching Barney. He helps me change his little sister's diaper and loves to teach her things. I don't care where he rates on a chart." As the words left my lips, the doctor started to grin. "Wow," she said, "your child is truly lucky to have you as a mom." I replied, "No, I'm the lucky one to have him as a son." My, I have come full circle.

Kate, Chris, and Joshua

For us, the biggest issue that we dealt with after trying to come to terms with Josh's Down syndrome was learning how to deal with the constant pressure to "treat him like a normal kid." Every one from doctors, to nurses, and therapists were telling us, "treat Josh like a normal kid and he'll be normal." Easy for them to say. They were constantly doing things to remind us how "not normal" he was.

What other kids have 5 hours of therapy each week? Even if it's a normal day, as soon as the physical therapist walks in and says, "Geez. He's still not developing sufficient ankle stability," or "He's currently operating at a 32% delay in gross motor skills," we are abruptly reminded that he's not normal. How can he live a normal life when every activity has a purpose? Chris and I pick puzzles that have a certain size knobs and think about how sippy cup brand X might affect his tongue protrusion that will ultimately hinder his speech. If we let him watch a cartoon that is not on the Public Broadcasting Service, we feel guilty because I wasted 30 minutes of learning in his life.

It sounds silly to people who don't live this, but before a therapist comes over, we find ourselves hiding the "bad" toys and setting out the "good" ones that they have recommended. One day, our developmental therapist saw a shape sorter sitting out. "Josh is way too young to be tackling that. You will confuse him if you don't put it away. He cannot worry about shapes until he has mastered colors," she said. I responded, "Well, he really likes this toy, and he's doing well with it." She looked at me with a disgusted look and said, "If he starts regressing on colors, don't say I didn't tell you so."

I was furious. What other parents have self-appointed toy specialists telling them what toys their children can and cannot play with? Luckily, Chris and I talked it over, and we switched therapists. We have the constant reminders of how Josh has Down syndrome with his therapists, but we surely did not need someone telling us how to parent too! We are glad we ignored her. Josh has now mastered three shapes and four colors.

Our instincts about what he could do were better than her training. Sometimes, to be normal, we just need to act more like normal parents and stop trying to please therapists. Slowly, we are realizing that if Josh is going to be as normal as possible, we have to start acting normally too. I find myself angry at them for controlling my life, and I have to stop and realize that I'm letting them do this and I have the power to stop it. Josh really benefits from his therapies, and I know they are invaluable. But I have to follow my instinct more, too, and speak up when I'm feeling uncomfortable.

Sheila and Kasey

Kasey is nearly two and learning how to be the best mom for her has been hard. People say "just treat her like you would any other kid," but there is a whole early intervention system of therapists that are set up to "fix her." The therapists we used were always trying to rate her, evaluate her, and tell me where she fit on a chart for development. When she was 9 months, they said her language scores put her at a five-month-old level, her gross motor skills at a four-month-old level, but her social skills were on track at a nine-month level. Overall, I was devastated.

Most of her scores put her at half of her chronological age. After talking to lots of mothers and finding a Web site called "Disabilityisnatural.com," I realized that Kasey doesn't need to be fixed. She is different, but all of us are in some way. I'm not so sure why everyone on our team is so concerned about making Kasey fit their mold rather than helping her be the best kid she can be.

I took control with the therapists. I told them to stop ranking and evaluating her. One therapist said, "Sheila, we have to rank Kasey so we can get her to normal levels. If we don't know where she is, we won't know how to get her where she needs to go." I realized she was trying to be helpful, but what she didn't see was that we kept focusing on all the things that were wrong with Kasey rather than her accomplishments.

The next week when she came, I was thrilled and said, "Look, look, Kasey can sit up on her own! Isn't that wonderful?" The therapist said, "Okay. Now can we get her to push to a four-point for crawling?" She did not stop for one second to applaud or say "that's fabulous." I was so proud to show off Kasey's new trick and I just felt deflated.

If she was a typical kid, I know this woman would have stopped to celebrate with me. The fact is that most therapists think their job is to fix Kasey and they don't understand that I don't see her as broken. Sure, she'll do things a bit slower than other kids, but she will do them. And, I want to celebrate each step along the way. Down syndrome is a beautiful thing. I feel grateful that I have been blessed by a child who sees beauty everywhere she turns. She is inquisitive and charming. I see a beautiful world through her eyes.

Stories like the above are prevalent in the Down syndrome community. There is often a love–hate relationship with doctors and therapists. Parents want their children to reach their full potential and know that medical professionals and therapists can help them. But evaluations and therapy sessions are also a constant reminder, even barrier, to leading a "normal" life for many families. Further, many parents also see therapists as failing to see and enjoy the development of the kids that they work with.

Jon, Carol, and Maren

We now have wonderful relationships with most of Maren's doctors and therapists.[4] In fact, even Maren eagerly awaits her speech, physical, and music therapy sessions. The relationships we have forged have taken work, though. After reading through story after story after story on online support groups about troubled therapist–family relationships, like the ones you have read about in this chapter, we took control of Maren's evaluations early on.

We told our providers that we would not allow Maren to be ranked in comparison with her 46-chromosomed peers and that we wanted to focus on goals for development, not delays she was experiencing. We also told them to try to refrain from using the word "normal". For us, like for many parents, normal is a strange word. It is often a painful word because it reflects an evaluative stance: Normal is Good; Abnormal is Bad. In its place, we prefer "typical" and "atypical."

Typically developing children progress at particular rates, and being atypical does not have such negative connotations. We similarly ask them to refrain from classifying Maren as "high functioning" or "low functioning." Though doctors and therapists find these terms useful, we seem them as needlessly evaluative. Honestly, we know that children who are high functioning are more acceptable to the majority of practitioners than kids who are not. We see these labels as simplistic and demeaning. We also believe that these labels serve to obscure a child's individuality and contribute to an overall assessment of a child rather than detailed attention to each child's strengths and weaknesses.

We have benefited tremendously from the mothers and fathers who have traveled this path before us. The labels may make life easier for the providers, but this is not about easy. It is about children who are loved by their parents and adored by siblings, and with the right support and help, chromosomally enhanced children will grow to be wonderful and productive adults.

DOCTORS' DEMEANOR

Jon, Carol, and Maren

In the process of learning our way through the therapy and medical communities, we have altered our therapy team members a couple of times and switched doctors. We insist on a provider's willingness to see our perspective, even if they do not agree with it. We are happy to be challenged, but we will not be ignored. We knew we had found the ideal doctor for Maren when, during our first visit, Dr. Baker simply listened to all of our concerns.

When she spoke, she began with, "As you will soon learn, if you haven't already, as a general pediatrician, I do not know everything there is to know about Down syndrome and cannot follow all of the latest trends and treatments. I will rely on you to correct me if I am doing something counter to your wishes and to keep me abreast of medical treatments that will affect Maren. You will be her biggest advocates and supporters, so don't be afraid of speaking up with me or any of her providers."

Needless to say, we are grateful that we found this doctor. We have been fortunate to be able to search out team members that could help us maximize our development. It is sad that we had to search, but realistic. Many of our friends relay horror stories of misinformed and verbally abusive doctors.

Christina, Dale, and Stephanie

Upon seeking an augmentative communication device to help our eight-year old daughter, Stephanie, who happens to be nonverbal (she has multiple physical problems unrelated to T21), we were told by her doctor, "It's probably a waste. You have no reason to believe your child would have anything worthwhile to say."

I cannot help but cry each time I think about that conversation, and Dale gets furious just thinking about it. We would have felt better if he would have punched us. . . . We could not believe he said that to us, and we were so stunned, we couldn't even say a word to him.

After we talked to four different specialists, many of whom were very negative, Stephanie received the device. Now, at 9 $1/2$ years old, Stephanie loves programming the pictures in the device to tell us about books she enjoys, the friends she is making, and how much she loves us and her sisters. She has so very much to communicate: feelings, ideas, beliefs, and thoughts, lots of thoughts.

After agonizing for nearly a year, I sat down and wrote a note to Stephanie's original doctor that said, "For some, a picture is worth a thousand words. For me and my family, it is worth our lives and our happiness. I'm sorry that you are unable to share in the wonder and joy that we know and experience every day and hope you will never keep another family from the joy you nearly kept us from. Stephanie not only has things to say, she has love to share." Not surprisingly, we have never received a reply from him.

Jenny and Catrina

Catrina had just turned 9 months old when she got very sick and was admitted to the pediatric intensive care unit for respiratory distress. She was diagnosed with viral pneumonia. On Friday, two days after being admitted, she was transferred to the pediatric floor, and we were visited by a second-year resident. It was obvious he had not reviewed her chart, as when he looked at her he said, "Oh, she's a Down's kid" and went on talking about how the chromosomes split and basically explaining T21 to me (like this was the first time I'd heard this in the nine months since she was born).

Well, believe it or not, he got worse. He started telling me that "Down's kids" are always sick, "you just can't keep them healthy" and that "they get everything." Keep in mind, this is a second-year resident! Where was he getting all of this information/experience to pass on to me? He continued by saying, "They will always be sick, their whole short lives," and "They get really sick and almost die; then they are fine the next day."

The entire time, he was not even looking at her or examining her. He was leaning against the rail of her bed spewing this garbage. Then he said something that astounded me. He said "Us doctors have a private joke (maybe it should stay private!). Down's kids, You just can't kill them." Can you believe this?!? He never examined her or talked about her condition.

I went off. I explained to him that his facts were wrong, that children with Down syndrome have an average life expectancy of 55 years. I told him that some do have significant health issues, but that others do not. I also told him referring to my daughter as "a Down's" was offensive, and that his joke was disgusting. He looked at me and told me I was getting all upset about nothing and that I was just "on edge" because my daughter was sick. He told me I needed to relax.

I wrote letters (as did at least 50 of my friends) to the hospital and the director of the residency program. The director apologized profusely, and I hope they can take care of that jerk. What scares me is that there are probably so many ill-educated doctors out there, and they can really make our lives tough. You would think they would know better. Obviously, they don't! Who is supposed to teach them? Where are they getting trained? Why isn't it working? That is what I want to know.

THE JOURNEY CONTINUES

Reading the scenarios in this case study, I hope that you can see some of the challenges that parents of children with T21 face when dealing with the medical and therapeutic communities. As a member of the T21 community for nearly two years, I have been shocked and saddened by all of the horrible things parents have endured from the medical community and therapists.

Conversely, I have friends whose lives have been enriched by those in the same profession. One dear friend, mom to a 3-year-old girl with T21, says, "My therapists and doctors make my life wonderful. They constantly help me strive for more for my daughter. They are her biggest cheerleaders, and I cannot imagine this journey without them! I'm grateful each and every day that I have a team who sees the beauty and brilliance in my daughter that I see."

As I have noted, I have had predominantly positive experiences, but I have had to work to develop the relationships we have and choose our providers carefully. In many ways, it is disappointing that so much work needs to be invested in finding providers with positive outlooks who are also willing to work closely with parents without feeling threatened or annoyed.

My daughter Maren is quickly approaching two years old. She takes swimming lessons, dances like it is going out of style, is addicted to Maisy, a children's television character, loves mangoes and french fries, and screams if an egg is headed in her direction. She loves teasing her older brother and kissing her younger brother when he cries. She even helps me change his diapers. She climbs the stairs as soon as you turn your back and, last week, she showed amazing resourcefulness. She went to the low cupboard where her cups are kept, grabbed one, and headed to the toilet. For curiosity's sake, I watched. She lowered her cup into the bowl, and scooped some water. She was thirsty. Luckily, she is never unsupervised.

Quite simply, Maren is a toddler. All of my friends with chromosomally enhanced children have similar funny, typical baby and toddler stories to tell. Many of them do not only accept Down syndrome, they celebrate it and feel blessed by the child they have. They frequently talk of learning the true meaning of unconditional love and speak of seeing the world through new eyes. Our children have an extra 21st chromosome; we know they have something extra special.

The late and much beloved Mr. Rogers hit the proverbial nail on the head with the quote used at the outset of this case: "No child is perfect in each and every way, and each child has endless possibilities for success" (Rogers, 1994). How we choose to evaluate children with different needs, orient toward them and their families, and talk about them, is a reflection of our own views and beliefs about their wholeness and their potential. If only health and therapy providers could truly understand that this journey into the land of Down syndrome, though unplanned for most, can be a marvelous adventure for parents, they might be better able to orient themselves to us in ways that reflect this understanding. They would be able to help us reframe our own experiences and look for the strengths and accomplishments of each individual child—and every child deserves no less.

RELEVANT CONCEPTS

Dialectical tensions: The contradictions, paradoxes, and/or competing demands that exist in interpersonal relationships.

Emotional support: The provision of empathic and responsive communication.

Framing: The way that we invoke models or perspectives to understand our experience. Frames are our basic organizing principles for seeing the world and making sense of our interactions.

Labeling: The process through which we give names to certain characteristics or traits that will have an effect on the ways that people orient themselves to those characteristics or traits. For example, it has been shown that students identified at the beginning of the school year to their teacher as either "slow" or "gifted," regardless of actual ability, will, at the end of the year, tend to perform at the level that corresponds to the arbitrary label.

Mindfulness: A term typically attributed to psychologist Ellen Langer represents a deliberate attempt to stress process over outcome and a conscious effort to open up one's mind to new information and alternative perspectives. Mindfulness is generally contrasted with mindlessness, the process of automatic, effortless thought.

Self-fulfilling prophecy: People often behave in ways that confirm the expectations of others, even if the behaviors would not have been present without the knowledge of those expectations. The end result is that the original prophecies get "confirmed," thus creating a cycle of expectation and confirmation.

Social construction of reality: Its fundamental premise is that knowledge and reality are not things to be discovered, but that they are achieved and created through interaction with others.

Uncertainty reduction: During relational development, individuals seek to minimize the ambiguity that is often present. According to uncertainty reduction theory, individuals are uncomfortable with uncertainty because it prevents us from accurately predicting interaction outcomes.

DISCUSSION QUESTIONS

1. As is frequently the case with struggles over language and terminology, it is possible you might be thinking, what difference does it matter if I call someone a "Down's" or a "Down's kid" versus "a child with T21?" If you have had that thought, close your eyes and think of a waiter. Describe that person in detail. Now, close your eyes again and think of a waitress. Describe that person in detail. Did you get two distinctly different images? How might that exemplify the differences between a "Down's baby" and a "baby with T21?"

2. How can parents manage the tensions of a normal life with a child with special needs? What role can providers play to make the balance easier?

3. What is "normal"? And what other concepts might represent the construct without the evaluative component?

4. If you were responsible for providing services to a child with a special need, what ways might you be able to point out developmental problems in nonthreatening ways?

5. One of the most common things parents report hearing when their child is first diagnosed (often at birth) is "I'm sorry." Why might providers, family members and friends refrain from saying this? What are some positive, supportive communication alternatives?

6. Consider the implications of some of the alternatives you generated above. What might be the downsides to those as well? Think about how "God doesn't give you anything you can't handle?" might reflect on the child and on your own views of T21. What about "Special people get special babies"?

7. Now, think about how responses, such as "Congratulations on your baby! I don't know much about T21. Is there anything I can do to help you figure all of this out?" or "Wow. You must have really mixed emotions right now. You've got a great new baby, but some unexpected news. Do you want to talk?" How might these be perceived?

8. Given that language is a powerful force in shaping the views of individuals with T21, how might parents go about educating family, friends, and care providers on the importance of their language when talking about T21 and their child?

ENDNOTES

[1] The interactions reported here are all based on real experiences. Identifying information of all parties, except my own family and poem contributor, Bob Lincoln, has been changed. Further, some cases are amalgams of several people's experiences.

[2] APGAR scores are infant assessments that help the medical team determine if a baby needs assistance adjusting to life outside the womb. The test is given twice, once 1 minute and another 5 minutes after birth. A score of 10 suggests the infant is completely healthy, and with any score lower than a 5, the baby needs immediate assistance in regulating his or her own body outside the womb. Though named for its inventor, Dr. Maria Apgar, medical trainees are often taught to remember the five parts of the test using the acronym (the letters of her last name): A = appearance, P = pulse, G = grimace, A = activity, and R = respiratory effort. A baby can earn 0 to 2 points for each factor; thus, 10 is a "perfect" score.

[3] Bob Lincoln has given the author permission to print his essay and his real name.

[4] When Maren was 2 days old, I posted on an Internet support group that is filled with other parents that are now among my closest friends. I have learned so much from them, including how I want to work with Maren's providers and what I can do to make the world a better place for her. I have also learned how many parents suffer without the information I garnered—information and support that providers could so readily provide.

REFERENCES/SUGGESTED READINGS

Drugan, A., Greb A., Johnson M. P., Krivchenia E. L., Uhlmann, W. R., Moghissi, K. S., & Evans M. I. (1990). Determinants of parental decisions to abort for chromosome abnormalities. *Prenatal Diagnosis, 10*, 483–490.

Hook, E. B., Mutton, D. E., Ide, R., Alberman, E. D., & Bobrow, M. (1998). The natural history of Down syndrome conceptuses diagnosed prenatally which are not electively terminated. *American Journal of Human Genetics, 57*, 875–881.

Langer, E. (1989). *Mindfulness.* New York: Addison-Wesley.

Rogers, F. (1994). *You are special: Words of wisdom from America's most beloved neighbor.* New York: Viking.

Smith-Bindman, R., Hosmer, W., Feldstein, V. A., & Goldberg, J. D. (2001). Second-trimester ultrasound to detect fetuses with Down syndrome. *JAMA, 285*(8), 1044–1055.

Stallings, G., & Cook, S. (1997). *Another season: A coach's story of raising an exceptional son.* New York: Broadway Books.

Stray-Gunderson, K. (1995). *Babies with Down syndrome* (2nd ed.). Bethesda, MD: Woodbine House.

Stuve-Bodeen, S. (1998). *We'll paint the octopus red.* Bethesda, MD: Woodbine House. (This is a wonderful children's book geared toward siblings and is an excellent first read).

Zukoff, M. (2002). *Choosing Naia.* Boston, MA: Beacon Press.

Additional Resources

http://www.ds-health.com: This is a Web site maintained by an M.D. who is also the father of a child with T21. This site has all of the latest news related to Down syndrome research.

http://www.ndss.org: This web site is sponsored by the National Down Syndrome Society and provides a wealth of information for providers, families, friends, and students looking for further information on T21.

17

Grieving Families: Social Support After the Death of a Loved One

Craig R. Hullett
University of Wisconsin–Madison

There is no need to debate whether the death of a loved one impacts the surviving family members. Questions regarding how to help people deal with their grief, however, are far from answered. There are no "silver-bullet" comforting messages; the experience of grief is sufficiently subjective to require competent supporters to adapt to the varying needs of individuals. The variance is increased by the differential capabilities of children to identify, express, and control their grief. Despite some parallels in emotional responses, the supportive needs of children and adult family members differ substantially, negating the potential for any one supportive approach to be effective for both children and adults. Over the last couple of decades, support groups in numerous communities have been established that are specifically designed to help all members of grieving families. These groups attempt to tailor their services to the specific needs of their members according to the ways in which grief affects family members of varying ages. This case focuses on one such facility, fictionally titled The Center.

THE EXPERIENCE AND EXPRESSION OF GRIEF

Individual reactions to the death of a family member vary, but generally include some common responses. Denial is possible for a period of time and is often experienced as a state of shock, but anger and depression are considered inevitable. Supporters may rally around the surviving family for a short time after the death, but soon, the survivors are often left feeling a sense of isolation and detachment. People may withdraw, and this period is when marriages are especially likely to suffer. Couples who lose a child often find themselves fighting more often, and their marital satisfaction suffers. Generally, adults enter The Center expressing a wide range of negative emotions, including depression, anger, guilt, anxiety, and isolation.

Children also show many emotional reactions to the death of a family member, and the reactions often depend upon the age of the child. Death is not comprehended fully by children under five years old, but the separation can still affect them. For the youngest children, there is often some regression exhibited, such as loss of toilet training. Most children after that age, and almost all children by age 10, can comprehend the reality and finality of death at both concrete and abstract levels of thinking. Children are likely to withdraw and become angry or depressed. Physiological symptoms, such as change in appetite, headaches, lethargy, and sleep disturbances, are common. Adolescents show strong reactions, including depression, anger, isolation, and decreases in school performance. Grief reactions may manifest in behaviors such as fighting, acting out, and getting into trouble at school.

THE CENTER: SUPPORT GROUPS FOR GRIEVING FAMILIES

The Center is a nonprofit organization dedicated to caring for grieving families. It accepts children ranging from age 3 to 18, as well as their parents or guardians. It was created because the community had no resources dedicated specifically to the support of grieving children. The Center does not charge for services, and it is nondenominational. The administration recognizes and encourages the spiritual side of the grieving process, but these two policies are designed to make the groups more accessible to a wider range of participants.

The treatment of grief is considered a family-based rather than individual-based endeavor, but differences in terms of child development and general supportive needs are reflected in the different groups formed for participants. Specifically, children attend support groups with other children similar in age (i.e., preschool, early elementary school, later elementary school, junior high school, and high school age ranges). The rules for group placement are not rigid, however, in that the incoming child's needs and capabilities are assessed in an attempt to match the child with the most appropriate group. Groups are also divided according to who died. Thus, children who have lost a parent are in a different group than children who have lost a sibling. Similarly, the parent groups are divided between parents who are grieving the loss of a child and parents who are grieving the loss of a spouse. These distinctions reflect an overarching goal of having a common foundation of experiences and needs within the groups. One additional advantage of this structure is that it also allows for some freedom of communication outside of the constraints of speaking in front of the remaining family members. Some might be "putting on a brave face" to protect the other members from more distress. The Center's administrators believe that talking about one's grief without such concerns is more liberating and beneficial.

The groups meet one evening per week. Before the sessions start, the group members and facilitators convene for a potluck dinner. This event is pleasantly noisy, much like a large family reunion. Name tags are affixed, friends formed over the past few weeks are greeted with hugs and smiles, and new members are casually introduced much like new friends are at any social gathering. No one goes into great detail about their past week here in the crowd—the time for that is just a little while away. After dinner, the participants break into their groups for sessions that last for about an hour and a half.

Support Group Structures

The activities within the individual groups vary according to developmental level and the person who died, but they all follow some common rules. All sessions start with a discussion circle in which members are encouraged, but never compelled, to talk about their feelings. Children and adults are reminded that what is discussed in group discussion is not to be discussed with people outside of the center as a means of protecting their privacy. However, children are also told that they should feel free to discuss anything with their family members.

There are many activities for the preschool children. The children are not presumed by members of The Center to be facile in expressing their grief. Therefore, the children spend much of their time with arts and crafts activities designed to allow the children to express their feelings in less explicit ways. The facilitators then help the children better identify the emotions associated with their reactions. Some children in these lowest age ranges have difficulty recalling or retaining pleasant memories of the deceased. Thus, there are several activities where the child is asked to tell stories about that person as a method for building memories.

The groups of children in middle school also allow for play and art-based activities. Memory exercises are still common, but these children have more concrete memories already in mind. They are typically much more cognizant about the permanence associated with death, and their discussions are correspondingly less abstract with regard to the loss. However, they frequently have difficulty controlling their emotions and behaviors, so activities are designed to help them identify emotions and their proper expression. One such activity involves having the children make drawings of how they feel. Another activity involves the children writing letters to their loved ones. The goals of such exercises are to get the children to attend to and express their grief, and also to open discussion about the appropriate outlets for their feelings. To that end, facilitators point out that the feelings themselves are natural and should not be labeled as "good" or "bad." They instead try to help the children understand the difference between the feeling and its expression, focusing on the latter as the element that needs to be controlled.

The adolescent groups operate like many adult support groups. Very little time is spent doing anything other than talking. Adolescents' parents note that these children suffer from substantial feelings of depression, anger, and isolation, and the adolescents' discussions frequently center on these feelings. Children from approximately junior high through high school are aware of their feelings and norms for their expression and, although some may have difficulty confronting their feelings, they are capable of identifying and discussing them directly.

The activities for parents are always discussion-based, differing substantially according to the person who died. Parents who have lost a child often focus on ways of maintaining their relationships, expressing the fact that the death has reduced their satisfaction with each other. Parents who have lost a spouse frequently discuss the practical and emotional losses associated with the death of a life partner. There are consistencies, however, in that all are concerned about the welfare of their surviving children, and all have their own grief as well.

With the above sketch of the support groups operated by The Center, we now consider the experience of two representative families as they proceed through their initial meetings with The Center.[1]

Case Family A: The Andersons

Steven and Linda Anderson have been married for 19 years. Both work full time, he as a middle manager at the local manufacturing plant and she as an accountant. Their son Mark, a junior high student, had always been a popular, extraverted boy. He did not do especially well in his classes, but his quick wit made it apparent to most of his teachers that he was a gifted student who never applied himself. Instead, he seemed far more interested in being the class clown and having fun with his friends doing anything other than schoolwork.

Five months ago, 17-year-old Audra, Mark's sister, was in the passenger seat of her boyfriend's car. It was a Saturday night, and they had just left the last party before school was set to resume after summer recess. Her boyfriend had had a bit to drink, but swore he was okay to drive. He survived the 45-mph impact with the tree eight minutes later, but Audra was thrown from the car and sustained severe injuries. Steven and Linda spent the following 51 hours at the hospital by their daughter's side. After consulting with their doctor, obtaining a second opinion, and taking a few minutes to say goodbye, Steven gave permission to end Audra's life support.

Case Family B: The Langdons

The Langdons have not been a very fortunate family for the past two years. The economy had been rough on manufacturing jobs and Thomas found himself on leave without pay from the plant for several extended periods. Michelle Langdon had done her best to work part time jobs at one of the local supermarkets, but that left her with little time and money to distribute to her three children. One of Michelle's sisters often helped by watching TJ, the youngest at four years old. Michelle also relied heavily on her daughters Tina (age 10) and Stephanie (age 16).

Thomas always had quite a cough from all of the smoking he did, and he figured the chest pain was primarily stress related. The rapid rate at which he dropped 25 pounds, however, convinced him it was time to visit the doctor. Despite the fact that he always joked about "cancer sticks," he was legitimately surprised when his doctor told him after his biopsy that he had small-cell lung cancer at an advanced stage. Six months of treatment did nothing to stop the course of the disease, and Thomas finally succumbed while in hospice care two months ago.

The Andersons' First Day

Steven and Linda Anderson both met with Susan, The Center's intake coordinator, early Tuesday afternoon. They were scheduled to begin attending the group sessions that night and needed to meet with Susan for the standard brief interview and orientation before they and their son could attend. At this initial meeting, Susan collects basic demographic information about each member of the family who will attend. She also collects information about the deceased, the way in which that person died, and the parents' perceptions of their children's reactions to that death. Finally, she asks what the family hopes to accomplish at The Center.

Linda answered most of Susan's questions. She informed Susan that they had tried to talk with Mark about how he's feeling, but felt that they were pushing him too much. Mark would always reply, either explicitly or implicitly, that he wanted to be "left alone." Linda said that they both noticed Mark was spending much of his time away from them these days, either out with friends or buried in his room with the music blaring. "We know that when a person withdraws that can be a sign of depression, but we just can't tell if he's acting like this because of his sister's accident or if he's just being a normal teenager. I mean, the music he keeps listening to sounds pretty depressing to us, but we got like that as kids, too." Linda went on to point out the fact that his behaviors were not all that different from their daughter's throughout adolescence, so they tried not to overinterpret the signs. On the other hand, Mark's semester grades indicated a severe drop in his coursework. A conference with his teachers indicated that Mark was now very sullen in the classroom—he was not making jokes, not participating in discussions, and just generally uninvolved overall. Most recently, Mark was suspended for getting into a fight. To Linda, the fight was the final indication that they needed to do something for Mark.

Steven and Linda reacted ambivalently when Susan asked how they were coping with the loss of their daughter. After looking at each other briefly, Steven finally spoke. He said, "It's definitely been rough. We don't really talk to each other all that much about it, though." Linda interrupted, "Not about us, at least. I'd say that whenever we talk about it, we talk about how Mark is doing." Steven nodded in agreement. When Susan asked if they noticed any differences in their relationship, they both shook their heads, but then Steven said, "I'd say we fight a lot more," to which Linda added, "about Mark."

Susan then asked what they hoped to accomplish at The Center. Steven was now quick to respond, stating that he did not want the people at The Center to try to "fix" Mark. "There isn't really anything *wrong* with him. He hasn't gone crazy or anything. He's just being a normal teenager, missing his sister." Linda remarked, partially toward her husband, "No one said there was anything wrong with him. We just want to make sure he's doing all right. He won't really talk to us, and I think that he needs to have someone he can talk to about this." When asked why they wanted to attend the parent sessions, Linda stated that they wanted to learn more about how to help Mark. Susan informed them that issues like that would be part of the discussion, but also that the impact of the death on their own relationship would be a frequent discussion topic.

That night at the potluck, the Anderson's were introduced informally by Susan to the facilitators for the groups they would be joining. When dinner ended, Steven and Linda followed their facilitator into the room marked "Parents," and Mark followed behind his facilitator.

Mark was surprised to see that his group was large. There were 13 other kids in the room, all of whom seemed to already know each other. Everyone sat in a circle around the perimeter of the small room. The meeting opened with the facilitator's announcement that there was a new member of their group this week. The facilitator had already asked Mark if he would like to introduce himself or if he would prefer to have the facilitator do it, and Mark had decided to introduce himself. He gave a small shrug, looked down toward the floor and said, "My name is Mark. My sister died in a car wreck a few months ago. I think that's all I'm supposed to say, right?" The rest of the members proceeded to take turns around the circle introducing themselves, stating who they had lost, and how long they had been attending The Center.

After all of the introductions were finished, the facilitator asked if there were any issues from the previous week's meeting that people wanted to continue discussing. One young man said, "I still get the feeling like I'm just supposed to be over it, you know? Like, 'Get over it because what's done is done.' People just want to pretend like it didn't happen, so I'm supposed to, too." A few others joined in, pointing out that not being able to talk about the death of their sibling made them feel alone, even in a large group of friends. Some pointed out that friends would say some of the most inappropriate things: "They say stupid stuff, like, 'Don't worry—time heals all wounds.' I swear to God I'm gonna crack the next person who says that to me."

Mark heard the facilitator ask something about what could be done to help friends understand better, but to him that was beside the point. The real problem was that people don't even try to understand what is going on. The only people who seemed to want to talk about Audra were his parents, and to him they don't even want to really talk about it. "They just want to know what's wrong with me and why I'm not working hard at school—same old thing. They just don't get it," he thought.

When he started listening to the group again, he found that the conversation had turned to talking about depression. Several were talking about how sad and depressed they were, and how just being able to talk with people at The Center who were going through the same thing made them feel better. Mark disagreed. He thought, "I'm not sad, I'm mad. This wasn't Audra's fault, and it isn't fair that she was the one who died." That was why people were bothering him at school, and why his parents were driving him crazy. To Mark, no one seemed to realize how angry they should be that that guy took Audra away. When the session finally ended, Mark rose quietly as he and the others filed out of the room. The same people who were talking to each other at the beginning of the session were still talking to each other on the way out. Mark walked out alone.

Steven and Linda's group had what seemed like 15 couples, but during the introductions, it was quickly apparent that not everyone came as a couple. Although none of these participants had lost a spouse, some were divorced and came alone, and others were still married, but their spouses chose not to come. For example, one participant named Sheila was still married, but her husband did not attend. Their 14-year-old son had committed suicide nine months ago, and she and her two remaining children had been attending the center for the last three months. Beth was another person who came without her spouse. She mentioned in her introduction that her daughter died of sudden infant death syndrome approximately eight months ago, and that she and her 4-year-old daughter had been attending since about one month after her death. Not all participants were alone, however. Tamara and Jeff had been coming to The Center with their 8-year-old son for over one year, since their 4-year-old son accidentally drowned. Overall, the introductions indicated that about 18 of the people were married couples, and the remaining, primarily female, participants were there without their spouses. Most had lost their children because of an accident, but several had also died from diseases, and a few children (primarily teens) had committed suicide. After the other participants introduced themselves, Linda took responsibility for their introductions, stating not only their names and describing briefly the loss of their daughter, but also mentioning that they were there hoping to figure out what they could do to help their son.

Rather than discussing how to help their children as Linda had expected, however, the conversation focused on the relationships of the adults. Several of the married people were especially eager to discuss what was clearly an ongoing topic of how to take care of a relationship in the aftermath of the death of a child. Sheila, for example, mentioned that she felt that the issue of blame was a continuing problem in her marriage: "I keep thinking that there must have been some kind of sign that I didn't see. Jack keeps telling me to stop thinking about it that way. He says there were no signs and that it doesn't do any good to keep beating myself up about this. I agree with him to a point, but I don't want to make the same mistake again with Andrea or Shane. I'm their mother, and it is up to me to make sure that this never happens again."

Beth added, "I have the exact other problem. I want to try to put this behind us as soon as possible so that we can get on with life, but my husband thinks I'm being too cold about it." As a number of people around the circle indicated recognition of both sides, the facilitator mentioned that these difficulties were all related to the notion discussed the previous week about the differences in how people react to death. Sheila then said, "Yeah, I know that we are going at different speeds in this, and I have been trying to do what you said about looking also at the ways in which our experiences are similar. But it seems like these are big differences between us—I can't just stop thinking about these things and he can't stay focused on it anymore."

Tamara replied, "That might be true for right now, but trust me, sooner or later you will have to stop thinking about all of these things. I know what it's like to keep asking 'what if,' but let me tell you, there will always be another what if. Some things just aren't under your control and the sooner you see that, the sooner you'll be able to stop all of those questions."

Linda finally spoke, asking, "Do you all also disagree about how to deal with your kids? I mean, not just the regular stuff, but about how to talk with them about what happened and how they're doing?" Steven crossed his arms and rolled his eyes, but the number of nodding heads around the circle seemed to convince Linda to continue. "I just think that we should try to get Mark to talk more about how he feels, but Steven thinks that might do more harm than good. I mean, I want to help him, but I agree that I don't want to make him feel worse. I just can't tell what he needs. I know that I would have needed to talk."

Steven interrupted, "But how do you know that's what he needs?" He looked around and directed the question to the entire group, "I mean, how do you know it isn't just some phase that every kid goes through?" The discussion quickly turned to the other parents' experiences, noting that they also had difficulty determining what their children needed. Several pointed out that grief was much harder to recognize in male children, probably because of social norms requiring them to hide their sadness. Interestingly, although the remaining conversation focused on the group members' differences in how they wanted to deal with their children and the importance of first figuring out what the child really needs before deciding on a course of action, the members did not acknowledge an additional point raised by Linda's question. Her question implied that she herself needed to talk about what she was experiencing, and perhaps that those needs were not necessarily being met at this point. No discussion resulted regarding the parents' needs, however; the focus remained on the children for the rest of the time.

The Langdons

The Langdons' first meeting was the following evening, and it started the same as the Anderson's. Michelle met with Susan to complete the intake interview. After describing briefly the details of her husband's death, Michelle described the reactions of her children. She started with TJ, "the easiest," because he really did not seem to be reacting to his father's death at all. Susan asked if there were any subtle signs like regressing, appetite or personality changes, or sleep disturbances, but Michelle had not observed any of those signs. Susan conceded that sometimes children under five years of age do not quite understand what has happened and therefore might not be experiencing grief, but added that TJ was still welcome to join.

Tina, the 10-year-old, was a much bigger concern for Michelle. In the short time since her father's death, Tina seemed to be unable to control her emotions. At some moments, she'd seem perfectly calm and then begin sobbing without any provocation. She was also very quick to lose her temper and was becoming aggressive in the way she expressed her displeasure. According to her teachers, these same behaviors were being exhibited at school. Tina had always received high marks in citizenship, but seemed no longer able to maintain her attention in the classroom. She would act out and would fight often with her classmates during group activities.

Stephanie, the oldest, worried Michelle in a slightly different way—she did not seem to be responding with any emotions. "Stephanie has always been my helper," said Michelle. "She has always helped take care of her little brother and sister, and she was a godsend during Tom's fight with cancer. I don't know what I'd have done without her." Michelle pointed out that Stephanie's behaviors showed no change after her father's death. "She doesn't cry, doesn't get upset. Every time I ask how she's doing she just smiles and says, 'Just fine,' and then changes the topic. I know she was very close to her father, and I worry that she isn't dealing with this at all and that it's going to eat her up inside."

When asked how she was doing personally, Michelle answered that she felt she was doing pretty well, "all things considered." She mentioned that the real shock happened when they first heard Thomas' prognosis, and since then, they'd had time to prepare. "It was hard, don't get me wrong, but at least we had the chance to say things that we needed to say and get some things done. It still feels like I think about him every minute of the day, but not all of my thoughts are depressing. We always had it rough even before he got sick, but he could still make me laugh. He sort of still can." She felt that she was lucky to have several family members nearby. She had always been active in church and was finding spiritual support to be especially comforting. What was concerning her was how to take care of her children, both emotionally and financially. She wanted to find out "how other people do it alone."

The Langdons' sessions began like all others. At the conclusion of the potluck, the children and adults went to their separate groups. Michelle had left TJ at her sister's house for the evening because she did not think he needed to be there.

Tina's group included eight other children. After the children were seated in chairs arranged in a small circle, the two facilitators, Jennifer and Deb, introduced themselves. Jennifer reminded the children that what people say in group is not to be discussed outside of group unless the children want to continue talking about it with their families, and then introduced Tina. She asked the remaining children to introduce themselves, after which she announced the evening's activity. Every child was provided a page of construction paper and a box of crayons as the children moved their chairs over to some low tables on which to work. The children were asked to draw pictures of themselves and their families showing how they had been feeling lately. As the children drew their pictures, the facilitators moved from child to child, asking what their pictures were and whether they wanted to share their pictures with the group.

Tina's picture was very simple. It was three stick figures representing her, her older sister, and her mother. The faces drawn on the figures were of Tina's mouth shaped as an inverted U, and the other two figures had faces with the opposite pattern. When Deb asked her what the faces meant, Tina responded, "I feel bad, but everyone else feels good." When asked to clarify what she meant by "bad," Tina said, "I don't know. I'm mad I guess." When asked at whom, Tina said she felt like she was mad at everybody and then added that she often felt bad because she would get in trouble for feeling that way. "I guess I'm just bad," Tina concluded.

When everyone finished drawing, Jennifer showed some of the pictures to the group, now seated in a circle again. Feelings of anger, sadness, and loneliness were depicted in several pictures, but one received particular attention. It was a picture of a person crying in a corner "where no one is supposed to see her." Jennifer began a directed discussion with the children about how some people feel differently on the inside than they show on the outside. "Sometimes people act happy when they are around others, but are really sad on the inside and they don't want others to know," she said. After several minutes of discussing why people may hide their emotions to protect the feelings of others, she turned the discussion toward why people are selective about the ways they act in different venues, encouraging the children to talk about the differences in the ways they are supposed to act in different places. "Think of how you are supposed to act in the classroom and how you can act on the playground. You might want to run and play in the classroom, but that is against the rules, right? Well, sometimes there are rules we need to follow for expressing our feelings. Let's talk about some of the feelings you drew in these pictures and see if we can figure out the rules for how and where we should express those feelings." The discussion continued with a specific focus on clarifying that when children were disciplined for their emotions, they should not see their feelings as bad but rather that it was because they chose an inappropriate way to express them.

Stephanie's group was small. There were just five other teenagers and one facilitator. Their discussion room had some comfortable old couches and chairs against three of the four walls, and the teenagers spread out in them in a semicircular pattern. Stephanie recognized one girl from school, but did not know her name. She was relieved to hear that there was an agreement to keep confidential everything said in the group, but she was a little uncertain about whether that was actually true. Everyone introduced themselves before Stephanie did, and their introductions were very detailed about who they were, who had died, and how long they had been coming to The Center. Two mentioned why they came, indicating that it was good to have someone to talk to who knew what they were going through.

Stephanie's introduction was rather brief, concluding with a statement indicating that she was there because her mother wanted her to go, "Otherwise, I just wish everyone would leave me alone about this." Allison, the teens' facilitator, asked Stephanie to elaborate on what she meant by wanting everyone to leave her alone. Stephanie then indicated that everyone, her mother, her aunts, and people at school only seemed to want to talk about her dad and how she's doing. "It's like every time I walk up to someone, they just get this sad look on their face and ask me how I'm doing. I feel like telling them I was doing just fine until they started acting like that. I just tell them that I'm fine, but I swear they just won't leave me alone. It's like I'm supposed to feel bad all of the time, but I don't want to. That's why I really didn't want to come here, where, no offense, everyone is just going to be crying about how bad they feel. I know it sucks that he's dead, but it happens. You've just got to deal with it and get over it."

Martin, a 17-year-old whose father had died 11 months ago from a heart attack, took issue with part of that statement. He said that group was not always about crying, "not that there's anything wrong with that if someone needs to let it out," but that they could talk about anything they wanted. The girl Stephanie recognized added, "Yeah, you're not the only one who gets mad at people about this stuff. We always end up talking about how other people drive us crazy. It's like sometimes you want people to understand that you're not happy right now and to give you some space, but you don't want people to always assume that you are feeling miserable." Others joined in, discussing the inability of others to fully comprehend what they go through because they had not experienced it themselves. Several personal anecdotes were told to illustrate that point. Rather than expressing anger at those people, however, the stories were told in joking ways showing some forgiveness of those inept but well-meaning attempts of others. At several times these members were also quick to add that that was the great benefit of coming to group. "We *have* been there and we *do* know what it's like, so it's kind of nice to be able to come here and talk with people who get it."

Michelle's group was large and primarily women. There were a few who were relatively new to The Center, like Cassandra, whose husband had died three months ago from a heart attack. Others, like Amy and Wendy, had been coming for just about one year. There was an obvious difference between the participants who had been attending for a long time and those who were relatively new. Cassandra's depression was obvious to any observer—her sullen facial expression, emotionless way of talking, and withdrawn posture were all consistent with the sadness of what she said. Amy, whose husband died of cancer 14 months ago, and Wendy, whose husband died at about the same time in a traffic accident, seemed comparatively happy. Their friendship was obvious, and they seemed almost to find some humor in what had happened to their lives. Not all of the long-time members were as jovial, however. For example, Dawn, whose husband had committed suicide 11 months ago, shared many of the depressive characteristics of Cassandra except for her obvious displeasure toward Amy and Wendy's behaviors. Dawn clearly did not see anything amusing about her situation. As the introductions continued, Michelle noticed that many of the people had lost their spouses suddenly, and that many of these deaths were rather violent, such as car accidents and even a couple murders.

Cassandra opened the discussion, mentioning her difficulty getting out of bed in the morning. "I lie there and feel like I'm not even strong enough to lift the covers off of me. I just lie there thinking about all of the things I've got to do alone for the rest of my life. My mind keeps flying in a million different directions. I know I've got a ton of things I need to do, but I just feel paralyzed there in bed. If not for the kids, I don't think I'd ever be able to get up." A few responded with encouragement about how they also had unbearably long mental lists of everything that they had to do and their ultimate discovery that they could take care of things on their own. Amy added, "I know what that's like. There were lots of times early on when I didn't think I could make it. But you'll be amazed what you can do when you have no choice. And that's just it—you don't have a choice. Now I feel like there isn't anything I can't do." Wendy joked, "Yeah, I thought it was pretty overwhelming at first, but then I realized I did all the work around the house *before* Harry died, so what's the difference?"

The discussion turned toward practical advice for writing a list of all of the things that need to be done rather than trying to remember all of them. This activity had been discussed in a past group, and several of the long-time members were familiar with it. They described it as a useful technique that helped them to take control of the anxiety associated with all of the responsibilities. Others also pointed out that they had adapted that exercise successfully in the past to add a column indicating whether there was anyone who could help with some of the list. They noted that there were numerous people who were willing to help with various needs and that often all one needed to do was ask. Dawn remarked to the contrary, however, that the exercise only reminded her of how alone she was. Still, Michelle found the advice to be very reasonable because she did have a number of family members nearby.

One interesting part of the discussion of that list involved the responsibility of taking care of the children. That was not a chore easily given to other people. Most of the parents were quick to agree that others could help out in terms of watching them, but that their emotional care was primarily the parent's responsibility. The only real exception for most of them was The Center. To many of the parents, it was the only alternative caregiver for these particular needs of their children. Those who had been attending for some time seemed especially comfortable talking about their own limitations in knowing what to do for the children, and the relief they felt in letting some "professionals" help. Some also noted that it kept them from feeling guilty for focusing on their own needs. They noted that to focus on themselves by going to their own therapy sessions would not feel right if it took their attention away from their children's needs. That burden is lifted, though, when they know that their children are simultaneously receiving the care they need. So The Center served as a place where they could get the support they need without feeling like they were neglecting their children.

UPDATE AND CONCLUSION

The preceding descriptions of each person's first night at The Center can only provide a small portion of the grief support group experience. The people with whom the families met represent group members at various stages of the grieving process, some of whom are benefiting from the experience. It is important to note, however, that the groups do not work for everyone.

Such was the case for Mark. He did not identify with any members of his group and quickly persuaded his father that The Center was not a place for him. Although Linda complied with their requests to let Mark stop attending The Center (thereby ending her and Steven's participation as well), a few more months of Mark's misbehavior at school even convinced Steven that something needed to be done for Mark. Mark then began individual counseling with a psychologist. Steven and Linda separated one year later.

Another interesting pattern emerged for Stephanie. Over the first few months at The Center, Stephanie found herself identifying more with her group members and became progressively more depressed about her father's death. It wasn't until the fourth month that she began to recover from those feelings. By the ninth month she was feeling "back to her old self" and found that she no longer looked forward to group. She then terminated her participation.

Tina continued to attend The Center for just over 13 months. Over that time, she showed continued improvement in the experience and expression of her feelings. Her feelings of sadness and anger diminished substantially over that time, and she no longer acted out aggressively at home or at school. She stopped attending The Center after telling her mother, "I just don't want to talk about it anymore."

RELEVANT CONCEPTS

Childhood development: Refers to the continuous physiological and psychological maturing of children from birth through the end of adolescence, focusing especially on the children's progression toward greater complexity in their ability to think, feel, and communicate with others.

Coping behaviors: Include the adaptive and maladaptive responses that people use in an attempt to overcome the stress associated with adverse events.

Grief: Refers to the suffering experienced as a result of the death of a loved one. It is a multifaceted construct that includes many negative emotional reactions to the loss.

Social support matching: Involves the provision of assistance that corresponds directly to the needs of the recipient.

Support groups: Organizations of people who come together in various settings to assist each other in dealing with the stress arising from an adverse event that each share in common.

DISCUSSION QUESTIONS

1. What factors led to Mark's decision not to continue attending The Center. What could or should have the group done to better serve Mark's needs?
2. How can you explain the pattern of Stephanie's emotions at The Center?
3. When should a person stop attending a support group?
4. How can you tell what type of support a grieving person needs?
5. Why might someone avoid or be resistant to going to a support group such as this one?
6. If you were a parent of these children, what would you do for them?

ENDNOTE

[1] These families are composites of real members of The Center. The names used are fictional, and the qualities of the individuals described are not meant to reflect any particular individuals. Instead, the modal and sometimes mean characteristics of these families and the group members with whom they meet are reflected in the following cases.

REFERENCES/SUGGESTED READINGS

Archer, J. (1999). *The nature of grief.* New York: Routledge.

Baker, J. E., & Sedney, M. A. (1996). How bereaved children cope with loss: An overview. In C. A. Corr & D. M. Corr (Eds.), *Handbook of childhood death and bereavement* (pp. 109–130). New York: Springer.

Burleson, B., & Goldsmith, D. (1998). How the comforting process works: Alleviating emotional distress through conversationally induced reappraisals. In P. Andersen & L. Guerrero (Eds.), *Communication and emotion: Research, theory, applications, and contexts* (pp. 245–280). San Diego, CA: Academic Press.

Naierman, N. (1997). Reaching out to grieving students. *Educational Leadership, 55,* 62–65.

Webb, N. B. (2002). The child and death. In N. B. Webb (Ed.), *Helping bereaved children: A handbook for practitioners* (Vol. 2, pp. 3–18). New York: Guilford.

18

Negotiating Communication Challenges While Experiencing Alzheimer's Disease: The Case of One Hispanic Family

Lyle J. Flint
Ball State University

Jim L. Query, Jr.
Alyssa Parrish[1]
University of Houston

As the 21st century continues to unfold, the United States is experiencing several health and cultural challenges. The health challenges range from physicians walking out of health care facilities because of exorbitant malpractice premiums, spiraling numbers of underinsured individuals, lack of a comprehensive prescription drug plan for seniors living on limited and fixed incomes, rising cases of AIDS, and a staggering rise in Alzheimer's disease (AD). In terms of cultural challenges, many parts of the country continue to engage in intense debates about the merits of bilingual education in Spanish, whether to mandate English as the official language, and a continuing influx of Hispanic immigrants transforming California into the first state to have a Hispanic majority.

One area where these challenges are evident is the intersection of AD and the growing Hispanic community in the United States. According to the Alzheimer's Association web site, 1 in 10 persons over age 65, nearly half of those over age 85, and a small percentage of people as young as 30 have AD. However, these statistics differ for Hispanic populations who, regardless of a suspected gene mutation, are twice as likely to develop AD as Whites by age 90 (Kukull & Martin, 1998). The strain of having a family member with AD, coupled with the challenges of being in a new culture, can become overwhelming for a Hispanic family. In addition, Hispanics in the United States tend to live three generations under one roof, often because of financial difficulties or for emotional support. According to census data from 2000, one fourth (26%) of all Hispanics in the United States are classified as living below the poverty level (Latino Mental Health, n.d.). Language difficulties, immigration status, and lack of education are interconnected factors that may contribute to the soaring number of Hispanics living in poverty. Poverty can also influence other social problems, such as insufficient health care coverage for old and young alike. Further compounding the unique challenges faced by Hispanic populations is the cultural belief that any form of dementia should remain a family secret and be managed by only the family while disregarding any formal assistance services offered by the community or medical industry. Such a belief not only has devastating effects on the family member afflicted with AD, but also places caregivers at greater risk of illness. Further, research indicates that Hispanic caregivers are at great risk because they tend to be younger, less educated, poorer, and in worse health than non-Hispanic White caregivers (Aranda, Villa, Trejo, Ramirez, & Ranney, 2003).

Because of the recent escalation in AD cases, having at least one member in either the extended or immediate family afflicted with AD is highly likely in an Hispanic family. And given the aforementioned unique challenges, combined with the Hispanic culture's apprehension or disentitlement of utilizing public facilities such as hospitals and social establishments, it is important to consider potential problems and outcomes when AD and culture collide. In this case, we examine a hypothetical, but typical, Hispanic family, the Gonzalez family, as they confront the challenges of AD.

THE GONZALEZ FAMILY

One is likely to find many families similar to the Gonzalez enclave when traveling to large southwestern and urban cities. Miguel is the oldest male at 60 years of age. His wife of 40 years, Consuelo, is 58 and a proud mother of three hijos—Cristabalita, Chuy, and Alejandro, all in their mid-30s—and the doting grandmama of their six grandchildren. Raul is the middle brother of Miguel at 50 years of age. Raul and Miguel have a sister, Reina, who is 48 years old. Their father, Ricardo, and his brother, Carlos, both died in their 40s, and few in the family seem to know what happened; or at least, none will talk about their deaths in candid terms. María Conchis viuda de Gonzalez, the widow of Ricardo and mother of Miguel, Raul, and Reina, is now in her late 80s. Although she is adamant about not discussing Ricardo's death with her immediate family, some close and honored friends, her padrinos (padrinos are close, lifelong friends considered to be part of the family, similar to godparents; see Cora-Bramble & Williams, 2000), Diego and Treva, know the truth and have kept her confidence for many years.

Revisiting the Early Days

Although Ricardo and María Conchis moved from their home in San Luis Potosi, Mexico, many years ago, it often seems like yesterday to María Conchis. She vividly recalls how afraid she was, how difficult it was to learn English, and wondering how they would make it financially. Ricardo was able to reassure her through his boundless enthusiasm. His heart was big, and his way with people was extraordinary, despite not having finished his formal education. Over the next 20 years, working 6 days a week and often 14 to 16 hours daily, Ricardo was able to translate his interpersonal skills and aspirations into a successful furniture business. And as the business prospered, Ricardo actively involved all members of his extended family who were able to work. As María Conchis relived those days sitting at the kitchen table, Miguel entered and sat down without breaking her reverie. After a few minutes, he gently broke the silence and placed his roughened hand on top of hers, "Ay mamá, you still miss him, don't you?" As María Conchis fought to keep from crying, Miguel moved closer and tried to reassure her. "I miss him, too mama. It also troubles me greatly that I don't know more about how he died and about how uncle Carlos would later pass on as well." Wiping away her tears, María Conchis decided it was time to finally let Miguel know the truth.

Sharing Heart-Wrenching Revelations

As María Conchis peered into her eldest son's eyes, Miguel noticed that her body tensed up as if some great emotional floodgate was about to be opened. "Tu papá [your dad] . . . well, one dark day, it was like the warmth of his soul had been replaced by a cold. At first, I just thought he was working too much."

Miguel replied, "I understand your words mamá, but I cannot believe papá changed overnight." As María Conchis reflected, she concurred with a sigh, referring to Miguel in a Hispanic mother's typical affectionate diminutive, "There had been signs, Miguelito. I just ignored them. Many times, he could not remember his regular customers' names . . . he could not remember what the store keys unlocked . . . he could not remember paying our suppliers. But these things happened slowly at first."

Miguel listened to his mother's words as he struggled to envision his vibrant father deteriorating into a feeble shell of a man. He consciously looked away from his mother to give her some additional time to compose herself and continue. Reestablishing eye contact, María Conchis proceeded: "I didn't know what to do . . . I could not explain it . . . So I talked to his brother, my mother, and our padrinos, Treva and Diego." Miguel nods; he understands that in the Hispanic culture, resolutions to problems often require the input of extended family and close friends. María Conchis resumed, "I asked them to visit without telling them my fears. That day . . . well, it was one of the worst in my life . . . Ricardo gave both of them the mal de ojo [evil eye]. . . . Sobbing, he uh . . . ay dios mío [Oh my God] . . . he then insisted they were federales sent to destroy our furniture business! And the more we all tried to tell him that was not true, the angrier he became. And it didn't matter what language we used, though we believed Spanish would be best because he was so upset. They finally had to leave, and I was a wreck—ataque de nervios [an attack of nerves and depression]. From that day on, your papá never spoke of them or to them again. He also stopped looking at furniture wholesale notices, the newspaper, and your little ones' homework. He no longer cared about the music on the radio, and he would often begin a conversation without ending it, or he would attempt to end someone else's conversation." Through the emotion of her words, Miguel was able to discern how much his father's condition greatly affected his mamá and La Familia.

Realizing that a great weight had just been lifted off his mother's shoulders, Miguel went to get her a cold ice tea. As he prepared her drink, he reflected on the information she had shared. His father clearly experienced losses in his short-term and semantic memory systems. Miguel also wondered if his father had realized that something was terribly out of balance and then began to create imaginary scapegoats (e.g., evil governmental agents). Miguel had heard of AD, but thought it only affected the very old, a widespread myth, especially when multiple family members contract AD. And Ricardo, along with his brother, Carlos, were very young when they died. Miguel was beginning to suspect that his uncle had also been afflicted with AD.

Primary Caregiver Memories Often Distorted

After taking a sip of her cold drink, María Conchis was composed and ready to begin sharing again: "Of course, Miguelito, you should also talk with our padrinos [Diego and Treva], as their memories may also fill in many of the gaps. And they can tell you about how your Uncle Carlos died. I will tell them it's OK." Miguel remembered hearing that caregivers can often distort events, and he made a mental note of this tendency in anticipation of talking later with their padrinos. He was very interested in gaining any additional information that would help him and the rest of the family understand Ricardo and Carlos' deaths.

Additional Symptoms and Symbolic Crisis

As Miguel contemplated the discussion, he remembered that there were more signs of atypical and problematic behaviors from Ricardo. These ranged from wandering away, becoming very agitated when the sun set (sundowner's syndrome), confusing the names of living relatives with deceased ones, and failing to recognize his own grandchildren. Longstanding communication patterns and meaningful relationships were irrevocably altered and transformed in ways that defied adequate description, thus triggering a symbolic crisis among the Gonzalez family. Miguel recalled some of these very disturbing behaviors more vividly now, and he wished he had known more about the warning signs of AD. Perhaps then he could have helped La Familia better understand and cope with what was happening to their beloved Ricardo.

María Conchis perceived what Miguel was feeling and thinking. "Ay hijo mío, ojalá que sí, sin embargo, no fue posible" [Ah, my dear son, only if it could be so, however, it was not possible]. She explained further, "One of the worst things in all of this was that none of us— your padrinos and me—could figure out what caused him to get sick, when Ricardo started to get what the doctors called Alzheimer's disease. And so, if we couldn't tell how and when it started, how could you or anyone else have been able to make a difference?" María Conchis lightly caressed Miguel's forehead to further reinforce the gentleness of her words and to help ease his guilty feelings.

Another chilling aspect of symbolic crises occurs when close family members attempt to compensate for the memory and behavioral difficulties of their loved one with AD. Miguelito now recalled numerous times when his wife, Consuelo, or uncle Raul, or aunt Reina would intercede and diligently try to smooth things over. He also remembered times when his children— Chuy, Alejandro, or Cristabalita—would cover for grandpa Ricardo as well, to help minimize potentially disruptive and explosive situations.

Rallying La Familia to Help with Caregiving Tasks

Eventually, however, the intensity of the symptoms escalated to where behavioral compensation and denial were futile in masking the underlying progression of the disease. As the level of dependency for the person living with AD increases, the caregiving burdens spiral astronomically. This pattern places primary caregivers at significant risk for illness and premature morbidity.

María Conchis acknowledged the great toll exacted by the seemingly endless caregiving process. "Miguelito, you may recall when I became very ill? I was sad a lot, lacked energy. I felt that my spirit was leaving me. If it weren't for the rest of La Familia coming to my aid, I don't know what I would have done. I, uh, I think I would have given up."

Miguel nodded his head and remembered that pivotal meeting among La Familia (everyone except his mother). Everyone agreed that she needed help, that they needed to show their love and respect to Ricardo and María Conchis for everything they had done for them over the many years. Although they were not told what was wrong with Ricardo, they all knew it was a grave situation. Only the eldest and most respected knew the truth and agreed to safeguard it for María Conchis and Ricardo's sake.

Learning About Carlos From the Padrinos

Diego and Treva had both lived in the same small town as Ricardo and María Conchis as they all were growing up. Although not biologically related, an outsider would have never deduced that. The four were practically inseparable. And although there were some minor "speed bumps" (i.e., slight disagreements) as they matured, it was as if they were already Familia. Powerful bonds were forged that would never be broken, except by death. As long as Miguel could remember, Diego and Treva were always welcome in their home and treated with great respect. Miguel still marveled, too, at how effortlessly Diego and Treva showed their deep love for all the children, despite not having any of their own.

After knocking on their door, it was soon opened by Treva, who gave Miguel a huge hug.

"Pásele Miguel. Adelante Miguel, lo esperábamos. Fíjate que Diego está en la cocina" [Come in, Miguel. Go forward, Miguel. We have been expecting you. Note that Diego is in the kitchen].

As soon as Diego recognized Miguel, he rose, and then shook his hand vigorously while also sporting a large smile. "You honor us with your visit, Miguel. Please, sit down."

Miguel could sense their deep love for each other and for his family. Those powerful, uplifting feelings helped ease his apprehension. For now, it was time to learn more about Carlos' death. Miguel began, "Mamá and I had a long talk about papá today. She told me the truth."

Diego and Treva exchanged knowing glances. "Miguel, we know. Tu mamá called Treva on the phone earlier. She asked us to talk to you about your father's brother, Carlos."

As a long pause filled the room. Treva then began, "Your family is really our family. We have always thought the world of Ricardo and María Conchis. We even knew, before they did, that they would be married."

Diego burst out laughing, "That's not entirely true. Treva knew they were soul mates. I only suspected they would marry eventually." Miguel chuckled as well. For all of them, the brief laughter and youthful memories were cathartic.

Diego resumed, "Even though the eldest of us eventually learned that Ricardo had AD, we believed it was an isolated case. Never in our wildest thoughts did we think that a few years later, Carlos would get it as well." As the conversation unfolded, Diego indicated they soon learned that there were two types of AD, early and late-onset.[2]

Diagnostic Difficulties

While Diego paused, Treva interjected, "With both Ricardo and Carlos, it took months and many tests before the médicos [doctors] were fairly sure they had Alzheimer's. But we didn't know for sure because the only way to know for certain was to look at their brains after they died."

Miguel nodded his assent and shared that he had heard AD was a diagnosis by exclusion and could only be confirmed by autopsy. That is, health care providers had to rule everything else out and then they could only be sure about 90% of the time. Further complicating Ricardo's timely diagnosis was his lack of formal education. Ardila, Rosselli, and Puente (1994) have reported that poorly educated or functionally illiterate Hispanic individuals often score low on traditional psychometric tests and then mirror the scores of a person living with AD.

Despite these diagnostic difficulties, after having seen what was happening with Ricardo, the padrinos soon knew with all their being that Carlos, too, had AD. Many of the symptoms were similar—short-term and semantic memory deficits, bizarre behaviors—and yet others were quite distinct from Ricardo. For instance, Carlos became very aggressive and confrontational.

Treva resumes, "Diego and I couldn't stand to see your family suffer again when the doctors told us about Carlos. And we couldn't let Carlos go to the home the doctors told us about— Carlos was La Familia. So we decided to take Carlos into our home and care for him. You might remember, we told many people that Carlos had gone sailing and never returned. Because our home is very large and not close to any towns, we were able to shield Carlos from the rest of the world. We realized also that some, when they found out, would blame us for lying. But we thought we had to lie because we wanted to protect La Familia. We knew that María Conchis had been working so hard with Ricardo that she was sick. And you and Consuelo had small children. We didn't think your family could give Carlos the help he needed—it would have been too great a sacrifice."

Miguel mused as he absorbed this latest information. Finally, he reached a conclusion, "Although I don't like to place words into the mouths of La Familia, I doubt that any will blame you for lying. You did it out of love and great respect. It would have been much easier to have let the doctors take Carlos away, or to have walked away yourselves. You both have great hearts."

Miguel took his leave, thanking the padrinos again for all they had done. More than ever, he realized that they are extraordinary individuals. His heart told him that his family was indeed blessed in the things that count the most.

Helping Their Adult Children Make Sense of AD

After arriving home, Miguel and Consuelo, su querida esposa (his beloved wife), had a long talk about AD and all it had done to La Familia. Miguel shared with her that AD has two types, early and late onset; that it kills twice (symbolically and physically); it proceeds at varying rates of speed; there are only some drugs that provide temporary relief and stability; that it can last from 5 to 20 years; and some of AD's risk factors include family history and educational levels (among several others; see Henderson & Jorm, 2000). They decided to call a meeting among their adult children, Cristabalita, Chuy, and Alejandro, now all in their mid-30s.

The young adults, with children of their own, still vividly remembered how their abuelito (diminutive of grandpa), Ricardo, was transformed from a strong, caring, devoted, and wonderful man into a "walking shell." Although no one ever told them what was wrong with abuelito, they soon observed many inexplicable changes that affected all of their relationships. As they awaited the talk with their parents, the "kids" discussed how their interaction with their abuelito changed. Cristabalita shared that she sensed something was terribly wrong when abuelito consistently could not recall or pick up a previous and recent conversation with her. Chuy chimed in that it became increasingly difficult to understand abuelito as there seemed to be no pattern concerning how he defined their relationship; some days, Chuy knew his abuelito loved him and other days, it was like he was a stranger. Alejandro concurred that he also felt distant from their abuelito many times, as there often was no mutual give and take during their abbreviated talks. Chuy then vocalized what all had been thinking. "I knew something was way out of balance. Yet, abuelito did not appear sick."

Alejandro shuddered as they revisited their changing interaction with abuelito Ricardo. "It's still too fresh, like yesterday. Abuelito would first make odd replies. Like when I would ask him how he was doing. He would often reply, 'Yes, and I like the hot weather,' or sometimes he would say, 'No, and I like the cold weather' to the preceding question."

Cristabalita nodded her head in agreement, "I know. It was so strange. For instance, remember how much abuelito loved his big watch and how much I liked to ask him the time? When he became sick, and I'm not sure when it began, I would ask him what time it was, and he would reply, 'Of course I know the time. Why don't you?'"

Chuy added, "One of the things that was most frustrating for me was constantly repeating the same information. I would tell abuelito that he didn't need to go work anymore numerous times and all in less than an hour."

Miguel and Consuelo sat down with Chuy, Cristabalita, and Alejandro. As each began to share the "hidden truth" about abuelito Ricardo and then uncle Carlos, the adult children indicated that they did understand better now. Moreover, they could move past mere awareness to now trying to help others "own" the disease and realize there was some quality of life possible for all concerned, albeit for a short time. It was so helpful to also have a name to place on the disease that robbed them of their abuelito querido (beloved grandpa). They all agreed that great patience and altered expectations were needed when interacting with a loved one having AD. And they realized the likelihood of their performing as caregivers in the future, given their family history. They knew that, throughout their time together, it was imperative to maintain the dignity of the person and demonstrate respect as much as possible (see Cora-Bramble & Williams, 2000), a goal that is very difficult to achieve in light of the many formidable communication challenges. Yet, they recognized it must be constantly pursued.

DISCUSSION

Alzheimer's Disease is an irreversible dementia that currently afflicts 4 million individuals and an estimated 19 million caregivers. Most authorities concur that, as the 21st century advances, the prevalence rates of AD are going to become alarming and trigger an epidemic tantamount to the AIDS crisis, especially in less-developed countries (see Henderson & Jorm, 2000). However, despite the risk faced by all, the Hispanic population faces even greater risks physically and socially. Further, the family dynamics of the Hispanic culture and the prevalence of poverty create additional burdens on the family members of a person afflicted with AD.

Although depression is common among all caregivers of persons with AD, María Conchis' "ataque de nervios" typifies the increased level of depression suffered by Hispanic caregivers. Perhaps one reason for the increased level of depression is the Hispanic culture's rejection of formal outside assistance, relying instead on family members as not only caregivers, but as the only means of social support. Communication scholars have examined the significant mediating effects of social support on depression and illness and, as social support options decrease, one would expect an increase in depression. Fortunately, researchers, and ultimately policy makers, are examining factors (such as native language use) that influence Hispanics' use of support services.

Researchers also report that Hispanic caregivers are not only frequently "newcomers" to a culture, but also newcomers to the long-term care system. It is, thus, an essential imperative that the care systems engage in "culturally sensitive delivery services," such as bilingual respite care, Spanish-language day care, legal consultation, and support groups, if the Hispanic caregiver is to take advantage of and benefit from these services (Aranda et al., 2003).

The primary caregiver of a person with AD in a Hispanic family is likely to be an adult daughter or the spouse of the patient. Although the majority of the daily burden will fall on the primary caregiver, the disease affects the entire family. This is particularly true in the traditional extended Hispanic family. One area where the family is most likely to experience great difficulty is coping with the changing roles within the family.

Most communication scholars agree with the symbolic interaction perspective of role negotiation. Individuals constantly redefine roles on the basis of how they interact with one another. Among Hispanics, however, roles are very ardently defined by their home culture; more so when considering family roles. When these cultural expectations are violated or seem to no longer function, as in the case of the Gonzalez family during Roberto's illness, individuals must negotiate interaction in an attempt to gain an understanding of the situation.

Chuy, Cristabalita, and Alejandro recount this challenging time as they discuss their interaction with their grandfather. Their recollections are consistent with Fisher's (1987) views about the quality of negotiated dimensions of interpersonal relationships. Cristabalita's concern that her grandfather could not pick up or recall recent conversations demonstrated a lack of *discontinuity*. Chuy was troubled by new and unpredictable patterns of interaction that demonstrated a lack of *synchrony* and *recurrence*. And Alejandro realized that the normal patterns of give and take that were previously apparent in conversations with his grandfather had all but vanished, indicating a lack of *reciprocity*. It is the dissolution of these four characteristics of interactional quality that first leads to what communication scholars refer to as a symbolic crisis and then ultimately to symbolic death—a change that has become so drastic that the relationship becomes unrecognizable. Yet, as drastic as the change is, it is a slow eventual process with no apparent starting point. As Wheeler (2001) notes in describing the paradoxical nature of AD, "Later it occurred to me that Alzheimer-type dementia does its insidious work as quietly and destructively as termites. It eats away at the core, leaving the surface seemingly intact. Before the damage is recognized, it is irreversible" (p. 5).

It is essential to realize that the hypothetical case presented in this chapter was that of a nondescript Hispanic family. This is consistent with much of the past literature and research that has examined the Hispanic culture, not only in terms of AD, but across a wide array of social and medical phenomena. However, researchers are beginning to caution against such research and have demonstrated the importance of treating Hispanic groups from different geographic regions as separate populations. For example, Umana-Taylor and Fine (2001) have identified a number of differences in self-esteem, autonomy, and familial ethnic socializations based on geographic region. In addition, biomedical researchers have recently discovered the existence of a gene that places Caribbean Hispanics (but not other Hispanics) at higher risk for early-onset AD (Athan et al., 2001). Certainly, future research will need to explore the differences that exist in caregiver characteristics and family interaction when examining Hispanic cultures from different geographic regions.

CONCLUSION

Currently, there is no cure for AD. There are, however, four "window of opportunity" drugs that temporarily stabilize some persons with AD. Unfortunately, however, these drugs typically only work for some months and they do not stop the disease or prevent its ultimate outcome—death.

Regarding early-onset AD, often called familial AD, the most prominent risk factor is a shared genetic history. In particular, as one's number of immediate relatives contracting AD increases, so too does one's risk. In contrast, in the case of late-onset AD, the most widely recognized risk factor is advanced age. Some research has implicated a lack of education as an additional risk factor (Henderson & Jorm, 2000). This finding appears particularly valid when daily abstraction and thinking processes are not being engaged in consistently.

As this chapter closes, we revisit the Gonzalez's family meeting. Miguel, Consuelo, Chuy, Cristabalita, and Alejandro hug each other, and tears flow freely. They all realize that together, La Familia did the very best they could for both Ricardo and Carlos. And united, La Familia can better combat AD if it strikes again. They also decide that once all family members learn the hidden truth, they should share it in their barrio. Only then may other frontline warriors—family caregivers—be empowered to ease the final journey of their loved ones with AD.

RELEVANT CONCEPTS

Alzheimer's disease (AD), early- and late-onset: A form of dementia that currently has no cure or known causes, although age and family history are significant risk factors. AD generally afflicts people over the age of 65 (late-onset) but may occur in individuals as young as 40 (early-onset).

Common AD symptoms: AD begins with minor memory loss but, as the disease progresses, there is an increase in memory loss and confusion, changes in personality, problems with language, emotional apathy, and an inability to perform activities of daily living, such as bathing and grooming.

Diagnosis by exclusion: The process of determining a specific illness by determining what it is not. In the case of AD, there is no sure diagnosis short of an autopsy, so health professionals diagnosis AD by ruling out other causes of dementia.

Discontinuity, synchrony, recurrence, and reciprocity: Characteristics of interactional quality. *Discontinuity* is the ability to pick up a conversation in the same place it left off during a previous period of interaction. *Synchrony* and *recurrence* are sensitivity to the established patterns of interaction. *Reciprocity* is defining roles in a complimentary manner.

Dysfunctional conversation: An ineffective form of communication that lacks an acceptable level of the characteristics of interactional quality; typical among the later stages of AD.

Hot and cold views of health: Health and illness are thought to be influenced by achieving an equilibrium among a person's blood (deemed as "hot"), phlegm (deemed as "cold"), yellow bile (deemed as "hot"), and black bile (deemed as "cold"). An imbalance is believed to increase one's risk for illness and disease (Cora-Bramble & Williams, 2000, p. 266).

La Familia decision-making approach: A typical method of decision making in Hispanic culture that includes all members of the family, both young and old.

Out-of-balance views of health: Many Hispanics believe that there must be an equilibrium (or balance) among social, physiological, spiritual, and symbolic dimensions of health. An imbalance among these dimensions is thought to increase one's likelihood of contracting some disease or chronic illness.

Padrinos: An Hispanic term for very close friends considered to be a part of the family, similar to godparents.

Symbolic crisis: Drawn from medical anthropology and communication literature, such trauma is the progression of three levels. The first level occurs when the ill person and his/her significant others view the catastrophic illness in dysfunctional ways that impede the delivery of sound health care delivery. The second level unfolds as ill persons, typically those experiencing an irreversible dementia, irrevocably lose their sense of relational histories. The third and final dimension involves the involuntary loss of self.

DISCUSSION QUESTIONS

1. Picture yourself in Miguel's position after having spoken with his padrinos. What would be going through your mind as you thought about what you would say to your wife? What specific communication strategies would you be considering as you approached the topics of caregiving and symbolic death?

2. Cristabalita, the daughter of Miguel and granddaughter of Ricardo, is in her mid-30s. Her grandfather died in his 40s, but her father is 60. Do you think Cristabalita should be concerned about early-onset AD? Is she at risk genetically? Is she at less risk because she is a female? What would you be thinking if you were in her place? What are some of the pros and cons of knowing if you're at risk?

3. Chuy is Miguel and Consuelo's eldest son. After the family meeting, Chuy wants to learn more about AD in general and specifically about caregiving. If you were Chuy, how would you go about getting more information? What sources on the Internet would be good to use? Are there any online government sources? What would you look for in the search engines?

4. Do you believe that hiding Ricardo and Carlos' disease was in the best interest for the remainder of the extended family? Why or why not? Do you think it could have benefited La Familia if the secret had been revealed? If so, in what ways? What would you do, given their circumstance, with your own family?

ACKNOWLEDGMENTS

The authors acknowledge the helpful comments from Corinne O'Brien, a Puerto Rican American, and Dr. María Jibaja-Weiss, a Hispanic scholar at Baylor College of Medicine.

ENDNOTES

[1] Ms. Parrish is a Hispanic American.

[2] Early AD applies to those 65 years of age and younger and can affect individuals as early as their 30s. Late-onset AD occurs as individuals become very old, especially in their 80s and older (Henderson & Jorm, 2000). Some recent examples of individuals with late-onset AD include former President Ronald Reagan, former Secretary of State Cyrus Vance, and former Senator Barry Goldwater.

REFERENCES/SUGGESTED READINGS

Athan, E. S., Williamson, J., Ciappa, A., Santana, V., Romas, S. N., Lee, J. H., Rondon, H., Lantigua, R. A., Medrano, M., Torres, M., Arawaka, S., Rogaeva, E., Song, Y., Sato, C., Kawarai, T., Fafel, K. C., Boss, M. A., Seltzer, W. K., Stern, Y., St George-Hyslop, P., Tycko, B., & Mayeux, R. (2001). A founder mutation in Presenilin 1 causing early-onset Alzheimer disease in unrelated Caribbean Hispanic families. *JAMA: Journal of the American Medical Association, 286,* 2257–2263.

Aranda, M. P., Villa, V. M., Trejo, L., Ramirez, R., & Ranney, M. (2003). El Portal Latino Alzheimer's Project: Model program for Latino caregivers of Alzheimer's Disease-affected people. *Social Work, 48*(2), 259–271.

Ardila, A., Rosselli, M., & Puente, A. E. (1994). *Neuropsychological evaluation of the Spanish speaker.* New York: Plenum Press.

Cora-Bramble, D., & Williams, L. (2000). Explaining illness to Latinos: Cultural foundations and messages. In B. B. Whaley (Ed.), *Explaining illness: Research, theory, and strategies* (pp. 257–281). Mahwah, NJ: Lawrence Erlbaum and Associates.

Fisher, B. A. (1987). *Interpersonal communication: Pragmatics of human communication.* New York: Random House.

Henderson, A. S., & Jorm, A. F. (2000). Definition and epidemiology of dementia: A review. In M. Maj & N. Sartorius, N. (Eds.), *Dementia* (pp. 1–33). New York: John Wiley & Sons, Ltd.

Kukull, W. A., & Martin, G. M. (1998). APOE polymorphisms and late-onset Alzheimer disease. *JAMA: Journal of the American Medical Association, 279,* 788–789.

Latino Mental Health. (n.d.). Census data. Retrieved September 6, 2003, from http://latinomentalhealth.net/census_data.htm

Umana-Taylor, A. J., & Fine, M. A. (2001). Methodological implications of grouping Latino adolescents into one collective ethnic group. *Hispanic Journal of Behavioral Sciences, 23,* 347–362.

Wheeler, B. M. (2001). *Close to me, but far away: Living with Alzheimer's.* Columbia, MO: University of Missouri Press.

Additional Resources

Alzheimer's Association. (2003). *Ten warning signs of Alzheimer's disease.* Retrieved September 6, 2003, from http://www.alz.org/AboutAD/10Signs.htm

Family Caregiver Alliance. (n.d.). Family caregiver alliance website. Retrieved September 14, 2003, from http://www.caregiver.org/

National Adult Day Services Association. (n.d.). NADSA home page. Retrieved September 14, 2003, from http://www.nadsa.org/

National Council of La Raza. (n.d.). Link to Hispanic resources. Retrieved September 14, 2003, from http://www.nclr.org/links/

Neighbor Care. (2003). The lending library. Retrieved September 14, 2003, from http://www.neighborcare.com/Services/Education/LendingLibraryVideos.htm

19

Finding the Right Place: Social Interaction and Life Transitions Among the Elderly

Margaret J. Pitts
Janice L. Krieger
Jon F. Nussbaum
Pennsylvania State University

As the life expectancy in the United States continues to increase, elderly adults across the nation are faced with the challenge of physical relocation because of increasing medical needs. However, finding the "right" place to move is not an easy mission. Some elderly adults may move in with family or friends. For others, the right place will be sharing a small, maintenance-free cottage in a retirement village with a spouse. Still others will find locations where medical assistance is available around-the-clock. In all scenarios, the process of relocation inevitably requires lifestyle changes. One such change that is often ignored during this process is the effect of relocation on social relationships.

Maintaining personal relationships is vital for good health among older adults. Family, friendship, and companion relations are essential ingredients to health and well-being throughout the lifespan. As we age, however, we enter new relationships and leave behind others. For many older adults, living facilities structure social interaction and help residents create, maintain, or disengage from these personal relationships. With this case study, we introduce you to Kris,[1] an elderly man who has recently experienced a myriad of life and living transitions. As an occupant of a modern, resident-centered long term care facility, Kris shares his experiences as he transitioned from living happily with his wife in an independent living arrangement, to living in separate assisted-living units, to her death, and to his permanent relocation to an intensive nursing care room. The community in which Kris resides prides itself on maintaining the dignity of its residents, offering an independent lifestyle, and providing ample opportunities for social engagement. However, our interactions with Kris revealed his personal struggle to create and sustain relationships and accept that he must now depend greatly on others for daily assistance. We hope that through the writing of this chapter we are better able to understand the process of life transitions ourselves and offer insight to the countless others who have a loved one experiencing similar transitions.

THE COMMUNITY

Walking through the sunlit corridors of Crystal Village, we hardly felt as though we were in the licensed nursing unit of a large retirement and personal-care facility. The hallways were buzzing with chatter among volunteers, nurses, and residents. Down one hall, bright blue and green lovebirds in a golden cage chirped away as an elderly woman spoke endearingly to them. The next hall housed a small indoor pond inhabited by dazzling orange and red koi and tropical plants. We stopped to speak with various members of staff and residents along the way. Everyone greeted us with a smile, perhaps because they remembered us from the weeks previous, or perhaps they were just friendly.

Crystal Village is a not-for-profit continuing care retirement community. This Quaker-directed facility encourages the health and well-being of its residents by providing, as written in their mission statement, for the "social, spiritual, nutritional, residential and health care needs of aging adults." As part of the Quaker philosophy, the members of the Crystal Village community strive to treat everyone with loving respect, regardless of circumstances or infirmity. One of their goals is to inspire a sense of community and inclusion among residents and staff. Included in their brochure are 10 "hallmarks of Quaker services for the aging." As this case unfolds, 3 of these "hallmarks" will become apparent as they play a significant role in Kris' life:

1. *Believing that all people have strengths and capacities that can be supported and nurtured.* Programs focus on a person's wellness and abilities rather than on needs, disability, or illness.
2. *Respecting the dignity of each individual.* Programs seek to understand and listen to the older person and to respond with care and flexibility. This respect is accorded all, regardless of infirmity or frailty.
3. *Involving participants in decisions about their own lives and surroundings*, including when they are infirm, as a way of recognizing independence and supporting the highest possible quality of life.

Many of the structural and environmental features of Crystal Village meet these expectations. However, as in Kris' case, not all of these expectations are met for each person because of physical and mental limitations.

Our guide brought us to a door half-ajar in the Honeyfield House intensive care unit and knocked. Honeyfield House is a 32-private-bed, licensed nursing care unit for residents in need of 24-hour professional health care service. Residents in Honeyfield are fairly dependent on the nursing and support staff for most of their daily activities. Yet, staff members in the Honeyfield unit continue to help residents maintain as much independence as possible. Honeyfield residents are not physically restrained, and Crystal Village attempts to provide for individual residents' needs with flexibility and availability of social and health care options. Though social interaction is somewhat restricted in this unit, guests may escort residents to the dining room or coffee shop for meals if they are physically able.

MEETING KRIS

On our first "official" meeting with Kris, he was lounging in his leather recliner in front of his television with his oxygen tank close by. His chair was positioned perfectly so as to have easy access to his desktop computer on his right, a sparsely decorated bookshelf directly behind him, and his bed not more than an arm's length away on his left. As the late afternoon sunlight streamed through the open curtains, we settled in on his small bed and wooden chairs that were squished between the desk and television. His room was furnished from floor to wall with belongings from his previous residences. A quick glance around revealed "how to" books for computers, mail, and weekly menus and social calendars for Crystal Village. Though we had met Kris before, this time, he shared part of his life with us, a life, he says, that should be written as a biography.

Kris is a 92-year-old widower living in an intensive care wing of an assisted-care facility. In the past five years, Kris has undergone several major life transitions. The most intense of these changes include his retirement from a lifelong career in civil engineering, his wife's cancer diagnosis and eventual death, and the rapid decline of his own cardiovascular and respiratory health. In addition to the stress inherent in each of these life transitions, Kris faced the additional burden of relocation as a result of each event. Compounding his difficulties, each relocation resulted in restricted access to social support from friends and family. Kris' experiences provide an illuminating example of how life transitions, such as severe health problems, retirement, bereavement, and weak family ties, can lead to social isolation and a feeling of despondency among older adults in assisted-living facilities.

Kris emigrated from Germany to central Pennsylvania just before the start of World War II. Kris was 25 and a recent college graduate when he arrived in the United States to work. He was employed in a small coal town in a rural portion of the state when he met a young woman named Carrie, a woman who would become his life partner. The couple settled permanently in Pennsylvania, and together they reared a daughter. Although Kris was consistently employed, he faced many challenges as an "enemy alien," including difficulty obtaining residence and work visas. Despite this difficulty, over time, his resumé included prestigious work as a civil engineer, professor, government employee, and consultant. He retired from his long-time university position and remained professor emeritus with a private office until his late 80s.

As Kris and Carrie grew older, Carrie actively looked into long-term-care options for their retirement. While conducting her research, Carrie was diagnosed with lung cancer. Her illness made the couple aware of the increasing urgency of this decision. After looking at various assisted-care facilities in their hometown, Kris, Carrie, and their daughter discussed all of the options. One option was for their daughter to assume a caregiver role. However, the couple knew it would be impossible for their daughter to fly in from Canada frequently enough to provide the kind of health care assistance they needed. Another option was for the couple to move to Canada to be closer to their daughter, but Kris and Carrie did not want to leave Pennsylvania. The family finally decided that Crystal Village Retirement Community was the best choice.

Kris and his family chose Crystal Village because it offered independent living cottages, as well as units inside the main facility where residents could receive varied levels of medical attention. Kris and Carrie lived a simple, but quaint life in an independent cottage. Their cottage had two bedrooms, a living room, a modern kitchen, and a small vegetable garden that allowed them the space and independence they wanted, without the necessary upkeep. In the evenings, they would meet acquaintances from the other cottages for dinner. They would even entertain friends and family in the cottage from time to time.

After a few years in the cottage, Carrie's cancer progressed. It became necessary for her to move into the main facility where she would have increased medical attention. Kris and Carrie moved from their two-bedroom cottage to a two-room residence inside Chester House, the personal care facility. Downsizing proved to be difficult and resulted in one of the biggest challenges and disappointments they had met along their life course. After choosing a few memory-laden items to keep, Kris and Carrie donated some of their furniture and other goods to Crystal

Village, transferred some to their daughter, and packed the rest in storage. Unfortunately, Carrie's cancer continued to spread. She was moved yet again to a smaller, intensive care room in Honeyfield House, where she spent the last year of her life, leaving Kris alone in the Chester House apartment. The couple's separation was accompanied by rapid physical decline for both Carrie and Kris; Carrie passed away within the year and Kris developed cardiovascular and respiratory problems. He was subsequently moved from the apartment to a small room in Honeyfield House where he currently resides. His only immediate family includes a daughter who lives in northern Canada and a sister who lives in Germany. Both live too far to visit often, though he talks to them periodically on the phone. He feels estranged by his family and secluded from his friends, and has had to relinquish all but a few remaining items from his lifetime of shared memories and rich experiences.

> So I ended up being alone in the apartment, and then I had some, well, heart and lung problems, and eventually they put me in here. I had to give up the apartment, and that was the real break, because, you know, that was the end. Especially with the medical diagnosis that I wouldn't go back there. So that meant disposing of, it was a two-bedroom apartment, and we had furniture, and pictures, and files, and everything. And I had to dispose of all of that. Abandon it. Lots of stuff I had to abandon.

SOCIAL INTERACTION AND AGING

Family, friends, and companions are pervasive sources of social support in the lives of the elderly. Although social support is extremely important, the availability of friends, companions, and even family diminished each time Kris moved into a new living situation. Friendship availability became constrained, as well as hours and methods of socialization. The time, desire, and energy available to Kris to devote to friendship development and socialization were also significantly reduced. His physical location and health status severely impaired his mobility and facility to maintain his social network, thus hindering his ability to tap into social support resources necessary for healthy living.

Particularly distressing for Kris were the transitions that took him from almost entirely independent living in the cottage to 24-hour care, where he no longer had access to various forms of social support ranging from active neighbors, close family, and friends from the larger community. While living in the independent cottages, Kris was able to participate in various community activities provided by Crystal Village. The Village encourages residents to play an active role in the community by initiating, directing, and planning their own activities. While living in the cottages and in Chester House, Kris had the opportunity to engage in various volunteer programs and serve on community boards and committees. Once Kris was relocated to Honeyfield, however, his movement and ability to engage in those activities was severely and permanently limited. He became dependent on the availability of staff members to assist him in those activities:

> Well, for instance, the retirees in the department have a monthly breakfast, and I can't go to that anymore . . . But uh, the main thing is that once you move out of the cottages to here, you get cut off from the world. Especially if you can't, well, theoretically you're not supposed to leave this floor at all. Only if you have somebody that watches you, you're okay. And I have been graduated, I can go around this place by myself, and I don't have to have anybody with me.

Social support among the elderly is often contextualized within the realm of health and stress, two salient factors in Kris' life. He converses at length about the decline of his physical health, as well as his wife's. Yet, he also emphasizes the importance of maintaining social ties with friends and neighbors and continuing with enjoyable activities as a means of sustaining good mental health. Previous to their move to Crystal Village, Kris and Carrie found it relatively easy to tap into various social support networks. For them, these networks were composed primarily of coworkers, friends, and neighbors. This aided Kris and Carrie in maintaining a healthy social life and reducing much of the stress present as they coped with declining health and life transitions. Research suggests that one of the major health benefits of having social support networks is the resulting "stress buffering effect." Social support played an important role in the lives of Kris and Carrie, but is something Kris expresses is sorely missed as he reflects on his current position in life. For Kris and Carrie, although they moved first from their large downtown house into the retirement village, they maintained many of their social activities and social networks, and became involved in new ones. As ill health restricted many of their previous social activities, their relocation to the retirement village enabled them to explore new options. They used the free transportation services provided by Crystal Village and engaged in many sponsored social activities. Kris describes his life after moving into the independent cottages as similar to when he and his wife owned their own home, but with a few changes in size and activities. But, as their health continued to decline, they became more and more restricted in their activities and reduced their level of social interaction and social support.

> Carrie was active in the Rose Symphony, and I had my business. I had an office until just recently in the civil engineering department. I think that was, it was not very bad compared with living here on your own. Of course, that was already a cut back when we moved out of our house, because we of course had an attic, and you have a cellar, you have stuff here and there, I had my little box of nuts and bolts. And various other things. And a power saw and so on. And you had a lot to garden, here you just had a little strip, but that was pretty much, initially, and you can have outside people in, and they would come fairly frequently.

Unfortunately, certain structural, social, and physical barriers may prevent older adults from enjoying social interaction when living in an assisted-care facility. Kris admits to needing additional support, both tangible and intangible, as he is aging, but he feels limited in the social support resources that are available to him in his new living situation. His major complaint is that he is no longer able to entertain outside guests as often as he would like, heightening his sense of loneliness and separation.

> And this place is more forbidding, I mean people don't come here as hastily as they did in the cottages. I don't have much social interaction. Yeah, I guess there's always somebody coming in or phoning or something, in fact people come in and they see me sleep, but they leave. Instead of waking me, they leave. Even though I encourage that [waking him].

Many factors determine the likelihood of an elderly person activating their social support network. Due to location, skills, and ability, access to this important resource is not equal for everyone. Because the psychological and social benefits derived from social support networks are contingent on accessibility to social networks, the environmental structure of nursing homes becomes very important. In Kris' case, the important interpersonal flow of resources provided by social support and social interaction are largely unavailable because of his physical location in the intensive care unit and his physical limitations. This is primarily because of two factors. His ill health does not permit him to walk far or engage in much physical activity. In addition, because he is in constant need of nursing care, he is located on a floor among others with equally limiting physical conditions. Additionally, the majority of residents on Kris' floor are significantly limited in social abilities due to Alzheimer's disease and other forms of dementia. As a result, Kris is lacking many of the benefits derived from informal sources of social support such as, among other things, affection, caring, material goods, and the opportunity to socialize.

THE ROLE OF FAMILY AND FRIENDS IN SOCIAL SUPPORT

A common assumption is that families of older adults will meet all or many of their social support needs. This is a result of a societal expectation that families should provide a certain amount of care to an aging individual. However, the family's ability to provide emotional and instrumental support depends on the environmental context of the family. Kris' main channel of social support is through mediated communication with his sister and daughter, either on the telephone or via the Internet on his personal computer. Though infrequent, this social support gives Kris a small sense of connectedness and well-being. He relies heavily on support from his daughter, equating her assistance and support with his ability to continue living.

> My daughter lives in Canada. We talk almost every second day on the phone. She was here for quite some time during my bad time. I became very ill. I think things would not have worked out without her.

For many older adults, distance hinders the amount and type of social support that family can provide. In Kris' situation, his frequent telephone conversations with his daughter and sister serve as a primary component of his social network. At the same time, the lack of family in close physical proximity has resulted in a great deal of stress for Kris. As each move forced him to relinquish more of his possessions, he is troubled by the reality that there is no one to whom he can pass on many of his most cherished belongings. Kris feels there is no one with whom he can share the memories of his life and continue his legacy:

> My daughter took some of the furniture, I gave some of it to Crystal Village, and the files are still in boxes and await my return. And cleaning them out, you know they're medical records of my wife, nobody wants those anymore. All the files and memories, photos, and books, and everything that we had accumulated through the years, suddenly went to nowhere. And that's of course another problem, because that means a lot of things that I will be leaving won't have any obvious takers. Basically you're cut off, you know, part of your life is chopped off.

It is important to note that family members are not the only type of social support available to older adults. Friends and companions are as prevalent in elder adulthood as they are in younger years, and the social support provided through these relationships differs in important ways from support provided by the family. For example, family members generally feel obligated to provide some degree of support, whereas support from friends and companions is offered voluntarily. Support from nonfamily relationships is usually provided when it is mutually gratifying. Certain life events may make finding relationships in which mutual gratification is possible more difficult. Although elder adults have some choice over their selection of friendships, they are nevertheless bound by physical and mental abilities, social conventions, physical location, social and environmental contexts, mobility, social skill, time, and accessibility. Changes in any one of these areas can transform the relational dynamics of dependence and independence. For Kris, the day he retired was a pivotal point in his friendships with his coworkers.

Well, I had a step like that when I retired. When I retired, the day before retirement, everybody was hopping when I said hop. And all of a sudden they didn't anymore! Meaning I had no control over things anymore, I couldn't use my stuff.

INDEPENDENCE AND SOCIAL SUPPORT

Social support networks are one way through which elder adults can establish a sense of independence in their lives. Nursing homes can facilitate this through supportive communication and providing environments and activities designed to increase residents' perceptions of control and competence. Crystal Village advertises that as a resident "you feel a genuine sense of welcome, support, and freedom from care as you enjoy your treasured independence." By offering a flexible and resident-focused facility, the Village attempts to offer as much independence as it deems prudent. Maintaining a sense of independence is of great importance to Kris. Yet, complete self-sufficiency is virtually impossible, stressing the need for Kris and other older adults to be integrated in a complex system of interdependent social relationships. In doing so, elder adults may find it difficult to maintain their needed independence *and* facilitate day-to-day living without assistance.

As Kris sits in his room with his oxygen tubes snaked through his nostrils, he has made it obvious that he perceives the dependency scale unbalanced. From removing his driving privileges to relying on others for Scotch tape, Kris realizes that he now relies on his friends and acquaintances for many things he used to do for himself and that he cannot provide such services to others.

There are all these complications that didn't exist before and many other enjoyable things are no longer available. I have somebody right now picking up some tape in the hardware store. Well, in the olden days I would have gone over there and gotten it, but now I gotta ask somebody. For somebody that used to do most of the things himself, that's difficult to do. And there are other little annoyances. They have a post office here, that's open for only two hours on Thursday. Well, most people don't have much and the ones that live in the cottages just go to the regular post office, so it's really for a limited number of people. Well, yesterday I was gonna go, but I plum forgot it, so now I've got to wait a whole week. You know these little things add up to quite some restrictions and so on. I can't go to the store to buy some sushi, and some of the people here wouldn't touch sushi with a ten foot pole (laughing). Even for consumption by somebody else!

Circumstances in an assisted-care facility pose a new dimension to social support, independency, and social well-being. Though Crystal Village has created programs and has attempted to structure its facility to increase and enhance independent living, many of the natural facets of nursing care facilities sustain and create a sense of dependence. Ultimately, dependency must be negotiated. However, in an assisted-care facility, a caregiver is charged with the responsibility of caring for the patient. The degree of care and dependency may not be negotiated in the same way as in other relationships. Complicating this matter is the North American preoccupation with independence and society's deeply rooted stereotypic beliefs and behaviors, which serve to underestimate the capabilities of older adults. As such, many older adults are vulnerable to feeling that their independence is threatened, hesitant to rely on others, and experience decreased levels of self-efficacy.

In fact, showing too much concern toward elderly persons can insult their independence, causing them to lose morale. In an assisted-care facility, caregivers and residents may have difficulty negotiating the extent to which residents require assistance. Although Crystal Village believes that the availability of tri-leveled medical assistance and lifetime care offers "invaluable peace of mind" and "a genuine sense of security," not all residents may value this approach.

As for Kris, he recognizes the good will of the caregivers, but simultaneously expresses his perception that some of the assistance he receives is trivial and quite possibly unnecessary.

> The service here is pretty good. Compared to what I hear from other people, this is a pretty good place. Some of the people around here are very helpful and look out for me. Of course, one thing—I have to wear compression stockings. I used to put those on myself, but I can't do that anymore, because bending down shuts off my air supply, and it just doesn't work. So, I get help here putting them on and things like that. Well, and they make sure that I don't forget to take my medications and things like that, but those are small improvements. I used to do pretty well myself.

The ability to choose when, with whom, and whether or not to pursue social interaction is powerful. One daily activity that Kris particularly relishes is socializing with other residents in the dining room during supper. This is the only area in which he feels he is given the freedom to pursue social relationships. In this way, Kris has reaped the benefits of Crystal Village's quest for flexibility, as he is the only person on his floor who has been given "permission" to leave his unit unescorted to dine communally with old friends and acquaintances from the cottages or Chester House each evening. The voluntary nature of these relationships enables Kris to experience some sense of control over his social life.

> No, not very much socializing. Well, that's one thing about social intercourse, of course all the people here are basically Alzheimer types, and there's not, there's nobody that I can really talk to. I do go out to the dining room for dinner, I have an oxygen machine up there, so I can enjoy my dinner and there I have interaction with people. I know a number of people, but friends I wouldn't call them, from out of the cottages and so on. So the dinner interaction is important.

It is important to offer the opportunity to socialize with compatible others to residents in retirement villages and nursing care facilities. Long-term care facilities attempt to provide these opportunities by developing age-segregated communities. The idea is that the likelihood of elderly individuals forming a supportive social network is greater among those who lived in age-segregated communities than those living in the multigenerational communities. This philosophy is illustrated by Crystal Village's vision statement:

> Crystal Village, a lifetime care retirement community, is a vibrant and caring community that encourages and supports older adults as they seek to live life fully and gracefully in harmony with the principles of simplicity, diversity, equality, mutual respect, compassion, and personal involvement.

For Kris, however, an age-segregated community means the loss of many interpersonal ties with younger coworkers, friends, and family members. Though Crystal Village practically guarantees that "you'll never feel as though you're 'out of touch' with whatever's happening," Kris feels otherwise. Despite his mental acuity and interest in creating social relationships with similar others, he resides in a social setting wherein many of the others are not physically or mentally able to create and maintain social relationships. In his own words, Kris suggests it is this very lack of social interaction that makes his daily living situation unbearable.

> It's irrational to feel that one steps down when one moves out of the cottages into this facility. But it's the truth. You do feel like a stool has been kicked out from under you. It's primarily the fact that you don't have any future here, and you can't do a lot of things. That's the main complaint and the main disadvantage. On the other hand, who knew that I was going to live 92 years (laughing)? So, one struggles along. I don't care what happens next week. Except that I hope winter ends and my daughter comes to visit me. And a couple other people that have said they would.

RELEVANT CONCEPTS

Lifespan communication: The study of change that occurs in the structure and function of communication across the life course.

Life transitions: Changes that occur throughout the lifespan, including changes in status, financial abilities, dependency, living arrangements, family and friend circles, and age cohort.

Nursing care: Paid health care services provided by trained medical and nursing staff to individuals unable to fully care for themselves.

Self-efficacy: A person's perceived ability to perform a particular task, including a person's perception of ability to accomplish everyday living tasks.

Social support: Tangible and intangible resources provided to a person to help her/him cope with stress present throughout the lifespan, such as comforting communication or financial assistance.

Successful aging: Positive attitude and healthful approach toward aging.

DISCUSSION QUESTIONS

1. The physical structure of a nursing care facility or retirement village can serve to facilitate or inhibit social interaction. If you were researching assisted-care facilities for a loved one, what environmental cues would you look for to ensure social interaction?
2. If you were on a committee whose job it was to help create a sense of independence and feeling of control for residents of an intensive care unit in an assisted living environment, what suggestions would you offer?
3. What ways can you think of to help ensure social support and well-being is available to nursing care patients who are in poor health and have limited physical ability?
4. People encounter multiple life transitions throughout the life course of varying degrees of significance and impact. What are some life transitions that might have the greatest effect on one's life and sense of well-being? What are some ways in which people can ease discomfort that often follows these transitions?

ENDNOTE

[1] All names and identifying information were changed to preserve the confidentiality of our participants. All of the data collected for this case study were obtained through in-depth personal interviews and observations in a well-established long-term care facility. Kris is a lucid, active, and extremely articulate 92-year-old widower living in this care facility whom we met while conducting this research. His narratives, as well our observations and informal discussions with other residents and staff, provide the basis for this case.

REFERENCES/SUGGESTED READINGS

Crohan, S. E., & Antonucci, T. C. (1989). Friends as a source of social support in old age. In R. G. Adams & R. Bliesner (Eds.), *Older adult friendship structure and process* (pp. 129–146). Newbury Park: Sage Publications.

Kahn, R. L. (1994). Social support: Content, causes and consequences. In R. P. Abeles, H. C. Gift, & M. G. Ory (Eds.), *Aging and quality of life* (pp.163–184). New York: Springer.

Nussbaum, J. F., & Coupland, J. (1995). *Handbook of communication and aging research.* Mahwah, NJ: Lawrence Erlbaum Associates.

Nussbaum, J. F., Pecchioni, L. L., Robinson, J. D., & Thompson, T. L. (2000). *Communication and aging* (2nd ed.). Mahwah, NJ: Lawrence Erlbaum Associates.

Poulin, J. E. (1984). Age segregation and the interpersonal involvement and morale of the aged. *The Gerontologist,* *24,* 266–269.

Samter, W. (2003). Friendship interaction skills across the lifespan. In J. O. Green & B. R. Burleson (Eds.), *Handbook* *of communication and social interaction skills.* Mahwah, NJ: Lawrence Erlbaum Associates.

Searle, M. S., Mahon, M. J., Iso-Ahola, S. E., Sdrolias, H. A., & van Dyck, J. (1998). Examining the long term effects of leisure education on a sense of independence and psychological well-being among the elderly. *Journal of Leisure* *Research, 30,* 331–340.

Williams, A., Giles, H., Coupland, N., Dalby, M., & Manasse, H. (1990). The communication contexts of elderly social support and health: A theoretical model. *Health Communication, 2,* 123–143.

Williams, A., & Nussbaum, J. F. (2001). *Intergenerational communication across the lifespan.* Mahwah, NJ: Lawrence Erlbaum Associates.

Additional Resources

Administration on Aging (AOA): http://www.aoa.dhhs.gov/
American Association of Retired Persons (AARP): http://www.aarp.org/
American Society on Aging (ASA): http://www.asaging.org/
The National Council on Aging (NCOA): http://www.ncoa.org/
The National Institute on Aging (NIA): http://www.nia.nih.gov/

V

Issues in Health Care Delivery

20

Role Negotiation, Stress, and Burnout: A Day in the Life of "Supernurse"

Julie Apker
Western Michigan University

Across the United States, spiraling health care costs, advancements in medical technology, and aging patient populations have transformed hospital health care delivery. Managed care— a system that strives to efficiently manage health care services and reduce medical costs—has driven many hospital changes. To remain competitive, more and more hospitals have been forced to do things differently through strategies such as reducing or limiting medical services, implementing shorter patient stays, downsizing staff, and restructuring employee roles. These changes have impacted the working conditions and professional practices of most hospital health care workers and, ultimately, have affected patient care.

Registered nurses (RNs) who work in hospitals often find themselves on the front lines of changes in their work roles, job responsibilities, and professional relationships. Today's nursing roles not only include traditional responsibilities, such as providing bedside care, but also new duties, such as team leading, administration, and supervising assistant personnel. Moreover, many RNs are taking on the tasks once done by allied health personnel and medical support staff. These role additions come at a time when nurses are pressured to "do more in less time" but without additional training, higher wages, or institutional support. Thus, nursing work is characterized by role overload, increased job complexity, and a lack of organizational resources. These workplace stressors can result in negative outcomes (e.g., physical illness, relationship conflict, and poor job performance). In some cases, role stress may actually cause nurses to burn out and leave their hospital positions for other jobs or even other professions.

THE HOSPITAL

City Hospital is a 900-bed, full-service teaching hospital located in a major midwestern city. As the flagship hospital of a large integrated health care system, this institution employs more than 1,000 physicians, nurses, allied health personnel, and support staff. Like many other urban health care facilities in the United States, City Hospital relies heavily on Medicare and Medicaid funding to pay for patient health care costs. Consequently, the hospital experienced a severe financial setback with the passage of the 1997 Balanced Budget Act—federal legislation that included substantial cuts in health care funding for elderly, poor, and indigent patients. In addition, managed care organizations continue to exert heavy pressure on the hospital to keep health care costs and insurance premiums down.

To curb multi-million dollar losses, City Hospital implemented a number of dramatic changes that directly affect the nursing staff and their patient care. First, the hospital eliminated hundreds of support personnel (e.g., respiratory therapists, phlebotomists, and patient educators) and assigned many of their duties to staff nurses. Second, RNs were given more patients to care for at the same time the hospital mandated shorter length-of-stay requirements. Third, nurses were required to supervise unlicensed personnel (nursing aides, housekeeping, and patient transport). In addition to these past changes, City Hospital has continued to experience a nursing shortage, and many of its medical services consistently run short of qualified nursing personnel. Nurses have felt the impact of many vacant RN positions firsthand which, in some cases, involves mandatory overtime. The combination of these factors has created a stressful work environment and negatively affected nurse morale.

THE NURSING UNIT

Three East—one of City Hospital's 26 inpatient units—is a 30-bed, general medicine unit made up of middle-age or elderly patients, usually with pulmonary-related diseases, such pneumonia, asthma, chronic obstructive pulmonary disease, and bronchitis. Three East employs about 50 full-time employees, of which 18 are RNs. Like all other inpatient nursing units in City Hospital, Three East functions 24 hours a day with three shifts of nursing staff, six nurses on each shift. The day shift runs from 7 a.m. to 3 p.m., the afternoon shift is staffed between 3 p.m. and 11 p.m., and the night shift is staffed between 11 p.m. and 7 a.m.

When entering Three East, a visitor immediately sees a small reception area with a comfortable visitor lounge instead of a large, central nursing station. Two glassed-in counseling areas located on either side of the lounge are used for private conversations between medical staff, patients, and their families. A small pharmacy is located behind the reception area, and social workers assigned to the unit have an office adjacent to the reception desk. Two wings branch off of the reception area. Each wing consists of a long hallway that houses patient rooms and two nursing ministations (also called pods). Each pod is "owned" by a particular health care team for the day, afternoon, and night shifts—the same RN and nursing aide cover the same six to eight beds every day. Each pod contains computer terminals, equipment, and supplies needed by the nursing and medical staff.

Communication is central to work life on Three East. In addition to wearing pagers, all nurses carry portable cellular phones—enabling constant, immediate communication on the floor among members of the health care team. Each pod has its own phone, which rings constantly, as other employees and individuals working outside the hospital contact nurses and doctors for patient care information. Further, medical and nursing staff communicate via multidisciplinary report sheets and patient documentation forms that are located in wall alcove chart stations. Nurses and doctors use these communication tools constantly to update each other on patients. In addition, they engage in dozens of face-to-face interactions during each shift in settings such as rounds, team meetings, and private consultations. Moreover, Three East nurses and physicians are consistently communicating with patients and their families as they perform their daily work activities.

THE NURSE

Rob Carter is a 35-year-old RN who holds a bachelor's degree in public health education and gerontology. Twelve years ago, he earned a diploma in nursing from City Hospital's School of Nursing. He has worked on Three East for his entire nursing career, including his two years of nurse training, making him one of the most senior staff nurses on the unit. Like many nurses, Rob describes his career as a calling:

> I always wanted to be a doctor as a kid, so I knew I wanted to be in the medical field. I found a job at a nursing home. I saw what the nurses did there, and I liked their focus on patient care. I didn't go into nursing for the paycheck. I went into nursing for myself, my own joy, to care for patients.

Rob supervises and coordinates the nursing care of six to eight patients that are assigned to Pod One. Rob works at the patient bedside and manages a nursing aide, Belinda, unit support personnel (e.g., patient transport and housekeeping), and senior nursing students, who are called externs. He describes his responsibilities:

> I lead the health care team to help our patients. I am someone who answers questions and directs other people to do their jobs effectively and efficiently. I pass meds to patients, document nursing activities, develop care plans, conduct patient assessment, and perform nursing interventions like dressing changes and drawing blood.

Rob takes his nursing role seriously, often working well beyond his regularly scheduled hours and skipping lunch to give "100%" to his patients. Below, he comments on his professional dedication:

> I have to know everything that's going on with my patients. If someone is going out the door, I better know about it. *Don't* take the patient off the floor before making me aware of it. It will mess up my whole day. I'm responsible. I have to be kept in the know. I like knowing that there's something I've done that's made an impact on my patients' well-being and their progress to optimum health.

Rob's comments typify the views of many care providers, professionals who see their jobs as a chance to make a difference in people's lives. Certainly, Rob's devotion to his patients should be valued, but there are significant human costs to his high levels of caring and commitment. As Rob suggests in the following quote, stressors such as workload, role conflict, and role ambiguity impact his nursing practice:

> I'm the king of stress. I can't handle a lot of stress ... everything and everyone at once. When the docs are all just pulling at me. It's 'Rob, Rob, Rob. Do this, do that, get this.' It just keeps eating at the stress level a little more. The docs push me too far. A lot of work falls on me to arrange at the last minute. Don't they know I have *my own* work to do? I can't be at their beck and call all the time. That causes me stress, and I'm not the best at coping with stress. I don't verbalize my stress. I keep it in. Some days, the stress makes me question whether I should work here. I wonder if I should just leave nursing entirely.

LIFE ON DAY SHIFT

During one eight-hour shift, Rob interacts with dozens of people (e.g., doctors, nursing aides, allied health personnel, patients, family members, etc.) on a wide variety of issues related to patient care. Although each of Rob's workdays is unique because of a varying patient mix, Rob's day always includes morning report, initial patient assessment, rounds, postround follow-up (which lasts several hours), and afternoon report.

7 a.m.—Morning Report

Report is a half-hour time period for the nurses to provide information from the previous shift about each patient's physical, emotional, and mental health. A typical day for Rob begins with him receiving morning report from Shirley, the Pod One nurse who works the night shift. Shirley and Rob review patient charts and visit patients so Rob can visually assess their conditions.

Today, Shirley tells Rob that Mr. Riordan, an elderly patient with chronic heart problems and pneumonia, has been particularly difficult to deal with during the night.

"Mr. Riordan keeps pulling out his feeding tubes and IV lines," said Shirley. "I was constantly in his room either checking on him so he wouldn't do it or putting the tubes and IVs back in when he did take them out. He's driving me crazy!"

"This is the guy who has depression, right? He has no friends or family who visit," replied Rob. "Maybe he's just trying to get someone to talk to him."

Shirley added, "You're probably right, but I just didn't have time to sit with him. It was a zoo last night."

"By the way, we still can't find a qualified nurse to work nights yet. The temps the nursing agency sends don't know what's going on. I don't have time to teach them, either, so they don't come back for a second night . . . I wish Mr. Riordan would leave well enough alone!"

"I'll talk with Mr. Riordan and ask Dr. Ryan to order a consult from psychiatry. About the temps . . . that's a tough one. We need their help, but we don't have time to train them. It's a no-win situation," sighed Rob. "What else is going on with our patients?"

Shirley sighed, "Well, they're the same group as yesterday. Their health status is unchanged, as you see in their charts."

"On a side note, I had difficulty stocking our supplies last night because of the staffing problem, so I couldn't get to it. To add to it, the computers are crashing again. We had to reboot them four times last night. That was fun—it takes even longer to document patient information! I've called tech support twice, and they say they'll be here as soon as possible, but I doubt it. You can't count on that department ever since the hospital downsized half of their technicians. Same goes for the supply department. It's ridiculous that we have to stock our own supplies!"

"Ever since the hospital got into debt, we've had to do more with less," said Rob. "Take the housekeeping situation. Last week, I had to leave the floor to go get clean towels because housekeeping couldn't spare anyone to deliver them to the unit! Last time I looked, delivering laundry was *not* a part of my job description! Next thing you know, they'll make washing laundry a part of our jobs. Unbelievable!"

"Well, all I know is that I have at least an hour of charting to do before I go because I didn't have time last night," Shirley responded. "The patients are all yours. I hope your day goes better for you than it did for me, Rob."

"Thanks, Shirley. I'll see you tomorrow," Rob said.

Rob asked Belinda to stock the pod before she starts her regularly assigned tasks. "Please look for the cell phone while you're at it," Rob told Belinda. "I think it was lost on afternoon or night shift."

"Rob, I keep telling you, you're not responsible for everything that goes on in Pod One," Belinda replied. "They lost the cell phone, not us."

"I know, but our unit can't afford to replace the phone again," Rob said. "They told us at the last staff meeting that if a cell phone is lost or stolen, we have to do without. I tried to tell the nurse manager that using the cell phones is the best way for the docs to reach us on the unit, but it doesn't matter. Administration doesn't understand that it makes our jobs more difficult when we can't communicate with each other. They just don't get it."

"I'll look for the phone. It probably was misplaced in the supply closet again," said Belinda. "After that, I'll start checking vital signs."

"Okay, in the meantime, I'll do our assessments and see what needs to be brought to the docs' attention during rounds. Mr. Riordan was giving Shirley some problems last night, so I'm going to spend some time with him to find out what's the matter."

7:30 a.m. to 9 a.m.—Patient Assessment

Today, Rob hurries through his assessments so he can spend time with Mr. Riordan. Rob enters Mr. Riordan's cramped room, which is filled with medical equipment and smells of disinfectant, and sits down next to the bed.

"How are you feeling today, Mr. Riordan?"

"Not good. These damn doctors won't give me a straight answer! They just keep running tests. One day, Dr. Andre tells me I need surgery. Then, the next day, she says no. Which is it? I've got so many tubes running in and out of me that I can't sleep and that stupid night nurse won't give me enough medication for the pain. A dog would get better care at a vet's office! That's how I'm feeling!"

"Mr. Riordan, it won't do either of us any good if you yell. Maybe I can help," responded Rob calmly. "I looked at your chart, and you're scheduled for surgery tomorrow. Dr. Andre will tell you more about it when she comes by at 9 o'clock for rounds. I'll be there too, and we can talk after the doctors leave in case you want more information about the procedure. The doctors have a lot of patients to visit in a short amount of time, but I'm here all day."

Mr. Riordan grumbled, "Well . . . okay. But what about the other nurse and these tubes? I want to be moved to another hospital where I'll get better treatment!"

"I'm sorry that you're unhappy with your care here," Rob said. "The tubes are there to feed you, give you fluids, and reduce your pain. You have a number of health problems, and it's important that you don't pull out any of the tubes. If you do, that just means that you'll be in the hospital longer. Shirley is a good nurse, and she's just trying to help. I understand how you're feeling, and I'll try not to bother you today any more than I have to, okay?"

"Oh. I don't mind you. I like talking with you. Lord knows my family doesn't come by to see me. I'm just tired of being here, that's all," sighed Mr. Riordan.

"I like talking with you, too, and we'll talk more after rounds, okay? I need to get back to work, now. Everything is going to be okay, and you'll be outta here in no time!" said Rob.

After leaving Mr. Riordan's room, Rob sighed and thought, "It really bothers me when patients complain about their care here. Most of the nurses on Three East really try to give 110% to their jobs, but lately, it doesn't seem to be enough. We don't have enough staff and supplies to do our jobs properly, and it affects patient care. It's so frustrating when we can't help the patient because the hospital is in the red financially."

"Hi Rob. What's going on in Pod One this morning?" asked Cathy, the nursing extern assigned to Rob's supervision for the past few weeks.

"Hi Cathy. We have a lot on our plate today, as usual. Ready to get to work?"

"What should I do first?" asks Cathy.

"Check on Mr. Riordan's IVs. I think he needs a new one."

"Rob, would you show me how to start one again?"

"I don't have time to help you now. I have to document morning assessments before rounds or the docs will complain. You're gonna have to start it on your own and call me *only* if you run into problems. You'll be taking your boards soon, and it's about time that you do a few things by yourself. It's how we all learned."

"Rob, don't some hospitals still have phlebotomists on staff who start and change all of the IVs and do patient blood draws? Why do the staff nurses have to do them here?"

"We used to, but a few years ago, the hospital decided to cut all that out to reduce costs. Phlebotomists, respiratory therapists, and patient educators all got downsized, and most of their jobs became part of nursing. We didn't have a say in it, it's just what we have to deal with now. Anyway, I have to get this charting done, and you need to do the IVs. After that, start passing meds. Remember that I have to check every dosage before you give them out."

Rob starts to document his patient assessments while simultaneously answering the now-found cell phone and responding to questions from Belinda, Cathy, and the other nurses on the floor. Time passes quickly, and Rob is surprised to see a team of physicians arrive for rounds. "It's 9 a.m.? Where did the time go?" he wondered aloud.

9 a.m.—Rounds

A senior physician, also called an attending, leads a group of five medical residents and one student to each patient room during rounds. Residents update the attending on their patients and nurses listen in to learn more about patients' conditions and discharge status. Today, the team begins with patients in Pod One, so Rob joins the rounding team immediately in the room of Mrs. Sims, an elderly patient who has a pulmonary-related disease complicated by asthma. She was brought in two days ago because of a severe asthma attack. Mrs. Sims is wide-eyed with surprise as six people enter her room and surround her bed, so Rob winks and smiles at her from his position in the doorway to relax her. Dr. Ryan listens as Dr. Andre summarizes Mrs. Sims' condition. After asking the group a few questions, Dr. Ryan concludes that Mrs. Sims should be discharged today and placed in a nursing home for continued treatment.

"Rob, make sure that the social worker knows to set up a nursing home for Mrs. Sims. She's well enough to leave the hospital, but it's too soon for her to go home. Tell her relatives that she can leave this afternoon." His decision surprises Rob, who thought Mrs. Sims' condition was still serious enough to require a day or two more of inpatient care.

Hearing this news, Mrs. Sims turns her head, her forehead furrowed and lips pressed hard together with worry. Her hands tremble, and she tries not to cry. The rounding team quickly files out of the room, the doctors oblivious to Mrs. Sims' emotional reaction because they are already conferring about their next patient. Rob stays behind.

"Mrs. Sims, it's okay. This is good news. The doctors think that you're well enough to leave the hospital," said Rob.

"Rob, I don't want to go to a nursing home. Have you heard the stories about what happens to people in those places? Besides, my husband and I can hardly make ends meet with our Medicare coverage now. How are we supposed to pay for a nursing home?" asked Mrs. Sims.

"I know, Mrs. Sims," Rob said, squeezing her hand reassuringly. "The thing is, though, that you have improved so much that you don't need to be in the hospital anymore. We have patients who are really sick who need our beds."

"I'm scared, Rob, about what's going to happen to me."

Rob responded, "There might be something I can do. Let me do some checking with the unit social worker about arranging for a visiting nurse who can stop in a couple of times a week at your place rather than sending you to a nursing home. This should be okay with Dr. Ryan. I'll call your daughter, Jan, and let her know about you being discharged."

Rob dials the room phone. "Hello, may I speak with Jan Ferris? Jan? This is Rob Carter at City Hospital. No, your mom is just fine. The doctors asked me to tell you that she's ready to be discharged. Can you or your dad drive over to the hospital this afternoon to pick her up? She should be ready at 4 o'clock. We're working on arrangements with either a nursing home or visiting nurse. A social worker will call you later today with more information. Here's your mom."

Mrs. Sims takes the phone from Rob and begins to talk with her daughter. Rob leaves the room and walks quickly to catch up with the rounding team down the hall. He thought, "I really hate having conversations like that. A few years ago, we could have kept Mrs. Sims here for a few more days for observation, but now we don't have that luxury. Insurance companies and the government will only pay us so much money to provide care for a particular patient's condition. Once that money is spent, we start going into debt. Ultimately, we could close if we don't watch expenses closely and send patients to outpatient care as soon as they're ready. It seems like now more than ever, we just patch 'em up and send 'em out. I just hope Mrs. Sims doesn't bounce back here and become one of our 'frequent fliers.'"

"Rob. Hey Rob! Could you do Mr. Hardy's breathing treatment? I got a late start because of stocking supplies, and it's time for him to have one," yelled Belinda from down the hall.

"Belinda, I'm in the middle of rounds right now," said Rob. "I can do it later."

Belinda, hands on her hips, responded, "Rob, you know that right after rounds all of the docs swarm you with questions. It's always 'Rob, help me with this. Rob, who do I call? Rob, where is this or that?' There will be no time for you to help me with Mr. Hardy!"

"I know, I know. But it's important for me to hear what the docs are saying during rounds. You know that. Get Cathy to help you."

"She's got her hands full starting and changing IVs. I'll do it myself, but I don't want to hear complaints from you that I'm behind on my work this afternoon. Not after I had to spend 30 minutes stocking and looking for that stupid cell phone," snapped Belinda.

"I love hearing the joy in your voice, Belinda," said Rob, trying to lighten the mood. "It makes coming to work the more worthwhile."

"Whatever," said Belinda sarcastically, as she enters Mr. Hardy's room with the breathing treatment equipment.

Rob joins the rounding team in Mr. Riordan's room just as Dr. Ryan begins to question one of the residents on a confusing diagnosis. Robs spends the next 45 minutes shadowing the doctors as they complete their Pod One assessments and discuss orders. He jots notes about the comments pertaining to nursing interventions and occasionally joins in their discussion.

11:00 a.m.—Postrounds

Rounding is barely concluded before food service carts line the hallway, filled with patients' lunches. Visiting hours begin, and friends and relatives flood the unit to visit loved ones. Noise on the floor increases to a low roar, as doctors, nurses, nursing aides, allied health personnel, and students crowd into Pod One to talk and review patient information. Ringing pagers and telephones, beeps and squeals from medical equipment, and animated hallway conversations fill the unit. Medical residents, who are rushing to finish their work from rounds before lunch, bombard Rob with questions, just as Belinda predicted.

"Rob, what form do I use for this order?"

"Rob, what is the phone number for Pod 1?"

"Rob, who should I talk to in radiology to schedule an x-ray for Mr. Riordan to be done ASAP?"

"Rob, why didn't Leigh complete this order that I wrote for Mr. Hardy? It was supposed to be done yesterday during afternoon shift."

"Rob, I need to call a clinic on the west side of town to schedule outpatient care. Which one would you recommend?"

A blur of activity dressed in hospital "whites," Rob is constantly on the move as he answers these questions, visiting patients having lunch, charting, and answering his pod's phones. On several occasions, Rob has two or more people waiting to speak with him as he rushes between patient rooms, assessing patients, supervising Cathy's activities, and talking with Belinda about their patients. Ignoring the tension in his neck and shoulders and a knot of anxiety growing in his stomach, Rob tries to respond to the many questions and requests as calmly as possible, but his answers get more and more abrupt with each conversation. His patience finally ends with the arrival of Dr. Ortega, a first-year resident who has a history of problems with the nursing staff.

"Rob, you need to call dietary and physical therapy NOW. Mrs. Flynn goes home *today*, and we need to schedule her outpatient treatment," ordered Dr. Ortega. "Dietary can wait, but PT needs to be on the floor within the hour."

"Dr. Ortega, why didn't this get taken care of last night? Why did we wait until the day Mrs. Flynn has to go home? If you told me yesterday, I would've had it all lined up! There's no way I can get PT and dietary here this afternoon on such short notice!" Rob exclaimed.

"Listen, I don't care how you do it. Just do it! Mrs. Flynn is ready to go home, and she leaves today," said Dr. Ortega as he turned his back on Rob and walked down the hall.

"Is that right! What about the other five patients that depend on me, Dr. Ortega? What do I tell them when I can't take care of them because I'm hunting down PT and dietary?" said Rob in a loud tone of voice. Then, under his breath, he said, "How would you like to change an IV for me while I take care of your dirty work?"

"Rob, stop," cautioned Belinda. "Saying that stuff will just cause problems with the docs. It's not worth it."

"I don't care! The docs are always pushing and pulling at me after rounds so they can go take their lunches on time. I rush, rush, rush so they can have time off. I can't spare a minute to sit down, much less take a break myself. I've had it!"

Suddenly, Mr. Riordan's call light blinks and Rob remembers he promised to check in on him during lunch. Somewhere down the hall, a resident calls to him "Rob, can you come here? I can't find the number for the lab. Where's the hospital directory?" Cathy suddenly appears at his elbow asking, "Rob will you verify this medication for me? It's for Mr. Bower. He needs it right now." At the same time, Mrs. Sims' husband and daughter walk out of her room and approach Rob. From the puzzled expressions on their faces, he knows that they have lots of questions for him, most likely about her leaving the hospital and outpatient care options.

Rob thought, "Damn! I didn't follow-up with the social worker about a visiting nurse. I was so busy with the residents that I completely forgot. Now these two will have questions I can't answer, and I'll have to go over again why Mrs. Sims can't stay another day here. I can't deal with this right now!"

Rob turns away, red-faced and angry, clenches his hands into fists and stalks down the hall to the reception area. His chest feels tight, as if it will explode any minute.

"Hey Rob," greets Teri, the Three East receptionist. "What's the matter?"

"Everything! The docs. Patients. Everybody wanting something different from me! I can't stand it sometimes! I only have so much time in the day to do my job. I can't take it anymore! I had to have a quiet scream down here!"

"Rob. Rob. Calm down. Take a deep breathe. You don't get paid enough to get this upset. It's lunchtime. Go outside. Some fresh air will give you a new perspective," said Teri.

"Teri, in the last five years, when have I ever had time to take a lunch? I hardly have a chance to use the restroom once during a shift. No one cares, they just expect me to be happy and cheerful and do it all perfectly. I feel like I'm having a meltdown!"

"You're doing a great job, Rob. Everybody says so. That's why they call you Supernurse."

"Ha! Supernurse. That's me alright, especially today," responded Rob, calming down slightly. "I'll be fine once Dr. Ortega gets off my back. The jerk! Has he left the floor? I may say or do something I'll regret if I see him now."

"Yeah, he left a few minutes ago. You can go back to work."

Still feeling upset and overwhelmed, Rob returns to Pod One. He tries to calm down as he calls the physical therapy and dietary departments to make arrangements for Mrs. Flynn, but he gets an earful of frustration from both Denise the dietician and Joan the physical therapist. After much begging from Rob, both promise to "do him a favor" and visit Mrs. Flynn. As Rob hung up the phone, he turned to Cathy, and said, "Are you sure that you want to be a nurse? It's a job that doesn't pay well, there's mandatory overtime, you're going to be constantly short on supplies and staff, and you'll be pulled in 20 different directions at once. It's not too late to change professions, you know. A nursing degree can be applied to a lot of other jobs."

"Geez, I don't know, Rob," said Cathy.

"Well, you better think about it because you could be me in about two years!"

"I'm sorry you're having a bad day, Rob."

"Me, too," said Rob sharply.

With this comment, Rob sighed and walked into Mr. Riordan's room to explain what the doctors discussed during rounds. Rob thought, "This is the last thing I want to do. There is so much work left! Breathing treatments. Charting. I'm supposed to teach Mrs. Beverly how to use her new asthma inhaler. There's no way I'll be done by 3 p.m. I'll be here until 5 o'clock for sure, and I promised Brenda I'd be home on time tonight, for once. It's our anniversary. She's gonna kill me."

"Hi, Mr. Riordan. Did you catch what the docs said during rounds? Let me tell you what their plans are for you . . . "

After visiting Mr. Riordan, Rob checks in with Belinda. While he listens to her report on her morning assignments, Rob also eavesdrops on the conversation of Dr. Hiroshi, a third-year resident, and Dr. Miller, the hospital's drug-dependency specialist, as they confer about the status of Mr. Bower, a 60-year-old patient who has a failing liver and chronic heart problems. Because the doctors often don't have time to update him on patient developments, Rob has found that listening to doctors' hallway conversations is one of the most valuable ways he can gather patient information.

Dr. Miller: "An open container of alcohol in Mr. Bower's room? He's the guy waiting on a liver transplant, right?"

Dr. Hiroshi: "That's right. Mr. Bower insists that he didn't drink any alcohol. He claims a visitor brought the container into the hospital and drank it in his room, but he won't tell who the person is. I don't believe him, personally. That's why I called you"

Dr. Miller: "Well, it certainly doesn't look good. If he has violated hospital policy by drinking alcohol, he'll be dropped to the bottom of the organ donation list."

Rob suddenly interrupts after overhearing this part of the conversation.

"Dr. Hiroshi, Dr. Milller, excuse me," said Rob. "I've been on the floor since 7 a.m., and I've visited Mr. Bower several times. If he'd been drinking, I would've known about it. He's completely sober."

Dr. Miller replied, "How can you be so sure, Rob? Where there's a will, there's a way. You'd be surprised at what some patients will try to get away with!"

"The last time I saw Mr. Bower, his wife was visiting him, and she was slurring her words and weaving back and forth. It seemed to me that she had been drinking, not him," said Rob. "Listen, have you checked his labs for alcohol?"

Dr. Hiroshi said, "I never thought to do that! That would give us a definite answer. I'll order a urine test for Mr. Bower right now."

Dr. Miller added, "Good catch, Rob."

Later, Dr. Hiroshi thanks Rob for his help. "Rob, the test came back negative for alcohol, so Mr. Bower still has his spot on the organ list. I appreciate you telling me about Mrs. Bower."

"Happy to help. Some docs in this hospital would have ignored me, or, more likely, bit my head off in front of everyone," said Rob.

"Rob, I know that things on Three East can get tense sometimes, especially between the medical and nursing staff. Still, we need more nurses to take the initiative and speak up."

"Thanks." said Rob. He turns his attention to Joan, who has arrived to work with Mrs. Flynn on her physical therapy and needs his help getting Mrs. Flynn up from her bed.

"You know, Rob, I just can't drop everything when one of your patients need PT," said Joan. "I have a schedule to follow and patients to see, too."

"I know that Joan. Let me tell you what happened earlier with Dr. Ortega . . . "

1 p.m.—Patient Crisis

After lunch, the frantic activity decreases on Three East as doctors leave the unit, dietary carts are cleared away, and patients rest or leave the unit for tests or other medical services. Rob uses this "down time" to review his notes and document his care team's activities in patient charts. After spending about 30 minutes hand writing notes and entering the same information into the Pod One computer, he looks at his watch and remembers he needs to teach Mrs. Beverly how to use her new asthma inhaler.

As he grabbed the inhaler and supplies from a cabinet, Rob thought, "A few years ago, a respiratory therapist would have taught Mrs. Beverly this information. Because the hospital all but eliminated the respiratory therapy department last year, it's now my job! I never would have thought, when I first started as a nurse, that I would be charge of so many aspects of patient care. Supervising, training, transporting patients, planning discharge, taking admissions. On and on. The nursing job keeps getting bigger and bigger, but we don't get higher wages or any help."

Rob shakes his head and rearranges his facial expressions into a smile when he enters Mrs. Beverly's room. "I've got to be positive in front of my patients," he thought.

"Hi, Mrs. Beverly! How are you feeling this afternoon? Was your lunch okay? Did you see that I sneaked a few extra packages of crackers for your soup? I remembered how much you liked them," said Rob loudly to accommodate Mrs. Beverly's hearing impairment.

"Thank you, Rob. I hope I didn't get you in any trouble."

"No trouble at all, Mrs. B. Finances might be tight here, but this hospital can spare a few extra crackers," joked Rob. "Now that you're done with lunch, it's time for me to teach you how to use your new asthma inhaler. Are you ready?"

"As ready as I'll ever be," Mrs. Beverly responded.

"Okay. The doctors want you to use this whenever you have difficulty breathing. One of the biggest mistakes that people make is they overuse the medication and don't breathe in deeply after taking a puff from the inhaler. You only need . . . "

"Rob, how is everything going at home? How is that dog of yours? Did he do anything funny lately? You tell the best stories about him!"

"I'll tell you all about Scout when we're done here, Mrs. B. It's really important that you pay attention so you can do this yourself at home. Okay, you should only need one or two puffs to help ease your breathing. Watch me demonstrate."

"How about your wife? She's an architect, right? How did you two meet, anyway? I've been wondering about that."

"Mrs. Beverly, we really need to focus on using the inhaler. I don't know when I'll have a chance to work with you on this again before you go home. Come on, you try." Rob handed her the inhaler.

"Rob, I'm embarrassed. I wasn't paying any attention to what you were saying. Could you repeat it?"

"Come on, Mrs. B. I know you're smarter than that. You just want someone to visit with you a bit, don't you? I'll try to come back after my shift is over and talk with you. For now, you try to use the inhaler properly and I'll coach you through."

"Okay. Okay," Mrs. Beverly sighed, disappointed that Rob couldn't stay to socialize.

Suddenly, their conversation is interrupted by a voice on the hospital loudspeaker. "Code Blue. Three East. Code Blue. Three East." Belinda appears at the doorway. "Rob, you better come quick. Mr. Riordan is coding! It looks like some type of seizure!"

"Mrs. B, I gotta go. I'll be back later," Rob leaps from Mrs. Beverly's bedside and runs across the hall to Mr. Riordan's room. Nursing aides quickly move out extra furniture to make room for the unit EKG machine and crash cart. A small crowd of onlookers, mostly Three East staff members, gathers outside the room to watch the crisis. Dr. Hiroshi rushes into the room, pushing people away from the door to get to Mr. Riordan's bedside.

"Break the cart!" ordered Dr. Hiroshi. Debbie, another nurse on the unit, grabs the crash cart and breaks open the seal that indicates it's sterilized and ready for use.

"I'm going to have to intubate him. You. You, Dr. Ortega," said Dr. Hiroshi, looking at one of the first-year residents, "Call for an emergency respiratory consult. Now!" Dr. Hiroshi puts his head down and begins to insert a tube down Mr. Riordan's throat. Out of the corner of his eye, Rob sees Cathy, watching wide-eyed and open-mouthed, staring in disbelief at the scene.

"Rob, start the chest compressions while I hold the Ambu bag. Debbie, push the IV meds. Helen start recording notes about what's going on," ordered Dr. Hiroshi.

"I got it," replied Rob as he stepped over to the bed. "Cathy, come over here and watch what's going on here. You'll be in this situation sooner or later and you might as well learn now. It's important to count the compressions. One, two, three . . . "

"Where the hell is the consult?" shouted Dr. Hiroshi after a few minutes passed. "It's been well over five minutes!"

Rob thought to himself, "I didn't see anyone move toward the phone when Dr. Hiroshi ordered the consult. I don't think anyone made the phone call! Dr. Ortega is already mad at me about our confrontation earlier today, but I have to do something!"

"Cathy, take over the compressions," said Rob. "I'll be right back. Keep counting."

Rob quickly steps out into the hall and uses his cell phone to call respiratory. "We need someone down here now on Three East. We have a patient coding. I think its cardiac distress."

Rob reenters the room, takes over from Cathy, who looks at him with a fearful expression, shaking a bit from the drama of the code. Minutes later, Dr. Marshall arrives and takes over from Dr. Hiroshi. Soon, the crowd of hallway onlookers drifts away as the excitement dies down, and Mr. Riordan's body becomes still. His heart monitor returns to normal, beeping quietly and at a regular rate.

"Okay, people. He's stabilized," said Dr. Marshall. "Let's get him up to the intensive care unit. Who will take him to ICU?"

"He's my patient. I'll do it," said Rob. "Belinda, will you grab his chart for me? Thanks. Debbie, will you cover my patients while I'm gone? I should be back in 20 minutes. I just need to update the ICU staff. I'll call Mr. Riordan's family later and tell them what happened. They need to know that his condition has gotten worse and he's in the ICU."

Setting the charts down near Mr. Riordan's feet, Rob rolls the bed out of the room. Rob walks down the Three East hallway toward the reception area, and he is joined by Dr. Hiroshi.

"Rob, I saw what you did in there. Thanks for making the phone call and getting the respiratory guy down here. It was touch and go there for a while. Those residents were like deer in headlights. They didn't make a move! I don't know what would have happened if Dr. Marshall hadn't arrived in time."

"I think that was the first code many of the residents have seen. They got a little freaked out and froze" said Rob. "But Dr. Marshall got here, and everything is fine now. Do you have any orders that I can take with me up to the ICU staff?"

"I'll contact the docs up there in a minute. Thanks for taking the lead."

"I just hope that Mr. Riordan will be okay," responded Rob, as he wheeled the bed into the unit elevator and pushed the 5th floor button for ICU.

"I wish I could tell you that," said Dr. Hiroshi, glancing down at Mr. Riordan. "It's really too soon to tell. The next few hours will be critical. I'll see you later."

The elevator doors close on Dr. Hiroshi's concerned expression.

Rob returns to Pod One at 2:30 p.m., after spending several extra minutes giving report on Mr. Riordan to the ICU nurses. With a sigh, he sits down heavily on a stool next to the computer terminal. This is the first time all day he has had a chance to sit down, catch his breath, and rest.

"Geez," Rob thought. "2:30? It seems like forever ago since rounds. This has been one long day. I need to hurry up on charting now so I can get out of here on time." Rob hunches over the keyboard and types in notes about Mr. Riordan. After a few minutes, he picks up the phone to call Mr. Riordan's wife. Rob feels someone staring at him. He half turns around, expecting to see Belinda, Cathy, or a resident waiting to talk to him. Instead, he sees a woman in her mid-30s, dressed in a business suit, glaring at him.

"Are you the nurse in charge of Ms. Taylor?" the woman demanded.

"Yes, I'm her nurse," said Rob, in a voice drained of all emotion.

"Well, I need to talk with you about the care she's received at this hospital."

"Listen, can I talk with you in just a couple minutes? I need to finish writing up these notes," said Rob.

"How many minutes?" the woman replied angrily. "I've got to go to work!"

Rob looks at her and thinks, "Oh no. Not this. Not at the end of the shift." He tells her, "I'll be with you in two minutes."

Turning quickly on her heel, the woman steps back into Ms. Taylor's room, but she stays just inside the doorway, glaring at Rob. He can feel her eyes burning holes in his back as he finishes his charting. He stands up, walks into Ms. Taylor's room, and looks at the woman.

"Who are you? I haven't seen you here before" he said.

"I'm Ms. Taylor's granddaughter, Nellie, that's who! Who are you? I haven't seen you around before!"

"I'm her nurse, Rob. What can I do for you?"

"My grandmother wants to get out of bed," said Nellie.

"Really? She told you that? She hasn't been able to talk to anyone for days."

"Well, she only feels comfortable talking to *me*. She just told me that she wants to sit up. It would make her feel better. I'd like her down the hall in front of the window."

"Well, that's not easy to do, given her condition. It will take some time and a couple of people to move her. I have to take care of a few things first."

"How long?" snapped Nellie.

"Ten or 15 minutes. Is there anything else bothering you, Nellie?"

"*Ms. Hill* to you. I don't like seeing my grandmother in the hospital in this way, and I don't appreciate being questioned like I'm some stranger who never visits! I've been here every day, in the evenings. Who do you think you are, anyway?"

"It's hospital policy for us to ask a visitor's identity before giving out any patient information," said Rob, a defensive tone creeping into his voice. "It's for patient security."

"Fine. I work for an insurance company, and I know what you people at the hospital are trying to do. You just want to get her out as soon as possible. You don't care if she gets better or not, just so she's not costing you more money!"

"Ms. Hill, I assure you, we're not trying to get your grandmother out of the hospital before she's ready to go home," said Rob, grimly. "She's unconscious. She can't hear what you're saying, and she can't speak. I think you heard a sound and thought it was a request."

"Don't tell me what I heard! I know what I heard!" yelled Ms. Hill. "My grandmother was just fine two weeks ago when she arrived here. You've been trying to pinch pennies, and now she looks like this! I've seen all of the horror stories about this hospital on the news. I know how you've had to cut back and patients suffer." She storms out of the room. "I'm talking to a doctor to get some results. When I get back, my grandmother better be moved or you'll have a lawsuit on your hands!"

Rob sighs and calls Belinda into the room. "Belinda, get Carl."

"Rob, are you crazy? We can't just drop everything and move Ms. Taylor. It will take half an hour to get her into a wheelchair and roll her down the hallway. It's almost time to go home, and we have a million things to do before the afternoon shift comes in for report," responded Belinda. "I can't stay late tonight, again. We both have family stuff to do this evening, remember."

"Belinda, what am I supposed to do? Tell Ms. Taylor's granddaughter that, no matter where we move Ms. Taylor or what we do, she's never going to be the same person who walked into this hospital? She could be right, you know, about the cutbacks."

"What do you mean?" asked Belinda.

"It's all over the news. How patients aren't getting the proper care because we can't afford the staff or services. I've wondered if we haven't been aggressive enough with Ms. Taylor's care because it costs too much and she's on Medicare. I've wondered if her condition would be different if she had private insurance."

"Okay, Rob, okay. Let's not go down that road. You win. I'll tell Carl to get a wheelchair," said Belinda wearily. "Let me help you."

Rob untucked Ms. Taylor blankets and sheets. Belinda put slippers on her feet and wrapped her in a bathrobe. As they worked, Rob told Belinda:

"Did you know, when I first started years ago, on night shift, we were able to give backrubs to every single patient on the floor before they fell asleep? The patients would talk about their fears, their hopes, and their feelings. We had so much time back then! Now, I'm lucky to be able to teach Mrs. Beverly for 10 minutes about her asthma inhaler. Patients like Ms. Taylor here may not be getting the best care available because of money. It's too much. This isn't the kind of environment I want to work in."

"Enough, Rob," said Belinda. "We need you. The patients do. I do. You can't leave!"

"I'd be lying to you if I said that leaving City Hospital isn't becoming more appealing every day," said Rob, as he, Belinda, and Carl carefully transferred Ms.Taylor from her bed into a wheelchair. She was so fragile, Rob was afraid she would break a bone in the move.

"My friend Mary used to work here as a nurse, and now she's employed in pharmaceutical sales. She's earning at least $100,000 a year. That could be me!"

"You would miss the patient contact," commented Belinda.

"Maybe, but all those dollar signs would make getting over it a lot easier."

"Rob, let's talk more about this later. We can take care of Ms. Taylor here and hand off our work to Leigh and Kelly at 3 p.m., okay?"

"I'm done talking about it, Belinda. I just can't make any long-term promises to City Hospital." Rob pushed Ms. Taylor's wheelchair down the hall and parked her near the window. Nellie was waiting, tapping her foot impatiently on the floor and glaring at him as he locked the wheels in place and spread a blanket over Ms. Hill's lap.

"Okay, Ms. Taylor," Rob said gently. "Your granddaughter is here to look after you." "Let the *afternoon* nurse know if your grandmother needs something," Rob said curtly to Ms. Hill.

He returned to Pod One to finish charting. "This was not the way I wanted to end the day," he thought. "I should have called in sick today and avoided this place!"

3 p.m.—Afternoon Report

Rob gives the report to Leigh when she arrives for the afternoon shift. Rob and Leigh review patient charts and see all their patients. Once they've completed their visits, Rob and Leigh return to the pod.

"Before I leave, Leigh, I wanted to ask you a question about Mr. Hardy," said Rob. "Why didn't you notify his resident about the change in his condition yesterday afternoon? Dr. Norris asked me about that today. He went off on me for 10 minutes about it."

"Dr. Norris wasn't on the floor at the time," said Leigh.

"Well, wasn't he still in the hospital? You could have paged him," Rob said.

"Why should I have to notify the docs about everything?" asked Leigh, defensively. "It's the docs responsibility to come by the unit periodically and check their patients' charts."

"Leigh, you know it's our responsibility to notify the residents about any significant changes," explained Rob. "We can't expect the docs to have time to check the charts just to check them. We have to give them a reason to check the charts. That's our job."

"I didn't know that Mr. Hardy's condition needed resident notification. Besides, the docs should check the charts as regularly as we do," said Leigh.

"I don't want to get involved in this. You need to talk to Dr. Norris and clear up the misunderstanding ASAP."

"I'm not going to apologize! I've got enough to do. How am I supposed to remember to contact the residents on every little change in a patient?" responded Leigh angrily.

"Just don't make this mistake again. Page the docs."

"I gotta get to my patients, Rob. I'll see you tomorrow." Leigh grabbed some supplies and walked down the hall to talk with Tyrone, her nursing aide.

Rob glanced at clock. It was 3:30 p.m. and day shift was over, at last. He grabbed a stool from Pod Two and placed several chart books on the Pod One desk. He began writing his nursing notes for all of the interventions and assessments he and Belinda had completed during the afternoon. He noted changes in patient status and marked areas that physicians needed to review. After finishing this, Rob turned his attention to reviewing Cathy's charting. He made corrections to her work (making a mental note to talk with her tomorrow about the errors he saw) and signed off on every procedure she performed. He then reviewed all of the physician orders and jotted notes about questions to ask the docs during rounds tomorrow.

As his day-shift colleagues left for home, Three East became quiet for the first time all day. Rob could feel one of his infamous migraines starting, in his temples and behind his eyes. "Oh no, not tonight," he thought. "Not on our wedding anniversary."

"Have a good night, Rob," said Belinda, as she put on her coat and walked down the hall toward the unit entrance. "Don't stay too late, again."

"I'll try, Belinda," answered Rob. "I just need to do a little more paperwork. "

"Rob, don't get too involved, not like you usually do. Remember, you promised Brenda that you'd leave on time tonight. You have a wife and kids that need you at home. You can't be Supernurse 24-7."

"I hear you, Belinda," said Rob. "Just a few more things to do. I'll be out of here by 4:30."

"Okay, then. See you tomorrow."

"Have a good evening, Belinda. Say hi to Sam and the kids for me."

Rob watched Belinda leave the unit. He thought, "She's right. I need to get home earlier. The thing is that I'm torn in too many directions during the shift. I'm constantly on the go, doing two or three tasks simultaneously, talking to everybody, and trying to solve problems. I can't seem to get it all done, even when I skip lunch and breaks."

Rob closed one chart and opened another, thinking more about his job. "I'm constantly drained after a day's work. I get home and I just want to crawl into bed with exhaustion. I want to spend more time with Brenda and the kids, but I'm so worn out. I never thought that I'd burn out, but that's exactly what's happening! So much for being Supernurse."

Suddenly, the phone rings, startling Rob and interrupting his thoughts.

"Rob? It's Brenda. It's 4 p.m. Remember you have to pick up the sitter at 5:30 so we can be on time for our dinner reservations at 6 o'clock. You need to leave now if you want to get cleaned up and changed before we leave for the restaurant. Let's go!"

"Okay, I'm almost done. I need to say goodbye to my patients and I'm outta here. I have had a really long day," Rob told Brenda.

"We'll have plenty of time to talk about it at dinner. Just leave in the next 10 minutes, please," said Brenda. "Don't forget to pick up pizza for the kids' dinner. You promised."

"I won't forget, Brenda."

"And Rob, please try to talk with Rob, Jr., about his soccer game. He scored two goals yesterday. I know you couldn't be there because of working late again, but it would mean a lot to him if you asked him about it. He needs to know that you're interested in his life."

"I *am* interested. I just totally forgot the big game was yesterday. I leave for work so early that I don't see him in the morning, and I'm so tired after work that I don't feel like talking to anyone. I'll make it up to him this weekend."

"That's what you said last week, and it didn't happen."

"Don't get started on me, Brenda. Not today. It's our anniversary, for heaven's sake!"

"I'll see you at home, Rob. Goodbye."

"Bye."

Rob wearily hung up the phone and managed to stand up with considerable effort. His feet were killing him, and his back ached from leaning over the charts and computer. "How am I going to make it through our anniversary dinner tonight?" Rob thought. He walked down the hall and entered Mrs. Beverly's room to say goodbye for the evening.

RELEVANT CONCEPTS

Burnout: Chronic strain that results from work and nonwork pressures that can lead to reduced personal accomplishment, depersonalization of others, and emotional exhaustion.

Emotional labor: Jobs in which employees are required to display certain emotions to satisfy organizational role expectations.

Role ambiguity: Uncertainty that exists over role requirements.

Role conflict: A clash between two or more competing and/or divergent role requirements.

Role negotiation: Interactions designed to modify the expectations of others about how a role should be performed and evaluated.

Role overload: Having too many and/or too difficult work responsibilities within a given role.

DISCUSSION QUESTIONS

1. How would you describe Rob's role on Three East?
2. What work role or organizational issues were causing stress and burnout for Rob? How do his personal characteristics and/or family stressors contribute to his experiences?

3. What symptoms of burnout does Rob exhibit? How is this burnout seen in Rob's interactions with his colleagues?
4. What could City Hospital do to improve Rob's situation?
5. What are the professional barriers that employees perceive that may prevent them from taking advantage of organizational programs or policies designed to help them manage stress and burnout?
6. Is Rob's stress having an impact on the quality of patient care? Why or why not?

REFERENCES/SUGGESTED READINGS

Apker, J. (2001). Role development in the managed care era: A case of hospital-based nursing. *Journal of Applied Communication Research, 29,* 117–136.

Apker, J., & Ray, E. B. (2003). Stress and social support in health care organizations. In T. Thompson, A. Dorsey, K. Miller, & R. A. Parrott (Eds.), *Handbook of health communication* (pp. 347–368). Mahwah, NJ: Lawrence Erlbaum Associates

Finkelman, A. W. (2001). *Managed care: A nursing perspective.* Upper Saddle River, NJ: Prentice Hall.

Geist, P., & Hardesty, M. (1992). *Negotiating the crisis: DRGs and the transformation of hospitals.* Hillsdale, NJ: Lawrence Erlbaum Associates.

Miller, K. I., Joseph, L., & Apker, J. (2000). Strategic ambiguity in the role development process, *Journal of Applied Communication Research, 28*, 193–214.

Additional Resources

The Doctor (popular film, starring William Hurt).

The Making of a Doctor (PBS/NOVA documentary).

Episodes of television shows such as the drama *ER*, the drama/comedy *Scrubs*, or the reality show *Hopkins 24/7*.

NurseWeek.com: www.nurseweek.com

NursingWorld: www.nursingworld.org

American Organization of Nurse Executives: www.aone.org

Honor Society of Nursing, Sigma Theta Tau International: www.nursesource.org

21

Medical Care, Health Insurance, and Family Resources: Complications to Otherwise Good News

George B. Ray
Cleveland State University

It is well known that a gap exists in the United States between overall health for African Americans and European Americans. Perhaps no statistic reflects this disparity more clearly than life expectancy data. As of 1998, on average, European Americans' life expectancy was 76.7 years, whereas the comparable figure for African Americans was a full six years less (Taylor & Braithwaite, 2001, p. 6).

At every stage of life, from infancy to adolescence to adulthood, many African Americans experience greater health problems. Health conditions for African Americans are due to a myriad of circumstances, many of which are linked to inadequate health care. This case shows how a series of events takes a cumulative toll on the health of members of one African American family. The experience of the Edwards family illustrates how, even with the best of intentions, bringing a healthy baby into the world can become a stressful struggle with health problems that may become compounded, leading to potentially devastating effects.

A NEW MEMBER IN THE EDWARDS FAMILY

As Angela and Jeffrey Edwards drove to the clinic, their thoughts and conversation were filled with questions they wanted to ask the pediatrician. They had been married for over two years, and although they had often thought they would eventually want to have a child, they suddenly realized that it was going to happen now. They were going to become parents in nine months! The results of the home pregnancy test were positive, and now they were going to meet with a pediatrician who would conduct a more complete test and, if the pregnancy were confirmed, begin the recommended prenatal care. They were at once excited, anxious, and a little uncertain about what to expect. But they knew they wanted to have a baby.

One thing they had not thought about was health insurance. Angela had worked mainly in part-time jobs and had never had health insurance through her employment, but Jeffrey had worked for over three years for an auto parts manufacturer, and his benefits included heath insurance for him and his dependents. They were both in their early 20s and felt healthy. They had never used the insurance much, but as far as they knew, it was satisfactory.

As they approached the receptionist at the clinic, they were given a medical history questionnaire. Much of the information was already on file for them separately, but now an updated family medical history was especially important. Everyone in Angela's family was African American. All of her grandparents had died before the age of 70, two with heart disease, one with complications from diabetes, and one from lung cancer. Her mother was 60 and in good health, but her father, age 64, was in poor health, suffering from arthritis and anemia. Everyone on Jeffrey's side of the family was also African American. Jeffrey's grandparents had died within the last 5 years. One grandfather died as a result of prostate cancer, the other grandfather was killed in an automotive accident. One grandmother died of a heart attack, and the other died from pneumonia. His parents were both alive and in moderately good health, although they did not receive particularly good health care. As Jeffrey and Angela filled out the questionnaire, they were reminded that longevity was not a strong suit in either of their families. But at least both of them felt they were in good health.

Their names were called, and they went in to meet Dr. Reese, the obstetrician. Dr. Reese was European American and appeared to be just a few years older than Jeffrey and Angela. He was courteous, but seemed most interested in getting straight to the basic medical information. Right away, Dr. Reese wanted to know how serious they were about providing good medical care for their child.

"Do you know much about caring for a newborn?" asked Dr. Reese.

"Well," Angela replied, "I grew up around a younger brother and two younger sisters, and I have already started to read some books about child care." Jeffrey noted that he had never paid much attention to young children; his only sibling was an older sister.

Dr. Reese explained that the key to raising a healthy child was to take all the necessary precautions prior to birth, then to pay close attention to the child's early development. He stressed that nutrition, although all-important, was only part of what good parents needed to be concerned with. Equally important was the need for a stable home environment and a strong and nurturing relationship between parents and child. Angela thought Dr. Reese sounded like he was lecturing a little too much. The session reminded her of a health class in high school, full of caution and warnings. But he seemed careful, and she felt she could trust his advice. Angela was then asked to go with a nurse who would draw blood and urine samples. Within 30 minutes, they would have clinical pregnancy test results, and within 48 hours they would have some test results on blood sugar and basic profiles on protein, amino acids, and cholesterol.

Dr. Reese spoke to Jeffrey: "Do you know how old your grandparents were when they died?"

Jeffrey thought for a moment. He was never close to his father's parents and had never been aware of their health. "Well, I can't tell you much about my father's parents. They lived in Detroit, and I never saw them much. I think my Grandma Edwards was 68 when she died, and Grandpa Edwards was around the same age. On my mother's side, I knew the family better because they all lived around here. My Grandpa Smith had prostate cancer and never got treatment until it was too late. He was 66 when he died. My Grandma Smith died of pneumonia when she was 65, but she had problems with her lungs all her life. She smoked for over 10 years, but on top of that, she had asthma. One other problem was that she grew up not too far from a refinery. My mother always said the air was no good around her house."

Angela returned and Dr. Reese had some questions for her. "I see, Angela, that none of your grandparents lived past the age of 70. Is that correct?"

"Yes, Dr. Reese. My family has not enjoyed especially good health."

The pediatrician proceeded with a long series of questions, and it reminded Angela of an interrogation. It seemed appropriate, yet a little too formal; she would have liked the doctor to speak in a friendlier tone. Dr. Reese continued, "Angela, do you know of any particular reason your father has anemia? Do you know what form of anemia he has?"

Angela thought for a moment, "No, I'm not sure how his anemia developed or exactly what form he has. I think I first heard about it three or four years ago. He seems to be OK, but I know he gets tired easily, and he takes some medication for it."

Dr. Reese then finished up the meeting. "Well, I see no reason why you can't have a healthy, normal baby. However, to be perfectly honest, there are several risks present. Although the longevity of grandparents is only one risk assessment indicator, it does help us reach some initial guidelines on things to look out for. I'm pleased to see that neither of you use tobacco, consume much alcohol, or are taking any medications. But I want to learn more about your parents' health and also find out more about Jeffrey's grandmother's pneumonia. Can you please contact the staff here and give us the names of your parents' physicians, and, Jeffrey, please see if your mother knows any more about her mother's pneumonia."

The nurse returned, and Dr. Reese reported on the pregnancy test. "Angela, you are definitely pregnant. Congratulations!" Angela and Jeffrey hugged each other.

"Wow! That's great, Dr. Reese. Now what do we do?"

"Angela, for the time being, simply continue with your regular routine. You may keep on working and do everything as you would normally do. Of course, no, and I repeat *no* alcohol. Stay away from second-hand smoke, and eat a healthy diet. Until we check out your blood sugar, try to stay away from sweets, starches, and soft drinks, and get plenty of rest. Before you leave, we'll give you a pamphlet with information on diet and exercise, and a list of things to expect throughout your pregnancy. We'll call you about the blood work, and I will want to examine you in three weeks. Any questions?"

As they were leaving, Angela and Jeffrey spoke to the receptionist who announced, "According to your health insurance, Mr. Edwards, you owe $25 for today, and we will file a claim for the pregnancy, blood, and urine tests." Neither Jeffrey nor Angela had visited a physician during the past year; the last time Jeffrey had seen a physician the copayment was $10.

Jeffrey asked, "Are you sure about that $25 copayment?" The receptionist checked again and, yes, the copayment had increased. "Do you mean every time my wife has to see the doctor we'll have to pay $25 up front?"

The receptionist could only reply yes, "I'm afraid so, Mr. Edwards. Those are the terms of your health insurance."

BABY TALK

On the way home from the pediatrician, Angela and Jeffrey talked about Dr. Reese and what he had said, the baby, and all the preparations they needed to make for the new member of their family. They talked about names for the baby, whether or not they wanted to know the baby's sex, and some of the changes they would need to make in their lifestyle. They had not realized they would need to come up with an extra $15 for the office visit copayments, and now they saw a need to start a new budget for the expenses associated with the baby. Jeffrey was making a decent wage, but in their excitement over the baby, they had not seriously considered just how much it would cost to care for a new baby. They now had some added insight into the parenthood adventure they were about to begin.

Later that night, all Angela and Jeffrey could talk about was the baby. "Jeffrey, do you think the spare bedroom is going to work out well for the baby? Will it be big enough? We used to talk about finding a bigger apartment, and maybe we should move before the baby is born. This neighborhood is not really quiet enough anyway. And I'm not sure how good the schools are here. We need to start thinking about . . . ."

"Whoa! Angela, calm down. We need to take first things first."

The next day, Angela went to the department store, where she worked in the office. She liked her work in bookkeeping, even if it was only part time. She had worked part time for over a year and was hoping a full-time position would open up. She usually went to work at noon, arriving in time to join her coworkers for lunch. As she talked with her friends over lunch, she told them about the results of her pregnancy test. They were excited for her and wanted to hear all about the baby. She had been telling them she and Jeffrey wanted to have a child, and her friends had a feeling it was just a matter of time before a baby would come along.

"Angela, would you rather have a boy or a girl?"

"Well," Angela responded, "it doesn't really matter. I think Jeffrey would like a little girl, but I don't care."

Angela and her friends talked about what happens during pregnancy and how there may be some rough days ahead for her. "Angela," her friend Danielle said, "I hope your delivery goes better than mine did. I had 8 hours of hard labor, and my son weighed $9\frac{1}{2}$ pounds. It took me over a month to get my strength back."

The group, all females, talked about infants and their sleeping and eating habits. Angela's three friends all had had at least one child each, and among them, they had a wealth of advice. The information was a little overwhelming for Angela, but it was all so exciting. It felt great to know she was going to be a mother and start her own family.

As the first few weeks passed, the parents-to-be found they could not stop thinking about the baby. Even though they knew the baby would mean a lot of changes in their lifestyle, they felt ready for it. It seemed a little like getting married: Part of what made it so exciting was that there were new, unknown events and experiences in store for them.

Jeffrey asked about his grandmother's pneumonia and asthma. His mother was not sure, but she said her mother had breathing problems all through her adult life. She remembered hearing that, even as a child, her mother had to restrict her activities because of asthma. When she moved away from home, her breathing improved, but it was never normal. She also said that she, too, had experienced asthma as a child. Jeffrey had never known this about his mother. He reported all of this to the clinic.

EXAMS FOR MOTHER AND BABY

At the three-week checkup, Dr. Reese examined Angela, and everything seemed satisfactory. He then explained to Angela that, after 12 weeks, she and Jeffrey might want to consider some prenatal tests just to make sure the baby was developing normally.

"Angela, right now there is no sign of anything unexpected or unusual. The baby seems fine in every respect. However, after 12 weeks, the baby will have developed to the point that there are two tests that can indicate whether anything suspicious is going on. We can do an ultrasound test, and if there is anything that warrants further tests, we can do an amniocentesis on the chemical make-up of the fluid surrounding the baby. This test could show us if there are early signs of abnormal development."

Angela asked, "What exactly might the amniocentesis results show?"

Dr. Reese carefully explained, "Among other things, if various organs including the lungs are not developing properly, there are indicators of that in the amniocentesis. Because Jeffrey's grandmother and mother had some pulmonary problems, the test is something you might want to consider."

Angela inquired, "What if the test indicated a problem with the developing lungs. Then what?"

The doctor paused and then said, "We would have to consider what we know at that time. You might want to do nothing, or you might want to run further tests."

But Angela was puzzled. She wondered what she would do with the information from the test. Her instinct was that she would not want the test done because whatever the results, it would not affect her desire for the baby. She felt that, ultimately, the information from the amniocentesis would not be useful to her.

At 9 weeks and again at 12 weeks, Angela went in for checkups. Each time, the baby and mother seemed to be doing well. The baby was beginning to gain weight, and Angela could feel her body changing more and more. During the 12-week visit, Dr. Reese suggested they do an ultrasound.

Angela asked, "Will the cost be covered by our insurance?"

Dr. Reese noted that the ultrasound is fairly routine and almost all insurance policies covered its cost.

"Well, yes, let's do the test." The ultrasound was scheduled, and Angela and Jeffrey went to another clinic for this test. It was so fascinating and exciting to look at the image of the child and see its head, arms, and legs. The test showed that the baby appeared normal in its current stage of development. Now, even more, the new parents felt the baby was becoming a real person. The idea of a name seemed more important. They wanted to call their new family member something personal. They decided they did not want to know the sex, so they wondered what to call it for the time being. Jeffrey said, "How about Jessi?" They decided that for the rest of the pregnancy they would call the baby Jessi.

Two weeks after the ultrasound, the Edwards received a bill for $250.00 for the test. Angela and Jeffrey were surprised and upset because they thought the test was covered by insurance. They phoned Dr. Reese's office and asked about it. The clerk at the clinic explained, "The insurance company disallowed the claim stating that the test was not necessary." They could speak to Dr. Reese, but he was out of the office for the next 10 days. They asked the clerk if he could resubmit the claim and he said he would. Since Jeffrey took his present job he had never had a concern about his health insurance coverage, but he wondered if he would begin to find problems. Now, when it mattered most, was not when he needed to discover health insurance problems.

Over the weeks and months during her pregnancy, Angela began to feel more and more tired. She had swelling around her legs and ankles, she was very thirsty, and she had less and less energy. Around 5 months, she felt that her condition was probably not out of the ordinary, but she wanted to make sure her health was OK. At her next regular checkup she asked Dr. Reese about her swelling and lack of energy. Dr. Reese ran some blood tests and found elevated blood sugar levels, a sign she might be experiencing gestational diabetes.

"Angela," he explained, "during pregnancy, your body is constantly adjusting to the task of nourishing its own needs as well as the needs of your developing child. Your additional food intake is something that requires a big adjustment. Perhaps your body has not yet made enough of an adjustment. Now, the baby is gaining more and more weight, and you need to eat more and more. Your body may not be producing enough insulin to respond to the added food, especially the carbohydrates you're consuming."

Angela was confused and afraid. "What are you telling me? Are you saying that my life and the health of my baby are in danger?"

Dr. Reese tried to be understanding and reassuring. "Angela, we need to keep checking your blood sugar. This may just straighten itself out, as it often does. There is a form of diabetes that can occur with pregnancy, but if that's the case, we can treat it and it usually disappears after birth. All I'm saying right now is that this is something we need to keep an eye on. I want you to come in every week for a blood sugar test."

WHERE WILL THE MONEY COME FROM?

In her mind, Angela knew there was no question that she needed whatever medical care it took to make sure she and the baby were OK. But she immediately thought of the extra $25 copayments. At home that night, she told Jeffrey about the possible blood sugar problem. Jeffrey was irritated.

"Man, what next? We're beginning to run tight on money, and we haven't even started to get furniture or clothes for Jessi. And a guy at the factory asked me if I had thought about life insurance. What shape would you and Jessi be in if something happened to me? Right now, neither one of us has any. Angela, I hate to think about it, but I'm gonna have to get a second job to bring in some extra money. This whole thing is costing more than I realized."

Angela cautioned, "But Jeffrey, I need you here at night. And especially when the baby comes, there will be lots to do around here, and I can't do it alone."

As they talked, they both decided that, for the next several months, right up until the birth, it would probably be a good idea for Jeffrey to work a few hours at night. The next day after work, he started looking for a part-time job. After a few days, he found several opportunities, none of them appealing. The best choice seemed to be stocking shelves at a supermarket. The job paid only $6 an hour, but the hours were flexible, and he could count on at least 25 hours a week. This would mean over $100 a week extra in take-home pay. He started the new part-time job right away. He knew it was bad for him to be away from Angela so much, but they didn't have much of a choice.

The claim from the insurance company came back, again, disallowed for the same reason. Angela phoned the insurance company, whose claims officer explained that Jeffrey's coverage did not have very generous benefits. Angela protested, "But the doctor recommended the test. I was just going with his recommendation. What good is this insurance if it doesn't cover a basic test like the ultrasound?"

The claims officer explained, "Ma'am, I get this kind of claim all the time, and I'm treating you the same way as everybody else. When your doctor doesn't state the specific need for the test, then there's nothing I can do."

Angela tried to phone Dr. Reese. He was delivering a baby and would be out the rest of the afternoon. "Well," she stated firmly, "you tell him that this claim needs to get covered and he needs to do whatever it takes to justify why this test was done." She was told that the next time, when she came in for a blood test, she could speak to him herself.

It had been a week since Jeffrey started his evening job. The work wasn't too strenuous, but he was very tired at night and sometimes he was restless and not able to sleep well. It seemed that, on weeknights, there was too little time to talk, and both of them knew this wasn't how they wanted the pregnancy to go. Angela told him that the most recent blood test showed her sugar was still too high. Dr. Reese ordered her to strictly monitor her sugar and carbohydrate intake and to take a brisk walk for 30 minutes a day to see whether they could lower the blood sugar enough without having to take insulin. She had left another message asking Dr. Reese to specify the need for the ultrasound test and then resubmit the insurance claim. The bill was now over 60 days past due, and they had been getting calls asking what arrangements they could make for payments. Between the baby, the blood sugar tests, the insurance company, and Jeffrey's work at night, Angela was getting stressed out. It was bad enough for her to deal with the stress, but she did not want her stress to have any ill effects on Jessi.

One night, Jeffrey was working late and came home exhausted. He was able to put in over 30 extra hours that week, but the extra work was taking a toll on him. The next day, at his regular job, he did not feel rested or very alert. While walking in the factory, he slipped on a greasy rag and fell on his shoulder. He felt a sharp pain and John, a coworker, helped him get up.

"Jeffrey, are you all right?"

Jeffrey rubbed his shoulder and sat down. "I don't know . . . I think I better get my shoulder checked out."

John cautioned Jeffrey. "You know, a guy who used to work here had a little accident on the job and went to the company doctor. He had a broken arm and they put his arm in a cast. For 6 weeks he couldn't work and he got Workman's Compensation. Then, when he came back, he found the company had reassigned him to a new job in another area of the factory. He was taken off his daytime schedule and put on the 11:00 p.m. to 7:00 a.m. shift. And the new job was much harder than his old one. The boss made things so rough on him that he quit. I think the company doesn't want employees to use their health insurance. If you need this job, I suggest that you not tell the company about this. You might make it rough on yourself."

Jeffrey sat dazed and confused. Could his employer be so inconsiderate of its employees that they would look for excuses to get rid of people? But there was no union, and he knew the employees had little influence with management. He also knew that, right at this time, he could not afford to risk losing this job. It was not a great job, but he knew it would be very difficult finding a better one, especially on short notice and at the time he had a family depending on him. Jeffrey decided not to say anything to his boss about his shoulder. It was painful and he did not know how serious his injury was, but he toughed it out.

EMPLOYMENT, HEALTH CARE RISKS, AND FAMILY RESOURCES

Later, he told Angela about his accident. "What? You mean you are injured but you are not sure you want to have your shoulder examined? Are you crazy?"

Jeffrey explained, "Angela, I don't know what to do. If, after a couple of days, the shoulder feels worse, then I'll have to get it checked. But I need my job."

Right then, Angela and Jeffrey began to feel that things were getting out of control. All they wanted was to have Jessi arrive as a healthy baby. But their financial problems were backing them into a corner and making the pregnancy far too stressful. They considered asking their parents for some money, but they both felt their parents had little money to spare, and it would be a huge drain on their parents' savings to come up with enough money to help them. They both had grown up hearing stories about how hard it was raising a family. Their grandparents and parents never made much money and worked hard all their lives just to get by. They never had any extra money to put into insurance, investments, or real estate. In retirement, their parents' quality of life was OK, but they had no extra money. They got by on modest pensions and social security. Angela and Jeffrey realized they were living in a pattern that had gone back many years in their families. No one in their families had gone to college or acquired professional skills to make big gains in their earnings. Now, Jeffrey and Angela understood how this pattern kept perpetuating itself. How could either one of them find the time and money to go to college? How would they ever be able to own a home? How would they ever get ahead? How would they ever be able to provide a good life for Jessi?

It was Thursday night. Jeffrey decided that he would work the next day, but not work at the supermarket that weekend and rest up as much as possible. Then, on Monday, if his shoulder was no better, he would go on his own to see a doctor and pay for it himself. If he had insurance claims on top of the claims for the pregnancy, his employer might look for ways to make his working conditions difficult. He had no way of knowing if he was blowing his fears out of proportion, but he decided that he could not risk losing his job.

On Monday, Jeffrey went to work and Angela went in for a blood test. The results showed her blood sugar levels were still too high, and she spoke to Dr. Reese. "Angela, your insulin production is insufficient to maintain proper levels of sugar in your blood. Are you sure you're watching what you eat and walking every day?"

"Dr. Reese," Angela replied, "since you asked me to cut back on carbohydrates and sweets, I have strictly monitored my diet. And I take a 30-minute walk every day. Do you think I would fool around when my health and my baby's health are at stake?"

"I have patients, some of whom are overweight, who often eat snacks between meals, and they forget that even a few potato chips or a couple of cookies can make their blood sugar increase too much. When they think of cutting back, they don't realize that they need to completely eliminate all snack foods as well as greatly reduce their intake of bread, pasta, potatoes, and even vegetables like corn and carrots. I'm simply stressing as strongly as I can the need for you to strictly limit your carbohydrates and sweets. That's all."

"Dr. Reese, I don't know who you are referring to when you say you have overweight patients who carelessly eat junk food and starches. I know there are some Black people who eat the wrong food and who are overweight, and maybe you think I'm one of them, but I am not."

"OK, OK. I'm sorry, Angela. I didn't mean to upset you. I guess I have made myself clear on the need to maintain your strict diet. Right now, I don't think we have any choice but to put you on a prescription for insulin. But first we need to carefully check your blood sugar four times a day for three days. I will give you a packet of chemically treated pieces of paper and a box of special needles. Four times a day, morning, early afternoon, late afternoon, and evening, you will need to prick your fingertip, produce a drop of blood, and apply the blood to the test strip. The test strip will change color, and you then need to match the color on the strip to the color chart that comes with the strips. Each time you do the test, record the results. Also, record exactly what you eat each day. Here, let me do one test, and I can show you exactly how it's done. After thee days, come into the office, bring your records, and we will determine exactly how high your blood sugar is. Then we will know if you need to start injecting insulin and how much to control your blood sugar levels. Once you start insulin injections, we will then be able to control your blood sugar, and there will be no adverse effects on your baby's health. Do you have any questions?"

Dr. Reese then got a needle and pricked one of Angela's finger tips. He applied the blood to a test strip and recorded the color on the chart that matched the color on the strip.

"There. As you can see, it is quick and simple. Any questions?"

"Yes, I have a question, but it's on another topic. When you recommended that I have an ultrasound done, was there a specific medical reason for that? The insurance company says there was no medical reason given and so they won't pay the claim. I need to have that claim paid immediately."

"Angela, the ultrasound is usually not necessary, but in my practice, it is routine because it gives us reassurances that the baby is developing normally. If the insurance company needs a specific medical justification, I can provide that because of your and your husband's family medical history. I'll take care of that. Now, I'll give you the needles and test strips. You can begin testing your blood sugar later today."

On the way home, Angela realized that if she needed to start injecting insulin, the prescription would mean one more expense. The health insurance prescription benefit was quite helpful, but there was still a $12.00 copayment. Money was getting tight and, at some point, she would have to stop working at the department store, and that would mean even less income. But she was even more worried about Jeffrey's injury.

TAKING CARE OF JEFFREY

Later that day Jeffrey came home and Angela asked him about his shoulder. Jeffrey paused and slowly spoke. "Well, right now I'm in bad shape. I'm afraid there is something wrong with my shoulder. I talked to my supervisor at the supermarket and he said I can come in this week whenever I want to, but I don't have to come in this week at all. What's got me worried is my regular job. What if I need treatment or surgery or something? Then what do I do?"

Angela had done some thinking about Jeffrey's injury. "Jeffrey, we can't mess around with your health. We can't have some injury that never properly heals and becomes a long-term disability. I know you feel you will jeopardize your job if you see a doctor and there are some big insurance claims involved. But I have an idea. I talked with Margie at work, and she knows of a doctor who will see patients without health insurance or who have health insurance problems. She runs a low-overhead office and tries to provide lower-cost health care. Why don't you try to see her tomorrow and find out what she thinks. You can call in sick tomorrow. You haven't been out sick all year, and I don't see why that would be a problem. What do you think?"

"Angela, if you think it's worth a try, I'll go. I guess we don't have too much to lose." That night, Jeffrey slept in a reclining chair and got some decent rest. The next morning, he called in sick and Angela called the doctor and explained to the receptionist that they needed to get in to see the doctor that day if there was any way possible. Fortunately, there had been a cancellation, and they were able to get in during the early afternoon. When they met the receptionist, they told her they were prepared to pay cash or, if possible, by credit card. Then they met the physician, Dr. Holbrook, a middle-aged women who seemed friendly and caring.

"Well," said Dr. Holbrook, "what have we got here? Tell me what happened."

After explaining the nature of the injury, Dr. Holbrook examined Jeffrey's shoulder and found there was significant swelling, discolored skin, and some intense pain. She ordered x-rays, which fortunately revealed no fracture or dislocation. Jeffrey's injury was a very bad bruise and would probably heal in good shape if he could keep from using it for at least a full week. "But, Dr. Holbrook, I need to work. I don't have any vacation time coming, and my company's sick leave policy is, well, basically, there is no sick leave policy."

Dr. Holbrook was very understanding, but she could see no way the bruise would heal without extended rest. She explained that the bruise, in and of itself, was not extremely serious, and the main problem for now was the pain. However, if he kept trying to use his arm, and especially if he did any lifting, the shoulder joint would become further inflamed and then there could be a risk of separation. Without proper rest and rehabilitation, the shoulder bruise might not heal properly and would require surgery. She had a week's worth of a pain-killing drug, which was a sample from a pharmaceutical company, and she was willing to give it to Jeffrey for free. She also recommended at least a week of rest, keeping the arm and shoulder immobilized, and applying heat on the shoulder for several days.

Dr. Holbrook charged Jeffrey $125, which seemed reasonable considering, there were two x-rays in addition to the examination. On the way home, Angela and Jeffrey thought about what they could do. They wanted to be thinking and talking about Jessi, but they were forced to think about a lot of other things. They were still happy and excited about the baby, and they were glad they had each other, but in the first few months of pregnancy, they felt like they had been on an emotional roller coaster and they were not sure what was in store for them. Jeffrey thought about all the things he wished he had: a good job that paid enough so he did not have to work at night, a job that had good health insurance, an employer that could give him time off for sick leave, and some savings that he could use in a time of need. He wasn't sure what his options were, but he resolved that, once Jessi arrived, he was going to find a better way. There just *had* to be a better way.

RELEVANT CONCEPTS

Cultural stereotypes: Commonly held beliefs or generalizations about a group of persons who are assumed to share various characteristics. The beliefs are often mistaken, but are believed to be true based on first impressions, false impressions, hearsay, or images presented in popular culture.

Emotional stress: Anxiety or mental tension caused by one's feelings as opposed to reactions to one's physical condition. Emotional stress may be directly related to the physical health of oneself or a loved one, but may be exacerbated by other factors (relational, financial, occupational, etc).

Health care resources: The wide range of medical services potentially available to anyone needing health care. Such services may include traditional health care systems, public health agencies, low-cost clinics, and community health care organizations sponsored by nonprofit groups, as well as local, regional, and national government.

Physician-centered health care: Medical treatment that is oriented to the physician's agenda. The physician exercises control over the health care, dominates the decision making, and acts in what he or she believes is in the patient's best interest while expecting the patient to accept the prescribed diagnosis and treatment.

Physician–patient interaction: The primary communication features present in face-to-face encounters between a primary caregiver and one receiving medical care. Such interaction includes verbal and nonverbal behavior and constitutes an important variable in the quality of the medical care received by the patient.

Social support: Comfort and encouragement offered by one's family, friends, and coworkers.

DISCUSSION QUESTIONS

1. What does the case indicate about communication in the physician–patient setting? What did Angela mean when she stated that Dr. Reese was too formal in his communication style and that his questions to her seemed like an interrogation? What could she have done differently?

2. As Jeffrey' and Angela's problems multiplied, they experienced more and more stress. Did this seem like a normal reaction on their part? How could they have handled these problems differently?

3. Did Jeffrey overreact to the dilemma that arose when he injured his shoulder? What are some alternatives he did not explore?

4. The case illustrates how financial resources can become stretched, resulting in stress and anxiety in other areas of life. Before deciding to have a baby, should Jeffrey and Angela have sought out counseling to help them plan for the expenses associated with a baby? How could they have learned about the availability of resources such as counseling?

REFERENCES/SUGGESTED READINGS

Hecht, M., Jackson, R., & Ribeau, S. (2003). *African American communication: Exploring identity and culture* (2nd ed.). Mahwah, NJ: Lawrence Erlbaum Associates.

Johnson, F. (2000). *Speaking culturally: Language diversity in the United States.* Thousand Oaks, CA: Sage. (See especially Chapter 8, Discourse consequences: Where language and culture matter.)

Marger, M. (2000). *Race and ethnic relations: American and global perspectives* (5th Ed.). Belmont, CA: Wadsworth. (See especially Chapter 8: African Americans.)

Taylor, S. E., & Braithwaite, R. L. (2001). African American health: An overview. In R. L. Braithwaite & S. E. Taylor (Eds.), *Health issues in the black community* (pp. 3–12). San Francisco: Jossey-Bass.

22

Enhancing Culturally Competent Health Communication: Constructing Understanding Between Providers and Culturally Diverse Patients

Claudia V. Angelelli
Patricia Geist-Martin
San Diego State University

In this case, we meet Ramira. Ramira is over 30 years old and is pregnant. She is from a rural area in Mexico and speaks only Spanish. She does not have any children and is excited about their first baby. We take you to one of her prenatal appointments during the second month of her pregnancy. What we will discover is that during this appointment, the nurse attempts to inform Ramira that she has the option of having an amniocentesis to find out if the baby is healthy. In this conversation between Ramira, the nurse, and the interpreter, we see how interpreting language is not simply a process of translating the words that each participant speaks.

As we will see when this story unfolds, interpretation and communication about illness and disease, diagnosis and treatment, caring and curing often are complicated by the "collision" of cultural communities. Clearly, the differences in health care beliefs and practices of persons seeking and providing health care can lead to problems in communicating with one another (Geist-Martin, Ray, & Sharf, 2003). Members of these diverse cultural groups often conceive health, disease, pain, and health care practices differently. What we learn in this case is how essential it is to examine and understand why these differences may lead to breakdowns in communication.

A community emerges through communication; it is the site where culture gets made and re-made through emotional connection, a sense of belonging, and a common set of customs, rules, rituals, and language. Ramira shares this community with the nurse and Annette, the interpreter. As is evident from Ramira's story, complex layers of meaning accompany all of our conversations about health, wellness, illness, and medicine in any one of these cultural communities. The complexity multiplies in the health care setting when interpreters are needed to bridge the cultural communities of the provider (and medicine) and the patient, not only by interpreting the languages spoken, but also in seeking answers to questions that providers and patients raise at they communicate with one another. Research investigating this complex context of communication with interpreters indicates that the difficulties in interpreted conversations lie in the construction of reciprocal understanding, the accurate transformation of semantic and pragmatic content, and the role of the interpreter as linguistic facilitator (Davidson, 1998). For health care providers, the interpreter is the instrument that keeps the patient on track; for the patient the interpreter is a co-conversationalist.

As we will see in the conversation between Ramira and the nurse, the nurse asks the majority of questions and Ramira is mostly limited to supplying answers. The nurse wants to explain to Ramira some information that, in the nurse's mind, is important and valuable. Ramira wants to make decisions based on information that, for her, is important and valuable. The notion of important and valuable is not shared. Ramira and the nurse not only do not speak the same language, but they also come from different cultures.

This case study looks at the complex interactions of patient, nurse, and interpreter as they communicate about prenatal testing. We see first hand, in this transcript of the conversation, the challenges that arise in the borderlands of cultural communities.

THE STUDY

The larger study, of which this transcript is a part, was conducted in a county hospital in northern California during 22 months (Angelelli, 2001). Using an ethnographic approach, 10 Spanish/English medical interpreters were observed at California Hope (CH; the site).[1] The encounter discussed in this chapter comes from Annette, one of the 10 full-time Spanish interpreters at CH.[2]

The Site

CH is located in Conte, California, where residents speak more than 46 different languages (Conte Unified School District). At the time the study was conducted, the population was more than 800,000, including African Americans (4.4%), Asians or Pacific Islanders (18.7%), Hispanics (26.6%), White (49.6%), and other (0.8%). The population served by CH ranges from middle class to working class, but the average patient is poor. The community that uses the services of CH is made up of a diverse ethnic pool, with most of the patients being African American, Asian, and Hispanic. Since 1976, CH has forged a long tradition of service and dedication to the health of the whole community, including an open-door policy that guarantees access to needed medical care, regardless of ability to pay.

The Participants

Annette works between 9:00 a.m. and 5:00 p.m., Monday through Friday, for Interpreting Services (IS). She is 45 and has been interpreting at CH for two years. To work at IS, Annette met the following requirements: two years of experience in the field (as a medical interpreter, translator, bilingual medical assistant, etc.), bilingual ability, and the ability to pass the IS test. Annette, like all other interpreters at CH, facilitates communication between Spanish-speaking patients (mostly working-class immigrants) and English-speaking health care providers.

The segment we analyze comes from a conversation between Ramira, a Spanish-speaking working-class female patient, and Martha, a young female nurse at CH. The interpreter, who is working on the speaker phone removed from the room, facilitates the communication between nurse and patient who are face-to-face in an office. The interaction begins with Martha, the nurse (N) calling in for an interpreter (I) to communicate with Ramira, the patient (P).

Data Collection

During the data collection, an effort was made to minimize the intrusion of the researcher in the interaction and among the participants. Interpreters at CH were used to having "others" listening to their interpretations (but never recording) or going with them to do a face-to-face interview with a patient, because that is the way in which new interpreters get the training. Interpreters-in-training observed and asked questions and so did the researcher. Consent for recording and observing was requested immediately before the interpreting started.

Data Analysis

In this chapter, we present and analyze segments of one interpreting communication event (ICE) by Annette to explore just some of the complexities of communication in the process of interpreting the conversation between a patient and a nurse. We proceed to explore how the distance between Ramira and the nurse seems to increase, even when Annette is there to bridge the differences in language and cultures between them. Annette is there to bring them closer.

"SHE DOESN'T WANT TO TALK ABOUT IT": THE COMPLEXITIES OF INTERPRETING

Ramira comes to the visit in her second month of pregnancy. She is over 30 years old. The nurse wants to explain to her that she has the option of doing an amniocentesis to find out if the baby is healthy. During the explanation of the procedure, Ramira interrupts the provider (line 28) to indicate her concern about this test. Ramira also explains to the nurse that her doctor has already ordered a blood test for the AFTP.[3]

28 *P:*   Sí... esteee...... precisamente.... Ayer el doctor de allá de Gilroy... me mandó
a hacerme... a que me sacaran para hacerme el estudio para el mongolismo.
*/yes... ehmm... precisely... yesterday the doctor in Gilroy... sent me to... so that
they would draw from me to have the study on mongolism done./*

The interpreter seeks clarification. Because Ramira is not stating the type of test that was performed to her, Annette (line 29) explores if the test done was a blood test or some other type of test.

29 *I:*   OK Pero... ¿fue de sangre o de qué m'hijita?
/OK but ... was it a blood test or what kind of test my dear?/

Ramira is not clear that there are different procedures for finding out if the child has Down syndrome. When the interpreter seeks clarification on the test type, she replies that it was a blood test. Annette conveys this information to the nurse (line 31).

31 *I:*   OK. She said yesterday her doctor sent her for a blood test for that.

In line 32, the nurse attempts to clarify to both patient and interpreter that blood test and amniocentesis are two different tests that provide different information.

32 *N:*   OK. The blood test and this test are two completely different things. The blood test
is only what we call a screening test... ah... and it is called the AFP blood test.

The nurse explains to the patient that the amniocentesis is an option that patients have. It is not a required test, but health care providers need to present patients with their options. As the nurse explains, she refers to a diagram that shows places where the needle can be inserted. The nurse notices that Ramira is expressing disagreement shaking her head "no" (line 50). At that point, the nurse emphasizes that the patient has a choice. She just needs to explain the test.

50 *N:*   Now . . . she's shaking her head. . . she doesn't need to have the test but I just need to explain it to her.

As the explanation is reassumed, the nurse notices a breakdown in communication and seeks help from the interpreter in line 53.

53 *N:*   OK. When we insert the needle. . . I . . . don't know but they are trying to say something. . . I don't know what that is.

Lines 54 to 63 represent a dialogue between the interpreter and the patient. Ramira is explaining what the nurse is saying about inserting a needle to perform the amniocentesis test. Ramira is concerned about the consequences of this test on the fetus. She is beyond the second month of pregnancy. She has had miscarriages after two and a half months. Her doctor advised her against doing this test. Ramira explains all of this to Annette.

54 *I:*   ¿Qué fue?
        /What's that?/
55 *P:*   Es que lo que pasa es que me está mostrando aquí en una. . . en un dibujo.
        /What happens is that she is showing to me on one. . . drawing./
56 *I:*   Aja?
        /Aha?/
57 *P:*   Este. . . uno que le están metiendo la jeringa al bebé.
        /Ehmm. . . it is a drawing where they are inserting the syringe to the baby./
58 *I:*   No es al bebé. . . pero parece. . . Yo sé cómo dice.
        /No, it is not to the baby, but it looks like it, I know what you mean./
59 *P:*   O sea. . . es a la matriz. . . o sea dónde está él.
        /I mean. . . to the womb . . . or where the baby is./
60 *I:*   Sí. . . es para sacar un poco de líquido que le rodea al bebé.
        /Yes, it is to get some of the liquid that surrounds the baby./
61 *P:*   Aja. . . entonces yo le pregunté al doctor de allá de Gilroy. . . entonces como yo he tenido problemas con los demás embarazos. . . de que se me caen a los dos meses y medio.
        /Aha, so I asked the doctor from Gilroy, that because I have had problems with the other pregnancies, that I lose them after two and a half months./
62 *I:*   Mhm.
63 *P:*   El doctor me dijo. . . esteee. . . me dijo que no me conviene que me hicieran este. . . este estudio. . . .
        /The doctor told me that this study is not convenient for me./

Annette interrupts the patient's description at the point where the patient has indicated that the test is not the best for her and offers her recommendation to the nurse to not go any further with the explanation of the text because her doctor has recommended that she not have the test in line 64.

64 *I:*   Bien, me permite un momentito entonces, señora. . . .momento eh. . . .
/All right, just a moment ma'am, one moment please./

You may not want to go any further with this because she has had problem
pregnancies, the doctor and she have discussed this particular study. She said that
she's been told by the doctor because she has in the past lost pregnancies, that . . .
emmm. . . . It wasn't a good test that she should have. . . . It's not something that
he would recommend.

The nurse wants to verify that she understands the patient and show her that she is listening.

65 *N:*   OK. She told me that she had three miscarriages, all at about two and a half
months, is that right?

66 *I:*   Yes, that's just what she was just saying.

The nurse also wants to find out the cause of the previous miscarriages. She requests this
information from the interpreter on line 67.

67 *N:*   OK. Ever find a cause for those miscarriages?

Lines 68 through 82 provide clarification of previous miscarriages and lack of treatment.
Nothing was determined as a reason why those occurred.

68 *I:*   Señora, ¿alguna vez le han dicho el porque que perdió esos bebés?
/Have you ever been told why you lost those pregnancies?/

69 *P:*   Pues, en realidad no.
/No, not really./

70 *I:*   No.

71 *P:*   No me han dicho porque yo. . . . No he estado en tratamiento. . . después de. . . de
lo. . . . de. . . .
/I wasn't told why I . . . I have not been treated after. . . after. . ./

72 *I:*   De lo sucedido, ¿verdad?
/After what happened, right?/

73 *P:*   Aja.
/Aha./

74 *I:*   OK. She said no because she didn't continue the treatment after those occurred.

75 *N:*   OK. So they never did any testing on her or her husband to find out the cause of
the miscarriages?

76 *I:*   ¿Asique nunca le hicieron estudios?
/So you never had any tests done?/

77 *P:*   No.

78 *I:*   Ni a usted ni a su esposo para ver el porque, ¿verdad?
/Neither you nor your husband to find out the reason, right?/

79 *P:*   No, lo que pasa es que. . . en este el doctor. . . este . . . me. . . me . . . o sea ya llevo
más adelantado que de los otros. . . por ejemplo. . . ahorita ya voy a cumplir. . . casi
los cuatro meses. . . y en los otros, no. . . no. . . estee nada más llegaba a los dos
meses y medio.
*/No, what happens is that . . . in this one the doctor. . . ehmmm. . . I mean I am
further along in this one than with the other ones . . . . for example, now I am going
to be almost four months . . . and in the other ones I only reached two and a half
months.*

80 *I:*   She said no they haven't. She said even further. . . with this particular pregnancy she's progressed further than she has with any other pregnancy. She is four months pregnant or almost four months pregnant. And with the other pregnancies she never got beyond two . . . two and a half months. . . .

81 *N:*   OK. So they haven't done any studies, that's what I just wanted to know.

82 *I:*   No, they have not.

What we see in this portion of the transcript is the patient's attempts to explain the history in a way that sets this pregnancy apart from the others in how far along she is in carrying this child. We can see the gap growing between the nurse and the patient as the nurse's talk stays focused on testing without any direct question about the patient' perspective on this pregnancy. In contrast, the patient's talk continues to move away from the testing, with no direct question about the nurse's perspective on testing options, emphasizing her desire to continue the pregnancy, no matter what the nurse has to say.

On line 83, the nurse comes back to explain the test and reiterates that the patient does not have to have it.

83 *N:*   OK. I'm just gonna briefly explain this test of the amniocentesis and if they don't want to have it, that's fine . . . but . . . .

The interpreter interrupts the "interpreting" process to directly question the nurse's decision to continue explaining the amniocentesis test. Through this action, the interpreter confirms the distance we have seen developing in the perspectives of the nurse and the patient about the need for the test.

84 *I:*   Excuse me. . . I know you know your business much better than I . . .

85 *N:*   Aha.

86 *I:*   But . . . I think it'll just make her a little bit more uncomfortable because she has already, as you've noticed, shaken her head.

87 *N:*   No.

88 *I:*   . . . and said she's discussed it with her doctor and really doesn't feel comfortable with talking about it.

On line 89, we see the distance growing even more as a disagreement begins to develop between the nurse and the interpreter as to what the "no" means. For the nurse, no means the patient does not want the test, but that continuing explanation of the test is appropriate (and her professional responsibility). For the interpreter, no means the patient does not want to talk about this any more.

89 *N:*   Oh. . . she told you she doesn't want to talk about it.

90 *I:*   That's why she keeps shaking her head no. . . that she doesn't want the study. . . she doesn't want to go further.

91 *N:*   OK. She only shook her head no one time.

92 *I:*   Okayyyy.

93 *N:*   OK? Umm.

94 *I:*   I'll ask her if she wants you to discuss it with her.

95 *N:*   Please do.

The nurse wants to verify this information. In line 89, she asks the interpreter to clarify the meaning of this "shaking her head no." The interpreter willingly gives her own interpretation of Ramira's head shaking (line 90). The nurse needs to know exactly what Ramira's concern is. She only saw the patient shaking her head once (line 91). From the nurse's perspective, that information does not provide grounds for the interpretation that Ramira does not want to talk about the test any more. The nurse, becoming aware of the growing distance, hopes to find out what the problem is and, once again, asks the interpreter for help (line 95). By questioning the patient, we believe the nurse is attempting to close the gap in their perspectives. At the same time, the interpreter's intervention complicates this interaction, actually increasing the gap between the nurse and the patient. The interpreter now becomes more aligned with the patient, unintentionally amplifying the distance between the nurse and the patient.

Aware of the growing distance, the interpreter turns to the patient for help, attempting to clarify if Ramira wants to continue talking about the test. Ramira lessens the distance between the nurse and herself by acknowledging the help the nurse is offering by way of the test (lines 99, 101, 103, and 105). The interpreter does her part in reducing the gap when she explains Ramira's position to the nurse (line 108). The nurse does her part in diminishing this distance by acknowledging Ramira's desire in line 109.

96 I: ¿Señora?
      /Ma'am?/
97 P: Sí.
      /Yes./
98 I: Usted quiere que ella siga hablando refiriente a ese procedimiento o prefiere que no?
      /Do you want her to continue talking to you about the procedure or would you rather not?/
99 P: Pues, ¿el de la jeringa?
      /Well, the one with the syringe?/
100 I: Aja.
       /Aha./
101 P: ¿La jeringa en el ... estómago?
       The syringe into the stomach?/
102 I: Aja.
       /aha./
103 P: Esteee pues la verdad ... o sea yo les agradezco que me traten de ayudar pero ... este ... en este caso ... yo no quiero hacerme ese ... estudio ... o sea ... quiero que me hagan por ejemplo el ... el ultrasonido.
       /Ehmmm well, truly, I mean, I appreciate that they are trying to help me, but, ehmmm, in this case I do not want to have that study done, I mean I want to have for example the ... the ultrasound./
104 I: Sí.
       /yes./
105 P: De... eso... sí... pero el estudio este... de las jeringas... no.
       /Of... that... yes... but this study... of the syringes... no./
106 I: Es muy razonable... me (sic)permita?
       /It is very reasonable. Would you allow me?/
107 P: Sí.
       /yes./
108 I: She said she'd rather not go into further discussion with the particular surgery involving the needle. She said she is very grateful that you are offering her this assistance.
109 N: OK.

Later in the transcript, we begin to see how the three interlocutors start to work together to become closer and more aligned in their perspectives. However, the nurse's belabored description of the test and what information it offers interrupts these beginning stages of alignment (lines 115–137). In addition, as the nurse attempts to correct the patient's misinterpretations of what information the blood test can provide, any alignment they had developed dissipates (lines 121–125). As the nurse continues her explanation of the blood test, Ramira repeatedly affirms her comprehension of what the nurse is describing; once again, they seem to be returning to some form of alignment (lines 126–137).

115 *N:*   And... the blood test that she said she had done performed yesterday, the ASP blood test, is that what it was?

116 *I:*   El estudio que le hicieron de la sangre ayer para eso, ¿fue el ASP le dijeron? ¿o no dijeron?
/The blood test that she had done yesterday for that, was it the ASP? Did they tell you or didn't they?/

117 *P:*   Sí... o sea... si me dijeron que era para lo del.
/Yes, I mean, yes, they told me that it was for the.../

118 *I:*   de la proteína.
/for the protein./

119 *P:*   Del... me dijeron que era para lo del... mongolismo.
/They told me it was for the mongolism./

120 *I:*   Bien.
/Right./
She said that it was to determine whether or not the child would have mongolism.

121 *N:*   Yes. Well... The blood test is not going to tell her whether or not the child has Down syndrome.

122 *I:*   Dice... bueno, pero con ese estudio de sangre no le pueden decir si lo tiene o si no.
/She says, well, with that blood test they can't tell you if it is or not./

123 *P:*   Aja.
/aha./

124 *N:*   OK? What the blood test did, is... It's really designed for women under the age of 35... and ehmm it's a screening test... meaning it's not very accurate... but it's a screening test to see if somebody could be at higher risk to have a baby with Down syndrome or... another chromosome problem called trisome 18 or having a child born with a neural tube defect.

125 *I:*   Bien... dice que lo que realmente es ese estudio y no es muy (sic) acurado, o sea, no sale cien por ciento cierto lo que dice, es para determinar si hay posibilidad de la criatura de, por ver la cantidad de proteínas que está produciendo al nivel del embarazo que se encuentra usted, si vaya a tener problemas... o tener posibilidad, mejor dicho de problemas con.... O el mongolismo... o dos otras condiciones... una de las cuales incluye problemas con la espina dorsal, OK?
/Okay, she says that what that study is really about, and it is not very accurate, I mean, it is not a hundred per cent sure what it says, it is to determine if there is a possibility that the baby—by watching the amount of protein that you are producing during this stage of the pregnancy—may have problems, or to have the possibility, I mean problems with mongolism, or two other conditions one of which includes problems with the spinal cord, OK?/

126 *P:*   Sí...
/Yes./

127 *N:*   If the results come back abnormal, it doesn't mean the baby is abnormal.

128 *I:*   Si resulta el estudio de sangre que le hicieron ayer, anormal...
        /If the blood test you had done yesterday comes back abnormal.../

129 *P:*   Aja.
        /Aha./

130 *I:*   ...eso no quiere decir que su hijo vaya a ser anormal.
        /... that doesn't mean that your child is going to be abnormal./

131 *P:*   Sí.
        /Yes./

132 *N:*   OK? All it means is that her risk or her chance to have a baby with one of those three conditions I talked about... went a little bit higher... and then the next step will be to offer amniocentesis because that is the way to know for sure.

133 *I:*   Dice, eso solamente indicará que la posibilidad de tener usted un hijo con una de las tres condiciones que ella comentó... o sea ha subido un poquito más alto.
        /She says that they will only indicate that the possibility of having a child with one of those three conditions that she mentioned, has increased a little./

134 *P:*   Mhmmmmm.

135 *I:*   La única manera para poder determinar seguro... por cierto si vaya a tener alguna de esas condiciones es por mediación de amiocentesis... o sea del procedimiento con la jeringa.
        /The only way to determine for sure if the baby is going to have any of those three conditions it is by means of an amniocentesis, I mean the procedure with the syringe./

136 *P:*   Sí.
        /Yes./

137 *N:*   OK?

Ramira abruptly changes the direction of the discussion by appealing to the interpreter to explain to the nurse that, in a sense, all of what the nurse is saying is inconsequential for her because she would have this baby no matter what information the test provides (lines 138–152). Clearly at this point, the distance between the nurse and Ramira is magnified to an extent that seems irreconcilable. In line 150, Ramira reemphasizes her position not to terminate her pregnancy no matter what. The alignment between Ramira and the interpreter is enhanced in line 151, when the interpreter reassures Ramira that she had told the nurse not to continue speaking about the test.

138 *P:*   Pero... mire... yo... yo quiero que usted le explique... verdad... que yo no tengo hijos.
        /But, listen I, I want you to explain to her that, true, that I do not have children./

139 *I:*   Aja.
        /Aha./

140 *P:*   Ni un hijo
        /Not even one child./

141 *I:*   Aja.
        /Aha./

142 *P:*   Entonces es el primer hijo... y si se me llega a lograr.
        /So this is my first child and if I can have the baby./

143 *I:*   Aja.
        /Aha./

144 *P:*   Vamos a ver... que a mi me salga mal mi bebé... esteee.

/Let's see... and if my baby is not right ehmm./

145 *I:* Es su bebé, ¿verdad?
/It is your baby, right?/

146 *P:* Aja... en ese caso... ¿qué es lo que pueden hacer?
/Aha, in that case what can they do?/

147 *I:* Sí... yo se... y va a tener... determinar...
/Yes, I know, and you will have to determine./

148 *P:* Aja... o sea si me sale mal... ¿me lo sacaría?
/Aha, I mean if the test results are bad, would I get rid of the baby?/

149 *I:* Le darían a usted para decidir si sí o no...
/They would ask you to decide if yes or no./

150 *P:* No... pero no me lo sacaría yo...
/No, but I would not get rid of the baby./

151 *I:* Entiendo ... y por eso le dije que no tenia que estar ahi... hablando más...
pero... ya sabe... yo nada más soy una intérprete... ¿Me permite un momentito,
eh?
*/I understand, and that is why I told her that she did not have to continue speaking
about this, but, you know, I am only an interpreter. Excuse me for a minute, OK?/*

152 *P:* Sí.
/Yes./

Now, the distance between the nurse and interpreter grows more intense when the nurse challenges the interpreter, suggesting that she is not interpreting correctly (line 156). The nurse assumes that the interpreter is talking to the patient about amnio rather than the blood test (line 154) and the possibility of the terminating the pregnancy (line 158). As a result, the interpreter becomes defensive and explains to the nurse what she has told the patient by echoing the patient's resolve to have her child regardless of any abnormalities that the test may find.

The nurse initially moves to close the gap between herself, the patient, and the interpreter by saying that she respects the patient's decision not to have any testing. However, she minimizes that move by, once again, attempting to explain the purpose of the blood test (line 160). In a move that aligns her with the patient, the interpreter tells Ramira that the nurse does not trust the accuracy of her interpretation. Furthermore, the interpreter indicates that the nurse insists on continuing her description of the purpose of the blood test (line 161–163).

153 *I:* She said she'd rather not continue this conversation, she said... because, what would happen? If she had the test... she said... she has no children... any child she would have will be her child... If any test that you will give her would show that the child would be abnormal... what would... her options be...? To... maybe terminate the pregnancy?... she says... she's not going to do that... so she doesn't want to discuss it.

154 *N:* We are not talking about the amniocentesis... we are talking about the blood test.

155 *I:* She.... she's... she doesn't want to go further... she wants to have a child... whatever kind of child she has.

156 *N:* OK... hmmm... I don't think you are translating what I'm saying.

157 *I:* Yes, I *am.*

158 *N:* OK... I am not talking about termination here... I'm just talking about... what the blood test screens for.

159 *I:* Yes... And I did tell her that... but she asked further... she said... OK and I will tell you... she said... OK... what you are going to do... you are going to tell what the blood test screens for... and if you want to go further... what are my options

going to be. . . she said. . . ultimately my options will only be to continue or to
terminate the pregnancy. . . and I'm just going to continue with the pregnancy. . . I
do not have any children. . and I hope I can carry this pregnancy through. . .

160 *N:* Yeah. . . That's fine. . . we respect her decision not to have any testing. . . that's
fine. . . we are not here to force her into any kind of testing. . . we are just here to
give her choices. . . and. . . since she elected to have her blood test yesterday. . . if I
could tell her what that blood test is for.

161 *I:* Right. . . Señora. . . porque ella cree que no le estoy interpretando como me está
diciendo. . . Ella quiere que yo le aclare que solamente está diciendo el por qué
del estudio de sangre que le hicieron ayer.
*/Ma'am, because she thinks that I am not interpreting what she is saying to
you . . . she wants me to make clear it to you that she is only telling you the reason
for the blood test that you had done yesterday.*

162 *P:* Aja.
/Aha./

163 *I:* Yo le dije. . . que no quería usted saber más. . . pero. . . va a seguir hablando. . .
*/I told her, that you did not want to know anything else, but, she is going to keep
on talking./*

Finally, the nurse understands the patient's desire to end any discussion of testing. Even
when this situation appears to be resolved in lines 164 to 172, it may be impossible to resolve
the gap that was constructed because of the very different world views held by the patient and
provider.

164 *P:* Sí.
/Yes./

165 *I:* ¿OK?

166 *P:* Sí,
/Yes./

167 *N:* OK? So. . . then. . . she's scheduled to have an ultrasound today. . . does she want
to have that?

168 *I:* She has already said she does want the ultrasound.

169 *N:* OK. . . hmmmm. . . so that's all we'll do here today. . . and what I need for her to
do is to sign some other forms for me. . .

170 *I:* Dice lo que ocupa es que usted le firme una que otra forma más. . . para ella. . . le
va a hacer el ultrasonido hoy. . . ¿usted lo desea, verdad?
*/She says that what she needs is for you to sign one form or other for her, she's
going to do the ultrasound today. You want that, right?*

171 *P:* Sí. . . sí. . . lo deseo.
/Yes I want it./

172 *I:* Yeah. . . she does desire the ultrasound. . . and she'll sign.

DISCUSSION

What is this interaction telling us about health care provider–patient communication when both
parties do not share the same linguistic and cultural background? How much understanding
can take place even when there is a language broker present? Where do distances begin to
grow? How do they get constructed in the first place?

This interaction provides some insight into the complexities of distance/closeness among the nurse, patient, and interpreter. Over the course of this 35-minute interaction, we see a wide range of behaviors that influence the alignments among the patient, nurse, and interpreter.

- The nurse questions the interpreters' interpretation.
- The nurse repeatedly asks the interpreter to explain.
- The interpreter questions/challenges the nurses' decision to "force" the explanation on the patient.
- The interpreter repeats and reemphasizes what the patient says "she has already said."
- The nurse and interpreter dialogue without the involvement of the patient (with no interpretation).
- The interpreter and the patient dialogue without the involvement of the nurse.
- The patient appeals to the interpreter to explain her position to the nurse.
- The patient appears to do "repair" work in the end by thanking the nurse repeatedly.
- The interpreter does her part in the repair process by aligning with the patient, continuing to articulate the patient's perspective, even after being challenged by the nurse on the quality of her interpretation.
- The nurse does her part in the repair process by accepting the patient's decision and moving on to the ultrasound.

Clearly, we need to deepen our understanding of the health beliefs and practices of individuals in cultural communities to meet their diverse, and often unmet, health care needs and expectations. Nearly all examinations of health and culture reveal that "miscommunication, noncompliance, different concepts of the nature of illness and what to do about it, and above all different values and preferences of patients and their physicians limit the potential benefits of both technology and caring" (Payer, 1988, p. 10). Cross-cultural caring considers health care to be a social process in which professionals and patients each bring a set of beliefs, expectations, and practices to the medical encounter (Waxler-Morrison, Anderson, & Richardson, 1991). Negotiating understanding within and among these multicultural health and illness communities, amid the cultural and political systems, is complicated and challenging.

RELEVANT CONCEPTS

Alignment: A process whereby people communicate in ways that indicate that they understand each other's perspectives; individuals work together to become closer and agree more about the topic under discussion.

Communication gap: When people have a difference of perspectives that complicates efforts to communication; often leads people to communicate in ways that intensifies rather than lessens the gap.

Cultural communities: Emerge through communication; the site where culture gets made and re-made through emotional connection, a sense of belonging, and a common set of customs, rules, rituals, and language.

Interpreted communication: When two of the speakers (in this case, patient and provider) do not share the same language and need an interpreter to broker their interaction.

Linguistic and cultural gaps: Speakers who do not have the same language or cultural background generally experience linguistic and cultural gaps. It is the interpreter's job to bridge those gaps.

Negotiating understanding: Negotiating understanding within and among multicultural health and illness communities necessitates willingness on the part of providers and patients to communicate honestly to build a supportive, trusting relationship.

Patient–provider distance: Patients and providers generally come from very different speech communities. They have different world views. They hold different positions of power based on the social status assigned to each of them by society. Sometimes, patients and providers may have difficulties in communication, even when both may speak the same language. When communication between the two occurs across languages, the intervention of the interpreter impacts this distance, either increasing or decreasing it.

Three-way communication: Communication between three people. In this case, it refers to interpreted communication.

DISCUSSION QUESTIONS

1. What forms of interaction contribute to alignment?
2. What forms of interaction construct distance?
3. What role does culture appear to play in the way discourse is constructed?
4. What other moves could the patient, nurse, or interpreter have made to change the forms of misunderstanding?

ENDNOTES

[1] Angelelli recorded interpreter communication events (ICEs), took notes, interviewed the interpreters and the manager of Interpreting Services at California Hope using semistructured protocols, and collected artifacts. A total of 392 ICEs illustrated different instances of cross-cultural communication.

[2] All names of participants and places are pseudonyms.

[3] The patient uses the incorrect acronym AFTP instead of the correct acronym AFP which stands for Alpha Fetal Protein. This is a blood test utilized during the 15th–20th week of pregnancy to determine the level of protein in a pregnant woman's blood. The test is designed to detect birth defects in the fetus.

REFERENCES/SUGGESTED READINGS

Angelelli, C. (2001). *Deconstructing the invisible interpreter: A critical study of the interpersonal role of the interpreter in a cross-cultural/linguistic communicative event*. DAI-A 62/09, p. 2953, Mar 2002. Doctoral Dissertation, Stanford University, Stanford. Published by UMI.

Davidson, B. (1998). *Interpreting medical discourse: A study of cross-linguistic communication in the hospital clinic*. DAI-A 59/08, p. 2951, Feb 1999. Unpublished doctoral dissertation, Stanford University, Stanford, CA.

Geist-Martin, P., Ray, E. B., & Sharf, B. F. (2003). *Communicating health: Personal, cultural, and political complexities*. Belmont, CA: Wadsworth.

Kaufert, J., & Putsch, R. (1997). Communication through interpreters in healthcare: Ethical dilemmas arising from differences in class, culture, language and power. *The Journal of Clinical Ethics, 8*(1), 71–85.

Payer, L. (1988). *Medicine and culture: Notions of health and sickness in Britain, the U.S., France, and West Germany*. London: Victor Gallancz.

Prince, C. (1986). *Hablando con el doctor: Communication problems between doctors and their Spanish-speaking patients*. Unpublished doctoral dissertation, Stanford University, Stanford, CA.

Waxler-Morrison, N., Anderson, J., & Richardson, E. (1991). *Cross-cultural caring: A handbook for health professionals in Western Canada*. Vancouver: University of British Columbia.

23

The Patient in 4: Framing and Sense-Making in Emergency Medicine

Alexandra G. Murphy
DePaul University

Eric M. Eisenberg
University of South Florida

Kathleen M. Sutcliffe
Steven Schenkel
University of Michigan

Hospital emergency departments (EDs) operate under very trying times. The number and type of patient complaints can vary dramatically on any given day, making it routine to expect the unexpected. National trends, such as hospital overcrowding and nursing shortages, have further thrown emergency medicine into an increasingly complex, uncertain environment. Given these complicating factors, it is remarkable how well most EDs function. No system, however, is perfect. This case study explores how physicians and nurses working in an academic hospital ED, called here University Hospital, must discover and correct errors before they escalate into a crisis. Focusing on a single detailed case—a "near miss" with regard to a serious head trauma– we show how these individuals organize and make sense of their uncertain environment through interaction and how individual actions and outcomes can be linked to layers of communicative contexts, as well as how such a multilevel approach can yield a richer and more useful account.

In the following section, we describe the events of that day using three different sense-making frames. Our goal is to show how different kinds of information illuminate a deceptively straightforward set of individual and organizational actions that nearly resulted in an adverse event. Our presentation in three frames somewhat mirrors our sense-making processes as researchers, specifically, how we continually revised our interpretation of events as we encountered new information.

At the end of each section, after each telling of the case from a particular frame, we pose a number of questions about your interpretations given what you know at that time. After responding to these questions, please continue reading as we "rewind" the tape and go over the details again from a different, expanded perspective. After the three frameworks have been presented, the final section of the paper is an analysis of what we believe can be learned from this case about communication and health care.

THE CASE OF THE PATIENT IN 4

Frame #1: A Huge Mistake

Thursday, 5:55 p.m.   Standing in the hallway outside of Room 4, a resident physician named Rhonda is furious with a nurse named Nicki. "I don't think you understand. This is a *huge* mistake," she says to the nurse. Her voice is loud and she sounds exasperated. "He could bleed in his head. Do you understand that?" The nurse stares back at the resident, but says nothing. Carey, the Charge Nurse on duty, arrives and watches the interaction from a few feet away. In a softer voice, Rhonda goes on, "Look, I know you are new, but we could really have a problem since we just sent a patient with a head injury to the floor without a CT and with no doctor assigned." She pauses, then continues, "Look, I'm not mad at you." To which Nicki responds, "No, you're just standing in the middle of the hall yelling at me and waving your arms."

Moving away from Nicki, Rhonda pulls Carey aside and tells her, "Look, you need to get that patient back from the floor and do the head CT. And tell her [Nicki] I'm not mad at her. I just need this to be taken care of." Carey nods, and a few moments later, she tells Nicki what Rhonda said.

Nicki responds, "I don't really care if she's mad or not. I did my job. You told me the bed was available so I sent him up."

Discussion Questions

1. Who is responsible for putting this patient at risk?
2. How might you characterize the communication dynamics demonstrated in this interaction?
3. What could be done to avoid similar occurrences in the future?
4. Given the chance, what questions would you ask the players in this incident to better understand what happened?

Frame #2: A Resident Takes Action

Rewind. Thursday, Noon, the Same Day.   As often occurs today in U.S. hospitals, this day, there are no beds available in the hospital to receive admitted patients from the ED. Colleen, the Charge Nurse, and Alan, the Attending Physician, are discussing how they can move patients around to try to open up some room for the many patients still waiting to be seen. "I could move the strep throat over to the intermediate care area," Colleen says. "No, they're full," Alan tells her. Frustrated by the situation, Alan states, "We need to go on bypass."

While the ED can never literally close its doors, going on bypass means that they will not be able to take any more patients transferred from other hospitals. Colleen says, "There is no way administration is going to do that. According to them, there are still four beds left in the hospital." These beds still have patients in them, but they are ready to leave and waiting for their discharge orders. It will be several more hours before the beds are physically empty, cleaned, and available to the next patients.

The situation in the ED has hit a breaking point. A resident physician named Roy walks by the main workstation and complains, "It is overwhelming to have so many sick people here at once. There are two people intubated in critical care." These critical patients arrived by ambulance within 10 minutes of each other and needed to be put on respirators to help them breathe. They must be closely monitored and are awaiting admission to intensive care units (ICUs), but there are no ICU beds available. Frustrated by the lack of space, Roy continues, "Some of my chest pain patients, who should be on monitors, are even in the hall." In the meantime, Colleen becomes increasingly focused on finding beds for patients waiting to be admitted to the hospital so that she can open up space for patients in the ED.

Thursday, 1:30 p.m.   Amidst all of this chaos and overcrowding, a new patient arrives in Room 4 with a head injury. With his arrival, Rhonda has taken over his care. She can tell by looking at him that his condition is serious, and he will have to be admitted. She also knows that, in the ideal world, she would wait for all test results to return before "officially" admitting the patient, but that will take hours and she doesn't want this man to have to wait for a bed any longer than he has to. She knows from experience that getting him a bed will likely take hours. So she decides to work around the system and writes an order requesting a bed, called a bed slip, on one of the hospital floors *at the same time* that she orders the tests.

Ideally, putting in a bed slip is part of an orderly process. The slip itself is a single sheet of paper with the patient's name and hospital number. The slip asks to what service the patient will be admitted (for example, the trauma service, the neurosurgical service, or the internal medicine service), who is the attending physician in charge of that service (who will be the person ultimately in charge of the patient's hospitalization), what is the reason for the admission, and what is the level of care (a general bed, a monitored bed, or an ICU bed). After the resident gives the slip to the ED clerk, it is faxed to the admitting office, where actual bed assignment is completed. The resident's next task is to talk with the resident for the admitting service to smooth the transition of medical care from the ED to the new service. Likewise, the nurse will talk with the admitting nurse prior to the patient leaving the ED.

While Rhonda is in seeing the patient, Colleen, the Charge Nurse, approaches Nicki and tells her, "You need to take your break now. Sonya is here to cover you. Go, but be back in 15." But Nicki doesn't want to go on break. She is feeling behind on her patient orders, and new orders keep coming in. But in the end, she figures she had better go now because the way this day is going, she probably won't get another break for the rest of the day.

Rhonda leaves the patient in Room 4 and walks into the center of the main ED. She looks around and doesn't see Nicki. "Well," she figures, "she must be around here somewhere." Just then, Colleen walks by. Rhonda gives her a status report about what she has done with the patient in Room 4. "I know the guy in 4 is going to have to go upstairs, so the bed slip is in. But, just in case a bed magically opens up before the head CT is done, don't move him." "Yeah," Colleen responds. "Like that's really going to happen today."

Rhonda laughs, "I know. I know." Colleen notices that Sonya is standing close by. "Did you get that?" she asks Sonya. "Yeah." Sonya answers.

Discussion Questions

1. Who is responsible for putting this patient at risk?
2. How might you characterize the communication dynamics demonstrated in this interaction?
3. What could be done to avoid similar occurrences in the future?
4. Given the chance, what questions would you ask the players in this incident to better understand what happened?

Frame #3: A Lucky Man

Rewind. Thursday, 1:45 p.m. the Same Day.   Nicki returns from her break. "God," she sighs, "It is never long enough." She walks over to Sonya and tells her she is back. "Great," Sonya says, "I'd better see where Colleen wants me to go now. See you." Nicki checks over her charts and notices that a bed slip has been ordered for the patient in Room 4. "Guess he's ready to go up" she thinks to herself.

Thursday, 3:00 p.m.   Colleen is getting ready to leave. Her shift is over and Carey, the evening Charge Nurse, should be here to take over any minute. "Wait until I tell her what a crazy day it has been!" she thinks. When Carey Arrives, they move into the side hallway to discuss the patient overload problem. "It has been crazy here today, I'm telling you," Colleen explains. She also gives Carey some other bad news. "You are going to be short a couple of nurses this evening. I haven't had a chance to call anyone to cover." She hands Carey a list of possible nurses to call. "Have fun!" she grins sarcastically. "Great," Carey groans. "This is all I need."

Based on her briefing, Carey is immediately focused on two difficult things: finding patient beds in the hospital and calling nurses to come in and cover the evening shift. She is going to be very busy for the next couple of hours. She is not told about the patient waiting for the head CT in room 4.

Carey goes on what she half-jokingly calls a "scavenger hunt" to find beds on the floor. She discovers that, although there are empty rooms upstairs, there are no physical beds in them. She calls housekeeping directly and tells them to get some beds in these rooms immediately. At University Hospital, they have an arrangement whereby housekeeping responds directly to the ED charge nurses. "That way," Carey explains, "the floor nurses can't jack us around and tell us that there are no beds when there really are."

Thursday, 4:55 p.m.   Carey gets a call from housekeeping. A room is now available, complete with a hospital bed. She lets Nicki know the good news, that a room is ready for the patient in room 4. "Wow," says Nicki, "less than 4 hours. What a lucky man!" Immediately, she calls patient transportation and arranges for the transfer. The patient, unaware that he is missing a crucial step in his care, is delighted to be moved to his new private room and to be leaving the ED.

Thursday, 5:55 p.m.   Resident physician Rhonda learns that the CT room is ready and goes looking for her patient in Room 4. But he is nowhere to be found. She starts yelling in the hallway, "Where is my patient in 4?" The nurse tells her that they have already moved him to the floor.

Standing in the hallway outside of Room 4, Rhonda is furious with Nicki. "I don't think you understand. This is a huge mistake," she says to the nurse. Her voice is loud and she sounds exasperated. "He could bleed in his head. Do you understand that?" The nurse stares back at the resident, but says nothing. Carey, the Charge Nurse on duty, arrives and watches the interaction.

In a softer voice, Rhonda goes on, "Look, I know you are new; but we could really have a problem since we just sent a patient with a head injury to the floor without a CT and with no doctor assigned." She pauses, then continues: "Look, I'm not mad at you." To which Nicki, finally, responds: "No, you're just standing in the middle of the hall yelling at me and waving your arms."

Moving away from Nicki, Rhonda pulls Carey aside and tells her, "Look, you need to get that patient back from the floor and do the head CT. And tell her [Nicki] I'm not mad at her. I just need this to be taken care of." Carey nods and a few moments later she tells Nicki what Rhonda said.

Nicki responds, "I don't really care if she's mad or not. I did my job. You told me the bed was available, so I sent him up."

Discussion Questions

1. Who is responsible for putting this patient at risk?
2. How might you characterize the communication dynamics demonstrated in this interaction?
3. What could be done to avoid similar occurrences in the future?
4. Given the chance, what questions would you ask the players in this incident to better understand what happened?

CASE ANALYSIS

The role of in the ED is not set in stone, but most would agree that fundamental to this role is the completion of any emergently required studies and the safe disposition of a patient to an appropriate hospital service. In this case, the patient was moved from the ED before the completion of the pending test and without adequate communication with the admitting service. Indeed, without completion of the test, the admitting service could not be finally determined. Fortunately, the lapse was caught in time, and there were no adverse results. The patient was found and returned to the ED, the CT scan was completed, and he was sent back up to the floor, physically unscathed but very much annoyed. But what can be learned from this incident?

To the extent that the involved parties see the recovery of this close call as a sign of success—a sure sign of the resilience of the system—they are unlikely to take any lessons from these events. Alternatively, if they are able to construe the event as a "near failure" or a sign of potential danger, it would help them offset the common organizational bias toward feelings of invulnerability because of past successes. Even in high reliability industries, the main issue is not whether mistakes can be avoided altogether, as they cannot, but whether organizational actors can learn to be mindful of each other and effectively manage unanticipated events when they do occur. With these thoughts in mind, we now return to the events of the day to take a closer look at the "deceptively simple" set of organizational and individual issues that, in this case, triggered a set of unexpected consequences.

Frame #1 Analysis

From the perspective of the first frame, "a huge mistake" was made. The primary attribution for the CT oversight was the incompetence of one individual, specifically Nicki, the nurse assigned to bed 4. Taking this view, it seems reasonable that a well-trained nurse should have known not to transfer a head trauma patient without first verifying that a CT was done. Moreover, the whole situation would have been averted if the nurse, Nicki, had questioned the order to move the patient, had been suspicious of how quickly and easily a bed had been obtained on such a chaotic day, and/or sought out other opinions about the best course of action before making the move.

Individual scapegoating like this is pervasive in complex organizations. Unfortunately, it tends to divert attention from weaknesses in underlying systems and processes. All too often, organizational members blame each other rather than examine the system for flaws. In this case, the resident blamed the nurses and the nurses blamed the resident, and both had some justifiable grievances. The nurses did not pass information along to each other, and the resident stepped outside of the hospital protocol by ordering the bed before the patient was ready to be admitted.

Blaming the individual parties, however, only reinforces divisions between two groups that are already divided because of competing professional training and concomitant differences in social status and power. In sick systems, there is more than enough individual blame to go around. In this case, employees from a range of professions showed an inability to work well at a systems level, leaving a patient to fall through the "white space" in the hospital organizational chart.

Frame #2 Analysis

The second explanatory frame ("a resident takes action") suggests a very different set of interpretations. Entering the scene at noon on Thursday, we are struck by the overcrowding and seeming confusion. We learn that, although the needed information to stop the patient in 4 from being transferred upstairs did exist in the department, it was not widely shared among department employees or with the specific individual who most needed to know. Indeed, there were several times throughout the afternoon when the situation could have been avoided had the information been given to Nicki, the nurse covering Room 4. We know that when the nurse sent the patient up to the floor, she was following the explicit written orders issued by Rhonda, the very resident who then yelled at her for following them. Unfortunately, Nicki was unaware that verbal orders limiting the timing of the transfer had been issued while she was out of the unit.

Nicki was on a 15-minute break when the resident told the morning charge nurse (Colleen) about the situation. Colleen then told Sonya, the nurse who was covering for Nicki, but it is unclear from her response whether she understood the implications of the information (i.e., "Did you get that?" "Yeah."). When Nicki returned from her break, Sonya did not think to pass on the information. She likely assumed the charge nurse or resident would tell Nicki what was going on, and moved on to cover for another nurse going out on break. At the same time, Nicki did not ask for information about the patient in 4. Because she did not hear anything from Sonya, she likely assumed that things were safe. An important question is: What does it mean when there is no news? Are things going well, are they going poorly, or is it unclear how things are going? The default answer to that question tells us a lot about the degree of mindfulness in an organization or the extent to which people are working on autopilot.

This particular part of the case is further evidence of the emerging conclusion that handoffs—transitions from person to person across specialty or shift—can be especially risky. It suggests the need for much more emphasis on intra- and interdepartmental cooperation and communication. It also hints of the possibilities in developing and deploying an information technology system that provides all known records for patients that are accessible at any point in the process.

It is dangerous, however, to focus solely on improved information transfer as the solution to system failures. Instead, there is a need to describe and address the system itself, not simply its implementation. CTs and laboratory tests, even at their most efficient, do take a certain amount of time; in addition, these departments are often backed up with work and are slower in producing results that patients and providers want as quickly as possible. This frustrates everyone, not the least of whome are the physicians, and hence, there is a strong tendency to work around the system. To be sure, these workarounds are often done with the patients' best interests in mind. Faster transfers mean continuing care on the floor, where it is most appropriate, for people who need it and speedier medical attention for sick people in the waiting room. Most of the time, the ploy works just fine, and patients receive faster, more seamless service.

One observation we have about ED work in general is that lots of energy is spent propping up the current system and processes, essentially bypassing the bigger issues to get through another day. This case suggests a serious need to explore the places where informal practices deviate substantially from formal rules and procedures. If we can understand this gap, we can make changes in education, communication, or the rule iteself—that might help close it.

Frame #3 Analysis

In the third frame—"a lucky man"—we learn even more about the bed management problem in the ED and how residents and charge nurses have chosen to deal with it. A common problem facing EDs today is the overcrowding of hospitals; when combined with the shortage of nurses, this leaves few places for ED patients to go once they are admitted to the hospital. To avoid total collapse, employees engage in a range of workarounds to keep the system from failing. The most obvious of these is the placement of patients in hallways and treating these hallways as makeshift units. Not only does this diminish patient privacy and dignity, it adds to the confusion of the system, as it becomes difficult to track patients and problematic to carry out a physical examination.

But perhaps the worst (and best!) thing about these workarounds is that they usually work. Because they do, the system is rarely thrown into crisis, so organizational members are effectively keeping a bad system in place, limping along, due to their heroic efforts at compensating.

The charge nurse, Carey, discussed how she believes the nurses and physicians enable a "bad" system. She recently went to an international conference in Emergency Medicine. She said, "A nurse from the UK told us, 'We don't have this kind of wait in the UK. You nurses are in a position of power. There is a health care crisis and a nursing shortage. You should be shouting.'" The Charge Nurse continued, "Do you see anyone shouting here? No. We don't shout because 90% of the nurses fall into the 'enabling' category and doctors don't want to admit failure."

Of course, we must also pay attention to how power and hierarchy affect communication—both its meaning and likely transmission. The interaction between the resident and the nurse reflects the hierarchical arrangement of their respective positions. Given the authoritative stance the resident takes when speaking to the nurse and the relatively silent response the nurse offers, we can assume a strong sense of role clarity. Even the charge nurse defers to the resident, indicating her subordinate role. Some nurses have explained that they will not follow verbal orders from the doctors. They don't trust the doctors to back them up if there is a problem. This is a problem when the written order follows the prescribed system and the verbal order is meant to introduce the workaround system.

The main insight we garner from this third frame is a bigger picture of the patient flow process, which may very well be a key obstacle to improving the nation's EDs. Hospitals lack available beds, leaving sick patients in the ED longer than they either should or expect to be there. This in turn backs up the waiting area. The severity of this now-chronic problem is what has Rhonda doing a workaround with the bed slip and Carey going on scavenger hunts for beds. In process terms, a significant obstacle downstream is threatening the integrity of upstream activity.

MINDFULNESS AS AN INSTITUTIONAL CAPACITY

All organizations maintain a balance between formal rules on the one hand and informal practices on the other. Moreover, this tension cannot be resolved in favor of either extreme; some degree of formality is required to facilitate coordination, but there must also be room for improvisation when mindful employees sense that a literal application of the rules will have an adverse and unintended effect.

The problems hospital EDs face are similar to the types of problems that some organizations have managed much more successfully. These high-reliability organizations (e.g., air traffic control centers, nuclear power plants, power dispatch grid) operate under difficult conditions but experience less than their fair share of accidents. They face an "excess of unexpected events because their technologies are complex and their constituencies are varied in their demands—and because the people who run these systems, like all of us, have an incomplete understanding of their own systems and what they face" (Weick & Sutcliffe, 2001, p. 3). It is counterproductive, then, to define the success of the ED in terms of their ability to *eliminate* error; rather, it succeeds when it doesn't allow errors to disable it.

Effective high-reliability organizations are those that have the capacity to act "mindfully." Their challenge is in knowing when to maintain standard operating practices that embody knowledge and experience and when to abandon them and improvise workarounds that keep the system flexible and "resilient" in the face of unexpected events. But flexibility does not guarantee success. As seen in this case, the resident demonstrated flexibility and worked around the slow system, so when the formal system actually worked and went faster than she had anticipated, it resulted in a life-threatening problem. The problem, therefore, is erroneously identified as the workaround, not the standard operating practice. We now return to the discussion questions we have posed throughout, offering our own responses given all of the information we have reported in the text.

Discussion Questions

1. *Who is responsible for putting this patient at risk?*
Although it would be easy to blame an individual or two (Rhonda and Nicki come to mind), a better way of thinking about the answer is in terms of a shared responsibility to speak up and not follow procedures when there is significant doubt about whether to proceed. This was the main finding that came out of the analysis of the Challenger Space Shuttle Challenger disaster, and it serves as a useful guide for communication in high-risk organizations more generally. To counter the prevailing bias toward maximization and efficiency, all parties must have the authority and be willing to question any particular decision that makes them feel uncomfortable. Even if their concerns do not change the outcome, questioning the process moves these actions from unconscious to conscious thought, making it much more likely that potential problems will be identified and addressed.

From a corporate perspective, there may also be some value in assigning responsibility to the various managers and directors who oversee the ED, in that it is their job to ensure proper employee training and to encourage organizational processes, practices, and values that encourage questioning and learning to minimize the likelihood of small mistakes accumulating into adverse events.

2. *How might you characterize the communication dynamics demonstrated in this interaction?*
One word to describe the communication in this ED on this day is stressed. Time pressures, overcrowding, and the overriding feeling of being overwhelmed bring out the worst in people as communicators. Once a misstep has occurred, this stress is evident in the reactions of all parties, which include anger, defensiveness, and placing blame.

Moreover, this constant pressure minimizes communication (almost all of the interactions are on the fly) and causes people to use shorthand in relaying information. Like most other EDs, University Hospital uses a big board to keep track of patients, but there were many instances during our observations when information was either omitted from the board or abbreviated in a way that was incomprehensible. Overall, the twin feelings of being overwhelmed and on the run seem one cause of the lack of communication in this case. We find this to be a much more likely explanation than one that would find key players incompetent or negligent.

Another way to characterize the communication is "heedless." Heedless interrelating occurs when individuals simply do their job, ignoring what goes on around them. Heedful interrelating occurs when people perform their work with a conscious awareness of how their job fits with other people's jobs to accomplish the goals of the system (Weick, 2002). Interrelating done with heed increases the alertness and intelligence of the system rather than any single individual, which makes it easier to mobilize the capability to get on top of unexpected events.

3. *What could be done to avoid similar occurrences in the future?*

There are of course some obvious things that could be done to reduce future risk. The first involves a restatement of the importance of written orders and especially the need to document any changes to what has been written. Why the resident chooses to write some orders while only verbalizing others opens a new avenue for evaluation. In the case where written and verbal orders conflict (which was not exactly true here, because Nicki never received the verbal order to make sure the CT was done first), employees must be made to feel comfortable questioning the decision to go forward.

Organizations are especially vulnerable to this kind of mistake during hand-offs and shift changes. There should be a mechanism in place when outgoing professionals give report to their successor to flag these kinds of pending decisions. Especially in this instance, where Colleen emphasized the priority to be staffing, it is not surprising that Carey had her head down and was thinking of little else. Perhaps certain actions or events, such as being transferred to a room, should trigger a quick checklist review that, in this case, would have included the CT scan.

In addition to shift changes and the use of verbal orders, this system is also made vulnerable—and inevitably, less mindful—by the rigidity of the medical hierarchy of expertise. Nurses complain mightily that, although they know the patients best from spending so much time with them, physicians very often minimize their observations in making their diagnoses and developing a treatment plan. What results is a trained incapacity for open dialogue across functions and levels, and an unwillingness on anyone's part to communicate doubt or uncertainty. Consequently, routines of all kinds get put into place and take on a life of their own, and are difficult to stop, even when there are concerns about their appropriateness.

4. *Given the chance, what questions would you ask the key players in this incident to better understand what happened?*

We're interested in knowing more about the unique role of the charge nurse in emergency medicine, how it is constructed here and elsewhere, and its special communicative function in this environment. From this case, it appeared that these individuals had a tremendous amount of control over the department culture and might be key allies in developing a more open communication climate and culture of respectful interaction. Also of interest is how physicians regard this kind of "near-miss" in the ED, and to what causal factors they attribute the mistake. Finally, it would be most interesting to learn more about the patient's perspective, how the system appeared to him and what might be changed to satisfy his concerns.

CONCLUSION

This study began by conceptualizing emergency medicine as sense-making par excellence, quickly revealing how this work is done in a highly stressful, high-reliability context. Although mistakes and near-misses often prompt a knee-jerk search for the offending individuals, we introduced significant contextual material that revealed how the near-miss in this case could be traced to a range of systems problems. This material was presented in three frames, but others are possible; the key point is that there is no single frame that is "true." The more we examine the facts of the case, the more we become convinced once again that there is rarely such a thing as an isolated failure in a complex system. As a general rule, it is a series of unfortunate events occurring in just the right order that leads to a failure.

Failures cannot, however, be perfectly well predicted or avoided. Instead, it is the building a kind of robust, resilient, open communication climate that makes opportunities for meta-conversations and challenges to orders and routine. In an inversion of the traditional command and control model, the challenging of arbitrary orders is construed here as a strength, not a weakness. If mindfulness is essential to the successful operation of high-reliability systems, mindful practice is essentially communicative.

RELEVANT CONCEPTS

Collective mindfulness: Ability on the part of individuals in a group to better notice unexpected events as they happen and focus on ways of preventing or containing them.

Heedful interrelating: When people perform their work with a conscious awareness of how their job fits with other people's jobs to accomplish the goals of the system.

Resilient and flexible systems: Mindful organizational systems know when to maintain resiliency and when to exhibit flexibility in the face unexpected events.

Sense-making: The job of organizing involves "making sense" of the uncertainties in environments through interaction.

DISCUSSION QUESTIONS

1. What does it mean for organizational members to manage unexpected events well?
2. Is it possible to build a robust, resilient, open organizational communication climate? If so, what would this entail?
3. How could a collective state of mindfulness benefit the quality, reliability, and productivity of other health care organizations?
4. What are the benefits and drawbacks of yielding a multilevel-framed approach to studying an organizational problem?

ACKNOWLEDGMENT

This project was funded by a generous grant from the National Patient Safety Foundation. The case described here was drawn from the ethnographic portion of the study of two academically affiliated emergency departments.

REFERENCES/SUGGESTED READINGS

American College of Emergency Physicians. (1998). *The future of emergency medicine*. Dallas, TX: Author.

Kelly, R. (1999). Goings-on in a CCU: An ethnomethodological account of things that go on in a routine handover. *Nursing Critical Care, 4*, 85–91.

Weick, K. E. (2002). The reduction of medical errors through mindful interdependence. In M. M. Rosenthal and K. M. Sutcliffe (Eds.). *Medical error: What do we know? What do we do?* (pp. 177–199). San Francisco: Jossey-Bass.

Weick, K. E., & Sutcliffe, K. (2001). *Managing the unexpected: Assuring high performance in an age of complexity*. San Francisco: Jossey Bass.

Additional Resources

Web sites:
   National Patient Safety Foundation: www.npsf.org
Agency for Healthcare Research and Quality (AHRQ): http:// webmm.ahrq.gov/
Films/Videos:
   The Doctor
Groupthink: The Challenger Air Disaster

24

Reorganized Medical Practice: An Institutional Perspective on Neonatal Care

John C. Lammers
Kristin A. Lindholm
Heidi M. Hazeu
University of Illinois at Urbana–Champaign

Many case studies in health communication concern an illness episode, a set of events at a specific health organization, or a particular patient's experience with an illness over its trajectory. Most of these cases focus in some way on patients, illnesses, or communication between patients and providers. An equally important kind of communication remains hidden: exchanges and relationships between hospitals, doctors, clinics, and governmental regulators. This behind-the-scenes communication creates the setting in which other health communication takes place, yet researchers often overlook it. It is a rapidly changing world of regulations, contracts, and policies. To study this world, communication researchers need to look not only for patients, but for providers; not only for illnesses, but for the legal definitions of health conditions; and not only for interpersonal exchanges, but also for formal communication in contracts and government regulations.

This case concerns Dr. John Smalley (a pseudonym), a successful and popular physician who practiced neonatal medicine (the care of newborn infants) for 16 years as a member of a multispecialty medical group in a medium-sized Midwestern city. The events of the case involve many organizations: care for high-risk infants takes place in neonatal intensive care units (NICUs), state health departments stipulate licensing requirements for NICUs within hospitals, and neonatologists may belong to multispecialty medical groups. Neonatal care requires frequent communication between specialists and other providers. Additionally, it is a relatively expensive service for hospitals to provide, which can lead to price competition among hospitals and medical groups. Perhaps most importantly, this case involves the collision of a successful medical practice and the world of regulations and contracts.

Dr. Smalley's practice was abruptly closed when the hospital in which he saw patients terminated its contract for neonatal services with his medical group. The hospital chose instead to contract with a larger, regional medical group that, in turn, subcontracted with physicians to provide services. The regional group negotiated with Smalley to work as their subcontractor, but he eventually decided to practice in another city despite his strong ties to the local community.

This case takes an institutional perspective on health communication, focusing on the organizational, economic, and regulatory context in which patient–provider communication and individual health services occur. In addition, the institutional view places emphasis on previously understudied aspects of health communication: the formal rules that constrain communication between providers and nonproviders other than patients, such as administrators, managers, and contract officers. A complete understanding of this case, therefore, requires close attention to the history, regulations, and organizational relations surrounding neonatology.

The case is built on over three dozen press reports, 14 personal interviews with most of the participants quoted in those reports, archival research on state regulations, and both library and Internet research on physicians' contracts. The case is told through a series of reconstructed press reports that document events over a 16-year period during which Dr. Smalley's personal life intersected with organizational mergers and break-ups, changing state regulations, and professional contracts. We have altered the names of persons and organizations to protect the actual participants' privacy. As the facts of the case unfold, you may notice a bewildering array of organizations and relationships; therefore, we have included a diagram (see Figure 24.1) that depicts the major organizations and their relationships, which contextualized Dr. Smalley's life and practice in the small city of Suburbia in Central State.

THE DAILY COURIER, APRIL 12, 1986

Neonatologist Joins Linford Clinic Staff

Linford Clinic is pleased to announce a new addition to its staff. Dr. John Smalley comes to Linford from Children's Hospital in Atlanta, Georgia, where he was a resident in general pediatrics. Currently a specialist in neonatal–perinatal medicine, Smalley will serve as Director of Linford Clinic's Neonatal–Perinatal Department. Because of Linford Clinic's association with Midwest Medical Center, Smalley will also serve as Director of the Newborn Intensive Care Unit at Midwest.

Dr. Smalley, who has degrees in medicine and public health, developed an interest in newborns and premature infants during his residency in Atlanta. Smalley and his wife have three daughters who will attend schools in the Suburbia School District.

THE DAILY COURIER, NOVEMBER 14, 1991

Local Doctor to Head New AIDS Task Force

Governor Pat Brown recently appointed Dr. John Smalley to lead a new statewide AIDS task force. The task force, composed of 25 health care workers and citizens, will study issues related to medical professionals who have AIDS or are infected by HIV and perform invasive procedures. The task force will also address procedures that medical professionals should follow when treating patients who are infected with HIV or have AIDS. Smalley said that he is particularly concerned about the risks involved in neonatal and obstetric care because HIV-infected mothers transmit the virus to their babies at a rate of approximately 30%.

According to State Senator Jane Major, Smalley is a natural choice for the role. "Since his arrival in the area several years ago, Dr. Smalley has been involved in a number of community projects and has established a solid reputation with both colleagues and patients in the local community," said Major. At the present time, Smalley is a member of the Springdale County and Central State Medical Societies. Smalley, a practicing pediatrician for the last 11 years, was certified in neonatal–perinatal medicine by the American Board of Pediatrics last December, a recognition of his contribution to the care of newborn and premature babies.

THE DAILY COURIER, DECEMBER 5, 1992

New Neonatologist Joins Midwest's Neonatal Unit

Dr. Lily Savage recently joined Midwest Medical Center's neonatal unit. Savage, a practicing pediatrician for more than a decade, comes to Midwest from St. Peter's Hospital in New Jersey. Savage will be working with Dr. John Smalley, who has been serving as the director of the unit since 1986.

Savage's arrival is welcomed by Smalley, who has been the lone doctor working in the 12-bed unit. Smalley was philosophical about his working conditions before Savage's hire due to his previous experience at an Atlanta hospital, in which there were 100 beds in the neonatal unit. "There, you could run yourself into the ground and still be uncertain of the outcome for particular infants. Here, I have had to do absolutely everything, but at least I was sure everything was being done correctly," Smalley said.

Savage is not the only addition to the unit this year. In March, the $20 million remodeling of Midwest Medical Center was completed, and that remodeling included the 12-bed neonatal unit.

THE DAILY COURIER, JULY 29, 1993

Local Hospitals Join Forces to Create the Regional Level III Perinatal Center

Midwest Medical Center and Pearl Hospital formally joined forces today to receive joint designation as the Regional Level III Perinatal Center. Although Midwest and Pearl will each maintain a separate neonatal intensive care unit, health care providers from both hospitals will work together, sharing resources and transcending physical boundaries.

Designation for perinatal centers is awarded by the Central State Department of Public Health (CSDPH) on the basis of meeting various conditions concerning staffing, equipment availability, and level of patient intake. The Statewide Perinatal Advisory Committee, composed of 22 health practitioners, 2 members of the general public, and 6 representatives from various health-related committees and associations, advises the CSDPH and makes recommendations concerning hospitals seeking designation as perinatal centers. State designation as a Regional Level III Unit means staff at Midwest and Pearl are able to treat the highest risk expectant mothers and premature babies. The Level III designation satisfies a need for comprehensive care of mothers and infants that was identified several years ago by officials at both hospitals, and this joint effort represents the culmination of talks that began in the 1980s.

Dr. John Smalley, a neonatologist at Midwest Medical Center, and Dr. Ronald Davies, a perinatologist at Pearl Hospital, are codirectors for the program. A neonatologist specializes in the care of infants under 28 days old. A perinatologist specializes in care during the perinatal period, which is the time between conception and the end of the first month of life. A neonatologist is a pediatrician who specializes in the care of the infant, whereas a perinatologist is an obstetrician who specializes in caring for the mother.

Midwest Medical Center was formed in 1985 when Tringham and Saints hospitals merged. Midwest currently provides the facilities where many of Linford Clinic's 100 doctors schedule their surgical procedures. Last year, Midwest underwent a $20 million remodeling, which expanded its neonatal intensive care unit to a 12-bed capacity.

Pearl Hospital was established in 1920 and is staffed with doctors from Pearl Clinic's 300-member medical group. Pearl's neonatal unit has 14 beds.

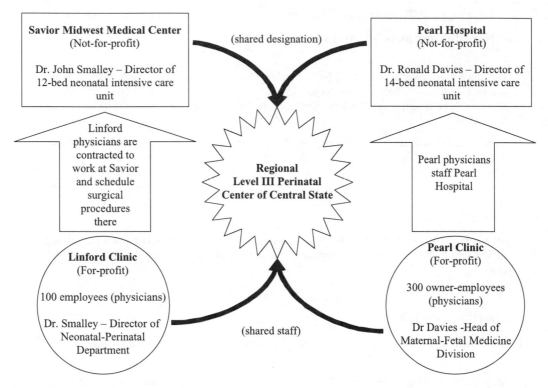

FIG. 24.1.   Structure of local health organizations with Shared Perinatal Designation.

THE DAILY COURIER, JUNE 23, 1997

New Name for Midwest Medical Center

Midwest Medical Center today became part of the Savior system of hospitals when Midwest's parent company, HelpCorp, merged with two other Catholic health networks to form Savior Health. Midwest Medical Center will now be known as Savior Midwest Medical Center.

Millie Smith, formerly CEO of HelpCorp and now Senior Vice-President for Savior Health, said, "For the past 25 years, HelpCorp has been dedicated to providing compassionate, quality care to needy people whatever their social standing. This merger will strengthen, not weaken, the ability of hospitals formerly associated with HelpCorp to provide efficient, quality care."

THE DAILY COURIER, MARCH 12, 1998

Local Clinic Sells Its Ownership of Insurance Program

Linford Clinic has sold its remaining half-ownership of PatientCare insurance to Savior Health. Linford Clinic used to be the sole owner of PatientCare, a managed care organization founded in the 1980s by physicians associated with Linford Clinic. In 1991, Linford Clinic sold its first half-ownership to the former Midwest Medical Center, now named Savior Midwest Medical Center.

Bill McNamara, CEO of Linford Clinic, said, "The sale of PatientCare insurance should enable physicians associated with our clinic to practice without any concern about a conflict of interest between their professional judgments and their compensation for providing health care. Linford Clinic's physicians are committed to providing high-quality care, and our Board of Directors felt it was in the patients' and doctors' best interests to sell our share of the insurance side of things."

THE DAILY COURIER, SEPTEMBER 18, 1998

Pearl Doctors Step in to Take Care of Linford Clinic's Cancer Patients

Following the departure of Linford Clinic's oncologist, Dr. Tim Chang, to a new position outside the state, oncologists from Pearl Clinic have stepped in to take over the care of his patients. Under the new arrangement, the Pearl physicians will take responsibility for the patients while Linford Clinic searches for an oncologist to replace Dr. Chang.

Dr. James Hesky, Medical Director for Linford Clinic, questioned whether this arrangement could signal the beginning of a merger of a number of services between Linford Clinic and Pearl Clinic. He also said that there had been positive feedback from physicians in both groups regarding the temporary arrangement, though it was too early to know how patients will respond.

This is not the first time Linford and Pearl have cooperated. The ophthalmology departments at the two clinics have been referring patients to one another over the past decade because of the areas of expertise represented by physicians in both organizations. The Regional Level III Perinatal Center, combining the resources of physicians from Linford Clinic and Pearl Clinic, was established in 1993.

THE DAILY COURIER, APRIL 1, 1999

Physicians Wrestle with Unionization

Suburbia's doctors are expressing mixed feelings about a Central State Medical Society resolution calling for them to consider collective bargaining and the formation of unions. Dr. John Smalley, a neonatologist at Linford Clinic, said that the details of the proposal are unclear. "Currently, the resolution is vague. We don't know for certain what the advantages would be. However, we do believe that collective bargaining could ultimately help patients by safeguarding doctors' rights."

Dr. Janet Bankey, a family practitioner at Pearl Clinic, thinks that collective bargaining makes sense in the current climate of health care. "More doctors are finding their practices affected by managed care contracts, agreements with particular multispecialty groups, and the economic realities of trying to keep their practices afloat," Bankey said. "Doctors might have had autonomy many years ago, but they currently do not. That's why this resolution makes sense."

Bill McNamara, CEO of Linford Clinic, is also giving his tentative support to the resolution. He believes that physicians need to have more of a voice in the issues that are affecting their ability to provide quality care to their patients. McNamara said, "There are several crucial factors that need to be addressed by doctors, and they have to have the ability to make their voices heard. Even medical groups are finding it difficult to negotiate effectively with larger health care organizations, like hospitals, if those organizations decide to contract outside of the local area or contract exclusively with particular groups."

THE DAILY COURIER, AUGUST 2, 2000

New State Regulations to Affect Perinatal Center

Central State legislators have approved more stringent requirements for Level III designation for state perinatal centers in the form of the Perinatal Health Care Code. The requirements will affect both Savior Midwest Medical Center and Pearl Hospital. The two hospitals jointly run the Regional Level III Perinatal Center, which is located in two separate physical locations but combines resources in the form of medical staff and equipment.

To be designated as a Level III facility, one that cares for the highest-risk mothers and premature babies, the perinatal center must comply with Central State Department of Public Health regulations concerning the level of medical care available. Hospital staff must be available to consult in various areas of expertise that include pediatric surgery, genetic counseling, anesthesiology, and neurological care.

A team of two medical directors must head the unit. One director, a pediatrician certified in neonatal–perinatal medicine, oversees neonatal activities. The second director, an obstetrician certified by the American Board of Obstetrics and Gynecology, oversees obstetric activities. These directors' services must be available at times when the directors are not.

Several specialized medical services and qualified staff must be available 24 hours per day to provide constant maternal–fetal monitoring. A physician or advanced practice nurse with experience in the care of ventilated infants must be on the hospital's premises whenever an infant is receiving ventilation. At least half of the nursing staff must have previous experience in a Level III neonatal intensive care unit (NICU). The NICU must also serve a minimum number of patients for a hospital to keep its Level III designation.

These changes will put extra pressure on the Regional Level III Perinatal Center to satisfy all service requirements. Perinatologist and Medical Director of the Center, Dr. Ronald Davies, commented on the new rules, "The coming months are likely to spell change for the center as we make adjustments to ensure all requirements are met. However, here at Pearl, we have a dedicated and broad array of staff who cover many specialties in the field of medicine, so we do not anticipate any major problems."

At Savior Midwest Medical Center, this sentiment was echoed by Dr. John Smalley, Davies' codirector: "Changes in regulations such as these have the potential to hit us hard. Fortunately, Savior's reciprocal relationship with Pearl allows us to combine resources and provide the best quality care possible for the local community."

THE DAILY COURIER, FEBRUARY 19, 2001

Community Prize for Local Doctor

Yesterday, Dr. John Smalley received the Community Caring Prize from Mayor LaKisha Ray in honor of his numerous contributions at the local and state levels. His efforts include organizing blood drives through the Rotary Club, raising money for health care research, and contributing to the March of Dimes. Smalley and his wife are also supporters of Suburbia's Children's Museum, which opened in 1995.

Smalley's contributions to medical students have been considerable. He has been a guest speaker for the State University Medical Student Organization, and he has mentored several medical students during the past decade.

Although Smalley works full time as Director of Linford Clinic's Neonatal–Perinatal Department and Director of the Newborn Intensive Care Unit at Savior Midwest Medical Center, he also volunteers his time to serve as a medical consultant on the state's AIDS Task Force. In awarding Smalley the prize, Mayor Ray said, "We are indeed fortunate and honored to have citizens like Dr. Smalley leading our community."

THE DAILY COURIER, JULY 22, 2001

Pearl Hospital to Run its Own Level III Perinatal Center

In the wake of new regulations for Central State's perinatal centers, Pearl Hospital has received Level III designation for its own perinatal center. This designation ends the eight-year partnership between Pearl and Savior Midwest Medical Center in operating a joint Regional Level III Perinatal Center. The state regulations involve new standards for care. Ronald Davies, Director of the Level III Perinatal Center at Pearl, explained, "The requirements include having several specific medical personnel available 24 hours a day, seven days a week. Pearl now has specialists in all required areas, and we have an outstanding team available for regional service."

The number of infants and mothers who are treated annually at Pearl's perinatal center has nearly doubled since 1993. Currently, the hospital handles nearly 300 cases per year. This increase in volume and the changing state standards led to Pearl's decision to become independent. Cynthia Gregory, CEO at Pearl Hospital, said, "Pearl and Savior are parting on friendly terms, and both hospitals will continue to provide excellent perinatal care for patients." No physical relocation will take place because the two units operated separately, each serving its own patients.

Savior Midwest Medical Center now faces the challenge of acquiring independent Level III status for its own perinatal center. According to Robert Bloom, Chief Operating Officer at Savior, the hospital will have one year to meet the state requirements for Level III status. In the interim, Savior will be able to retain its Level III designation. "Patients should see no change in the level of care they receive," said Bloom. "Yes, we had a joint designation with Pearl, but we have been operating our own neonatal intensive care unit for many years now. Dr. John Smalley has provided excellent leadership for us in the past. Currently, our focus is on recruiting the staff we need to have the best neonatal intensive care unit possible. We at Savior have full confidence that we will meet the state requirements well before the deadline."

THE DAILY COURIER, NOVEMBER 4, 2001

CARTE Challenges Savior Midwest Medical Center

Members of the health care advocacy group County Activists React to Exploitation (CARTE) organized an early-morning protest outside Savior Midwest Medical Center yesterday. Even though temperatures were well below the freezing point, about 100 people gathered to protest Savior's hiring and firing practices.

"All citizens should be concerned about the kind of health care that is available in our community, and the quality of that care depends on consumer choice," said Laura McMillan, organizer of the protest. "Savior Midwest Medical Center is hiring personnel in ways that inhibit free choice." McMillan and others pointed to recent examples of exclusive contracts formed between Savior and for-profit organizations that provide services in the hospital.

Paul Bartholomew, a representative of CARTE, claimed that Savior is forging relationships that are questionable. Bartholomew said, "Savior Midwest Medical Center and other nonprofit hospitals like it are sending money to their parent organization, Savior. CARTE believes that the parent group is then funneling that money into for-profit groups that it is associated with. Essentially, the nonprofit hospitals are giving money to the for-profit ventures. Doesn't that seem backwards?"

Savior's CEO, Nataly Satgian, expressed sympathy with the goals of the activists. "We all want to see quality care in this community, and I think the challenges provided by CARTE keep both Savior and Pearl on our toes," said Satgian. She denied any financial irresponsibility on the part of Savior and explained that Savior's commitment to quality care sometimes requires the hospital to look outside of the local area to find the best care at the best price.

THE DAILY COURIER, MARCH 3, 2002

Conflict Continues for Local Medical Center

Savior Midwest Medical Center has received intermittent public criticism from the health care advocacy group County Activists React to Exploitation (CARTE) during the past four months. Now Savior is receiving criticism from Linford Clinic. According to Savior's CEO, Nataly Satgian, the hospital has adopted a "vertical integration" approach that places various aspects of health care— hospitals, doctors, and insurance providers—under one ownership. This approach has brought with it problems for Savior's long-term association with Linford Clinic and its doctors.

"Hospitals have no business owning health plans, and physicians should not own them either," said Bill McNamara, CEO of Linford Clinic. "This arrangement keeps consumers from choosing physicians and specialists according to their needs." Linford Clinic formerly owned a managed care plan, PatientCare, but sold one half to Midwest Medical Center in 1991 and the second half to Savior Health in 1998.

According to McNamara, physicians with Linford Clinic are also concerned about Savior's recent contracts with physicians from outside the local community. Satgian defends Savior's recent choices. "Linford Clinic is a fine organization that Savior is proud to be associated with," she said. "At times, however, Linford may not be able to meet all of the needs of the hospital and the community. At that point, we are obliged to look elsewhere."

THE DAILY COURIER, MAY 15, 2002

Community to Say Goodbye to Popular Doctor

In a surprise to many members of Suburbia, Dr. John Smalley is leaving his positions as Director of Linford Clinic's Neonatal–Perinatal Department and Director of the Savior Midwest Medical Center's Newborn Intensive Care Unit at the end of June after 16 years of service. He has accepted a position as a neonatologist at a pediatric medical group working with a hospital in Capital City, about 75 miles away. Former patient Arlene Hardy expressed surprise that Dr. Smalley was leaving and says that Smalley will be missed. "Dr. Smalley was there for my husband and me when our son, Nathan, was barely hanging on to life. He worked tirelessly to help us, and now we send Dr. Smalley Nathan's school photo every year to remind him of our gratitude and the excellent work he does."

A neonatologist from the Metropolitan Neonatology Group will fill Smalley's position. Savior Midwest Medical Center offered the Metropolitan Group an exclusive contract to provide the personnel for Savior's Level III Perinatal Center. Tracie Riley, Vice President at Savior, announced the termination of the neonatology contract between Savior Midwest Medical Center and Linford Clinic. The new contract with the Metropolitan Group will go into effect later this summer. The new contract requires the Metropolitan Group to provide at least two physicians for Savior.

Several factors led to the change in arrangements at Savior Midwest Medical Center, according to Riley. First, Central State implemented new regulations regarding perinatal centers that were brought into force in August 2000. A second factor was Pearl Hospital's decision to end its commitment to the jointly operated Regional Level III Perinatal Center last summer. Pearl's decision put extra pressure on Savior to satisfy state requirements independently.

Dr. Lily Savage, a neonatologist at Savior, has been hired by the Metropolitan Neonatology Group and will remain in her current position. Dr. Bruce Race, a neonatologist, and Dr. C. E. Xiang, perinatologist, will join Savior at the beginning of July.

According to Dr. Smalley's recent farewell speech, he will be commuting to Capital City, the closest city with a Level III perinatal center. About Suburbia, he said, "This has been our home for 16 years. We've raised our daughters here, and we really don't want to move. So, for the time being, I'll commute."

DISCUSSION

Dr. Smalley's experience is only one physician's story, but his personal problem is quickly becoming a public issue. There are four larger issues that Dr. Smalley's experience illuminates: (1) the role of regulations as part of the communicated environment of medical practitioners, (2) the role of contracts in formal communication, (3) the rate and kind of organizational change occurring in health care environments like Dr. Smalley's, and (4) physicians' reactions to these changes.

The Role of Regulations as Part of the Communicated Environment of Medical Practitioners

Health care may be one of the most regulated arenas within which to work, with laws governing everything from the licensure of practitioners and organizations to health statistics reporting and financial reimbursement. Government regulations of medical care in the United States are so imbedded and pervasive that they are invisible to most consumers of care. It may be useful to distinguish regulations (a feature of government's role) from contractual provisions (a feature of private relationships between providers and organizations). Regulations stipulated by state and local governments in general are aimed at three issues: (1) quality and safety of services, (2) access to services, and (3) financing and reimbursement of services.

In Dr. Smalley's case, state regulations govern the terms under which a hospital can provide services to mothers and babies. The rules, enforced by the state health department, literally stipulate what equipment and personnel must be available for a hospital to provide a certain level of service. These rules protect public safety and offer best practice guidelines to organizations, but also place less wealthy hospitals like Savior in a precarious position. The only way that Savior could staff a legal "Level III perinatal center" was by contracting with a medical group from outside of the city, which had hired its physicians at extremely competitive rates. One local observer suggested that the changes in state regulations that led to hospital staffing alterations contributed to fragmentation in the local health services environment.

The staffing aspects of the regulations also intersect with financing issues in health care. Health plans, hospitals, and medical groups have attempted to "vertically integrate" their operations to assure a steady and predictable flow of patients into their systems. Vertical integration refers to an organization owning or controlling more than one stage of production, such as a factory buying a source of its raw material or a hospital buying an ambulance company. These efforts have met with mixed success because of the difficulty of resolving the conflicting missions of health plans and providers. In Dr. Smalley's case, Linford Clinic had initially tried to assure and manage an adequate flow of patients through its ownership of PatientCare, a health plan. As one of the participants in the case observed, however, ethical issues arise when the doctors and hospitals treating patients are also those who stand to profit from the success of a health plan—which may become wealthier by *limiting* care.

The Role of Contracts in Formal Communication

Like the regulatory environment, the contractual aspect of health communication is invisible to most of us. The vast majority of physicians in the United States (over 90%) contract with managed care organizations of one kind or another. In particular, physicians in the United States work with an average of about 13 contracts to secure their revenues. Fewer of those contracts in 2001 compared with 1997 were capitated contracts. A capitated contract is an agreement to treat all members of a population for a fixed amount per member per month; fee-for-service contracts are agreements to treat members of a population on a fixed-fee-per-procedure schedule. Therefore, for the physician, revenue is based increasingly on the number of procedures or examinations rather than agreements to see patients. Typically, managed care contracts between physicians or physician groups and health plans include clauses that stipulate the manner and rate at which physicians will be paid; clauses that limit referrals to laboratories, specialists, and hospitals; "gag" clauses that limit issues the physician might discuss with a patient; clauses that define the quality and availability of services to be provided to patients; and claim submission rules, among others. The contracts and the relationships that they stipulate have become the focus of much discontent among physicians, and in response, a number of state medical societies and the American Medical Association have begun to document their hassles on "Hassle Factor Reporting Forms." Physicians' belief that they are coerced or constrained to enter into these contracts also has led some to discuss unionization (Scheffler, 1999), as Dr. Smalley noted.

In addition to these contracts, many physicians (probably most, although no counts are available) also have employment or professional service contracts with the clinics, medical groups, or hospitals with which they work. Typical professional services contracts for physi- cians include clauses concerning compensation, malpractice insurance, outside employment or moonlighting, dispute resolution, causes for termination, and noncompetition after the contract ends.

In Dr. Smalley's case, the noncompete clause in his contract may have been one of the reasons that he sought work in another community when Linford Clinic's neonatal contract with Savior was terminated. His contract with Linford stipulated that if he should leave, he would not set up a practice that would directly compete with other local physicians. Noncompete clauses vary in their duration and the distance they enforce, and sometimes courts will even void them if their enforcement is not consistent with community benefits. In Dr. Smalley's case, circumstances left him with little option but to practice in a distant city.

Organizational Change in Health Care Environments

Both the regulations and the contracts described above play a role in the organizational changes occurring in health care today. When confronted with financial pressures, as Savior was, hospitals reduce staffing levels, reduce intensity of services (especially for patients whose payers reduce reimbursement), provide less charity care, limit public health and specialty services, seek new revenue sources, and face higher financing costs. These pressures led to the bewildering array of mergers, reorganizations, partnerships, dissolutions, and divestitures that occurred in this case. The 1990s, the decade during which most of the events of this case took place, witnessed 860 hospital closures and 820 hospital mergers in the United States. Hospitals were not the only health organizations to experience merger activity during the 1990s; merger and acquisition activity among medical groups, health plans, and behavioral medicine firms accounted for billions of dollars in financial transactions every year since the early 1990s. In Dr. Smalley's case, this translates into a tremendous amount of administrative activity during the time period covered by this case.

Physicians' Reactions to Changes

There is ongoing evidence that up to one third of physicians are dissatisfied with their careers, although for different reasons. Health maintenance organizations and other group practice physicians find time pressures high on their list of complaints, whereas reimbursement hassles and earnings are dissatisfiers for solo and two-physician groups. Especially for physicians out- side the well-established prepaid groups, like Kaiser-Permanente in California, administrative hassles are time-consuming and burdensome: "Documentation requirements [are a source of dissatisfaction]. I spend a good 25 percent of my day just documenting. Sometimes I spend more time documenting on a patient than I do actually seeing the patient" (quoted in Grumbach et al., 2002).

Our own interview research for this case suggests that physicians may not understand very well the contracts under which they work. Nor have the traditional expectations of physicians actually changed. Legal responsibility (and liability) for the practice of medicine still resides with the individual physician. For a variety of reasons, Pathman et al. (2002) found that more than one fourth (27%) of physicians indicated that there was a moderate-to-definite likelihood of leaving their practices within two years.

Hospitals, hospital systems, insurance companies, and health maintenance organizations are struggling to remain financially solvent or profitable, so many of the changes they make, such as forming or dissolving partnerships and offering new contracts to physicians or benefit packages to consumers, are made for financial reasons. These changes are confusing and disturbing to providers and patients alike, and frequently gain the attention of the media in the form of films like *John Q* (in which a fictional youngster was denied heart surgery) and the made-for-TV movie *Damaged Care*, the story of a health maintenance organization critic. In the meantime, the system is failing to meet adequately the needs of 40 million Americans, including 8.5 million children.

Indeed, the medical care system has evolved in such a way as to disadvantage both physicians and patients, many of whom do not understand how we have arrived at this point. Readers of this case may feel overwhelmed and confused by all the facts, organizations, regulations, names, roles, and changes in the case. It might feel frustrating not to know more about Dr. Smalley's actual medical practice, his patients, and the dyadic communication that occurred between them. This analysis has placed in the foreground instead what Robert McPhee calls the "explicit, authoritative, meta-communication" (1985, p. 162) of organizational structure. In this case, organizational structures in health care are explicit (they are written in rules), authoritative (the rules and contracts have the force of law), and metacommunicative (the regulations and contracts are communication about communication). In emphasizing structures, we hope to give readers a sense of just how confusing the health care system in the United States has become, not only for patients but physicians as well, and how deeply these structures have penetrated everyday discourse.

RELEVANT CONCEPTS

Capitation: A system of payment for health care where managed care plans pay doctors and hospitals a fixed amount to care for a patient over a given period (typically per month, though contracts can be written for any length of time). Providers are not reimbursed for services that exceed the allotted amount. The rate may be fixed for all members or it can be adjusted for the age and gender of the member. From a health communication point of view, capitation is a way of standardizing treatment.

Collective bargaining: A method of negotiation in which employees use authorized union representatives to assist them in bargaining for wages and benefits with an employer or group of employers, rather than having separate agreements for each individual employee. From a communication point of view, collective bargaining groups employees into formal structures.

Contracts: A binding agreement between two or more parties (persons and/or organizations) that is enforceable by law. Contracts are a good example of formal communication that becomes an unspoken part of doing business.

Fee-for-service: A traditional method of payment for health care services where specific payment is made for specific services rendered, usually contrasted with capitation. Payment may be made by an insurance company, the patient, or a government program such as Medicare or Medicaid. For physicians, this refers to payment in specific amounts for specific services rendered as opposed to retainer, salary, or other contract arrangements.

For patients, it refers to payment in specific amounts for specific services received, in contrast to the advance payment of an insurance premium or membership fee for coverage. This mode of payment would vary with each medical encounter.

Mergers: The combination of two or more commercial enterprises, increasingly common in health care today. Mergers often increase efficiency, but can create confusing changes for employees.

Neonatology: A branch of medicine concerned with the care, development, and diseases of newborn infants, most of which takes place in hospitals.

Regulations: The formal aspect of the institutional environment of organizations that also includes laws and standards, and which contrasts with informal rules, such as norms, habits, and customs. From an institutional point of view, participants in organizations act in accordance with such rules in their communication and choices.

Vertical integration: The absorption into a single organization other organizations involved in aspects of a product's manufacture from raw materials to distribution. In health care, hospitals seek to combine other aspects of health care, including medical groups, clinics, insurance or managed care, and even ambulances, physician and nurse training, and real estate, into one integrated health system.

DISCUSSION QUESTIONS

1. This case includes many organizations, participants, and regulations. What did you find most confusing? Why?
2. After reading the case, (a) briefly describe each of the organizations listed below, (b) draw a map of the organizations, and (c) identify the communication links between them. For example, is the communication formal or informal, positive or negative?

CARTE
Joint Level III Perinatal Center
Linford Clinic
Metropolitan Neonatology Group
PatientCare
Pearl Clinic
Pearl Hospital
Savior Health (HelpCorp)
(Savior) Midwest Medical Center
State Department of Public Health

3. The case states, "contractual communication is invisible to most of us." But one way that contractual communication is not invisible concerns the terms of the health plans that provide us with medical coverage. If you are employed, obtain a copy of your health plan (or if not, your parents' health plan) and see how it contextualizes the health care you receive (it's a contract!). Identify how many different health plans cover members of your class. What are the benefits or disadvantages of having multiple plans?
4. Choose two of the organizations in the case. For each organization, describe its values and goals as well as the specific problems it faces.

ACKNOWLEDGMENT

The authors wish to thank Lance Rintamaki for helpful suggestions on an earlier draft of this case.

REFERENCES/SUGGESTED READINGS

American Medical Association. (1998). *American Medical Association Model Managed Care Medical Services Agreement*. Retrieved April 8, 2003, from http://www.ama-assn.org/physlegl/legal/part2.htm
Bodenheimer, T. S., & Grumbach, K. (2002). *Understanding health policy: A clinical approach.* (3rd ed.). New York: Lange Medical Books/McGraw Hill.

Grumbach, K., Dower, C., Mutha, S., Yoon, J., Huen, W., Keane, D., Rittenhouse, D., & Bindman, A. (2002). *California physicians 2002: Practice and perceptions*. San Francisco, CA: California Workforce Initiative at the UCSF Center for the Health Professions.

Lammers, J., Barbour, J., & Duggan, A. (2003). Organizational forms of the provision of health care: An institutional perspective. In T. Thompson, A. Dorsey, K. Miller, & R. Parrott (Eds.), *The handbook of health communication* (pp. 319–345). Mahwah, NJ: Lawrence Erlbaum Associates.

McPhee, R. D. (1985). Formal structure and organizational communication. In R. D. McPhee & P. K. Tompkins (Eds.), *Organizational communication: Traditional themes and new directions* (pp. 149–177). Beverly Hills, CA.: Sage.

Pathman, D. E., Konrad, T. R., Williams, E. S., Scheckler, W. E., Linzer, M., & Douglas, J. (2002). Physician job satisfaction, dissatisfaction, and turnover. *Journal of Family Practice, 51*, 593.

Scheffler, R. (1999). Physician collective bargaining: A turning point in U.S. medicine. *Journal of Health Politics, Policy, & Law, 5*, 1071–1076.

Additional Resources

American Medical Association: http://www.ama-assn.org/

Burg, M. (Producer), & Cassavetes, N. (Director). (2002). *John Q.* [Motion picture]. United States: New Line Productions.

Managed Care Online: http://www.mcol.com/

Roessell, D. (Producer), & Winer, H. (Director). (2002). *Damaged Care* [Television broadcast]. United States: Showtime Networks.

25

Making Empowerment Work: Medical Center Soars in Satisfaction Ratings

Athena du Pré
University of West Florida

When Mr. S arrived in the telemetry unit at Baptist Hospital in Pensacola, Florida, he was not happy to be there. His discharge had been delayed, and he badly wanted to be at home. The delay was especially frustrating because it coincided with his wedding anniversary. Sympathetic to his distress, nurse Lynn Pierce had an idea. She and her coworkers organized a surprise, romantic celebration for the couple. "We all got together and went down to the gift shop. We bought his wife a present," she remembers. "Then we got the fancy dishes from the doctor's lounge and rolled in a romantic, candlelit dinner for them." The man, previously disgruntled, thanked the staff fondly before he left.

Similar stories unfold every day at the Pensacola-based Baptist Health Care system, where staff members pride themselves on going the extra mile. But that wasn't always the case. Morale was low in the mid-1990s. Patient satisfaction scores were lower than 80% of similar-sized hospitals',[1] and 30–40% of employees were leaving each year. Fierce competition added to the tension. Market analysts calculated that, with six large health care centers in a six-mile radius, Pensacola was oversupplied by about one full hospital. "We were in trouble," recalls Pam Bilbrey, now Senior Vice President of Corporate Development.

Confronted with these facts, the leaders at Baptist Health Care began to refocus their efforts. The result was a comprehensive cultural overhaul and a bold venture into employee empowerment. Since then, the Pensacola-based health center has been named by *Fortune* magazine as one of the 100 best companies to work for in the United States 3 years running ("The 100 Best," 2002, 2003, 2004), and it now consistently ranks among the top 1% of hospitals in the United States in terms of patient satisfaction.

This chapter describes Baptist Health Care's cultural transformation in terms of communication. More specifically, it examines how organizational members have used communication to establish heroes and villains, shared values, rituals and ceremonies, and active communication networks (Deal & Kennedy, 1982, 1999). Employee empowerment and satisfaction are central components in each area.

HEROES AND VILLAINS

As the culture has evolved at Baptist Health Care, organizational members have changed their minds about what makes a "good" employee. Often, communication skills make the difference between organizational villains and heroes. For example, years ago, an Emergency Room nurse at Baptist made a name for herself—as a tyrant. "She was mean as a snake," says Bob Murphy, the Vice President and Chief Operating Officer (COO). The nurse snapped impatiently at people and didn't listen very closely. However, she was highly skilled at the technical aspects of nursing. Murphy remembers:

> When we had conversations about her, we said, "She's mean. But she's a very good nurse." Ever had a conversation like that? We've had to change the definition of what it takes to be a good nurse. It's about providing good service, having a good attitude.

These days, organizational members are honored for providing physical care *and* compassionate attention. Employees are encouraged to listen to patients and respond to their unique needs. Thank-you letters from grateful patients and families circulate throughout the organization, and dozens of them are posted on the hospital president's bulletin board. One letter is from a woman whose mother was a patient in an intensive care unit (ICU) at Baptist Hospital. According to the letter, the ICU staff made it a point to get to know the woman and her family. When the staff learned how much the patient prided herself on her appearance, they took extra time to wash and comb her hair and even provided a manicure and pedicure. When they found out *Lawrence Welk* was her favorite program, they tuned her television to the program every Saturday at 7 p.m. Even after the woman was moved to another unit, the intensive care nurses came by to check on her and the family. The daughter writes: "They have all been so genuinely kind, professional, pleasant, supportive, and have always asked if they could do anything more. They never seemed inconvenienced to help even though I knew how busy they were."

The staff at Baptist Health Care says patient satisfaction began to rise when employees themselves became more satisfied. In 1996, Baptist Health Care employees were below the national average on 13 of 18 satisfaction indicators. Employees were especially *dis*satisfied with top management, job security, and compensation.

Faced with the dilemma of *being* the perceived problem, Baptist leaders deferred to leadership from within. The chief executive officer (CEO) surveyed everyone in the organization: "If we were to build a colony on Mars, what five leaders in this organization would you choose to lead it?" The greatest vote of confidence went to Eleanor McGee, an employee in the Finance Department who had been employed with Baptist for 22 years.

The CEO approached McGee with a simple question: "Would she lead the effort to build a leadership development program for Baptist Health Care?" McGee was flattered but initially hesitant about taking on so much responsibility. A single mother helping her three children overcome the recent death of their father, she already felt overwhelmed. "Then I asked myself, 'How many times in your career is the CEO going to call you in and say, 'I need your help to drive the culture of this organization'? Probably only once!" she says. She accepted the task.

McGee and her team soon realized that distrust was common throughout the organization. Like many hospitals in the 1980s and 1990s, Baptist was evolving into an integrated health system with the acquisition of additional facilities and service centers. The mergers brought people from diverse organizations together. It was easy to regard former competitors as villains, even though they were now on the same team.

"We went from 2,000 employees to 5,000 employees in 2 years," McGee recalls. "We didn't know each other. We didn't like each other. We didn't have a common vision. We didn't have a common mission."

McGee's team members set out to change that. They created the blueprint for a cultural revolution based on building strong leaders who could bridge the gaps that had fragmented the organization. Their initiative was an 18-month "Bridges" leadership development program that ultimately helped prepare more than 300 employees to assume leadership roles in the organization.

McGee became one of the first heroes of the transformation. Today she is Vice President of Finance and Controller for Baptist Health Care. "Eleanor is just really good about motivating people. She always has a positive outlook," says Sharon Shields, Accounts Payable Supervisor, who has worked with McGee for 20 years. "And she likes to have fun. She started a lot of the celebrations. Any time we reach a goal she would make sure we celebrated it."

Other heroes emerged as well. Leadership teams were formed to focus on key areas of improvement, elevating the involvement and visibility of many Baptist employees. The administrators who emerged from the transition also became heroes. The presidents and CEO's since the transformation began—Quint Studer, John Heer, and Al Stubblefield—are regarded within the organization as visionaries who inspired miraculous change.

Karen Smith, writer/editor in the Public Relations Department at Baptist, remembers the transformation first hand. "It was one of the most exciting years of my work career, just seeing what was happening," she says. Smith feels each of the top administrators brought something different to the transition. She regards Al Stubblefield, CEO, as the steady, guiding force behind it all. Without calling a lot of attention to himself, she says, Stubblefield has kept everyone oriented to the organization's values and potential.

Stubblefield recruited Quint Studer, whose charismatic leadership and decisiveness incited enthusiasm. "Quint was the catalyst," Smith says. "He's one of those people who, when you're 90 years old, you're going to still remember." On arriving at Baptist, Studer began visiting hospital units. "He would show up on all three shifts before people knew who he was and would sit around and talk to people. He'd ask, 'What bothers you?' and he would make it a point to address it right away," Smith remembers. When a nursing assistant told Studer the late-night shift had difficulty cleaning spills because housekeeping supplies were locked up at night, he had carts of cleaning supplies delivered to each nursing unit within days. Smith feels Studer's attention to frontline concerns brought the transformation to life at all levels of the organization.

In turn, Studer recruited his successor, John Heer, previously the COO at St. Bernard's Hospital in Jonesboro, Arkansas. Heer had helped the hospital raise patient satisfaction scores to the 97th percentile and had earned respect for the way he handled national media attention after the Jonesboro school shootings in 1998. Consistent with organizational values, Heer is a visible and popular president, Smith says.

In summary, in the early 1990s, it was tempting to point fingers. Employees given low marks by patients may have regarded the patients as ungrateful and overly demanding. Employees and administrators may have blamed each other for the organization's failure. In this case, however, the organization was saved from tailspin by a commitment not to simply assign blame, but to involve everyone in an organizational transformation. The emphasis shifted to listening both to employees and to patients. Leaders in the revolution became role models for a new set of values. Senior executives, once considered the villains, were within a few years regarded as heroes, along with scores of other new leaders.

SHARED VALUES

Heroes do not emerge in a vacuum. They are revered for the cultural values they represent. Because Eleanor McGee and others already enjoyed the high regard of their peers, they were promising role models in an otherwise discouraging environment. But hope without result is unlikely to endure. The most daunting task still remained—to create an organizational culture that could raise employee and patient satisfaction scores and keep them up.

Baptist leaders were convinced that gaining employees' support meant involving them from the beginning. However, not all employees were excited by the prospect. Stubblefield remembers that people within the organization were wary of yet another quick-fix program. "We had to convince them that this wasn't the program of the month or the year, but who we were going to be on a regular basis," Stubblefield says. "Delivering world-class service takes every single employee, 100% of your workforce. We needed everyone behind this."

Employees were recruited to become leaders by serving on one of seven service teams on issues such as measurement, standards, communication, and satisfaction among various stakeholder groups. Sometimes the goals were specific. "We formed an Irritants Team simply to remove things that were irritating our patients," says Pierce. Other teams were responsible for broader changes, such as assessing and elevating inpatient satisfaction.

"We soon realized we had a good staff who had not developed as leaders because we had not defined what we were all about," Bilbrey says. Books on culture, communication, and management began circulating through the organization. The staff borrowed ideas from the Ritz Carlton and Disney. Employee involvement became a central theme, not only of the reform effort, but of the emerging culture.

One of the first goals of unification was to redefine the organization's mission with input from employees. The mission that emerged reads: "To provide superior service based on Christian values to improve the quality of life for the people and communities served." This mission is built on "five pillars of operational excellence"—people, service, quality, financial performance, and growth—in that order. The mission and pillars appear on bulletin boards and displays in every department. People in each department set measurable goals for attaining excellence within each pillar and chart their progress throughout the year.

The Baptist staff felt from the beginning that achieving the mission would not be a simple matter of implementing a few programs. They wanted to *live* the mission. To make high-quality service a reality at Baptist meant behaving and communicating in new ways. Supporting values emerged as the staff began to embody the mission in everyday rituals and ceremonies.

RITUALS AND CEREMONIES

The staff at Baptist Health Care observes an extensive number of rituals and ceremonies supporting organizational values. Following are examples of rituals and ceremonies that exemplify the ideals of ownership, equality, selective admittance, continual development, service, and recognition.

Ownership Rituals

Many of the everyday practices at Baptist are meant to illustrate an ownership philosophy. Bob Murphy recalls the origin of a new ritual set when Studer became President of Baptist Hospital in 1996:

> His first day on the job, I walked with him through the hospital. He was picking up little pieces of paper on the floor and putting them in his pocket. We'd be talking and he'd say, "Hold on a second," and pick something else up. Well, I started walking just a little ahead, trying to pick up little pieces of trash before he found them!

The ritual gave rise to new awareness. "Suddenly I started noticing what needed to be picked up," Murphy declares. "I had walked there for 7 years and hadn't noticed!" Soon, other employees caught on. Now Baptist employees pride themselves on picking up any refuse they see in the buildings or on the grounds.

Studer also began what employees call the Baptist Shuffle. As he walked through the hallways, he made it a point to rub out scuffmarks by stepping on them and twisting his foot. As the current president, Heer is revered to have the best Baptist Shuffle yet, and he demonstrates it at workshops and new employee orientations, playfully displaying his technique by twist-stepping on a tiny sheet of paper without looking down or breaking stride.

The rituals are small in the scheme of things, but Murphy says they remind employees to be concerned with everything around them. Nothing is outside a person's job description if he or she "owns the place."

A sense of ownership has implications for the way employees behave. "What would you do if you owned the place?" asks Murphy. "For one thing, you'd be nice to your guests. I can give you directions from our boardroom to my office and you'd get lost twice, and it's not all that complicated. But what I need to do is take the time to walk you there. All our employees know that and they do it."

Pierce concurs. "We have this thing at Baptist that, if you encounter it—it's your problem. It doesn't matter where it started." This applies to a ringing phone (answer it), a patient call light (respond and arrange for assistance), lost guests (escort them), and any other service needs that arise.

A sense of ownership means going beyond job duties. When an employee at the Baptist-owned Gulf Breeze Hospital noticed an elderly woman standing alone in the lobby, she asked if she could help. The woman's family had dropped her off at the wrong location. She actually had an appointment at a medical center several blocks away. The employee personally drove the woman to the correct location. When the medical visit was over, the employee returned for the grateful patient and drove her back to the hospital to meet her family as planned.

Equality Rituals

Employee empowerment is evident in the lack of status markers at Baptist Hospital. Employees refer to everyone, regardless of rank, by first name. On employee name badges—including those of the CEO and president—the wearer's first name appears in boldface, a line above and twice as large as his or her last name.

With few status barriers, everyone is expected to pitch in. Dick Fulford, administrator of Gulf Breeze Hospital, decided before the hospital opened its doors 17 years ago that it would be a place where people never said, "It's not my job." He has reiterated this wish at monthly orientation sessions ever since. "The reason I think it sticks is people kid me about it," Fulford says. "They look at me and smile and say, 'Can I say it's not my job?' It's all in fun because we know what we're about." He tells of a physician who personally arranged chairs before a meeting at the hospital because, as he later told Fulford, he didn't want to be caught saying it wasn't his job.

Visibility also minimizes status differences. In many hospitals, top-level administrators occupy plush executive suites virtually off-limits to the majority of employees. By contrast, administrators' offices at Baptist are modestly furnished and located in the busiest area of the hospital. A large plate-glass window provides a view directly into the president's office. Visitors and employees walking down the hall often wave hello as they pass. The ritual of waving and observing "John" at work in an office no different than other employees' suggests he is not isolated from what goes on in the organization.

Selective Admittance Rituals

Murphy says that, to maintain a service culture, it is imperative to select employees well suited to the culture, empower them to make a difference, and reward and recognize their efforts.

Every potential employee of Baptist Health Care is interviewed by peers as well as leaders in the organization. No one is hired who does not meet the approval of his or her potential colleagues. One person was recently interviewed by 17 people before receiving a job offer. To make sure hiring is conducted fairly and effectively, quarterly training sessions are provided to prepare peer interviewers.

"Does it take a little longer to do it this way? Yeah," says Murphy. "But I have time. What I don't have time for is an employee who doesn't care and doesn't try. What we do is too hard to work around somebody with a bad attitude all the time."

Continual Development Rituals

Once hired, Baptist Health Care employees have opportunities to continue learning and contributing. Murphy calls himself the poster child for advancement at Baptist. He began as a trauma nurse 13 years ago. With the support of the organization, he has steadily advanced in the ranks to become a vice president and COO while simultaneously earning a law degree and a master's degree in public administration. "There's a saying at Baptist that, if Murphy can do it, anyone can," he jokes.

Education is offered inhouse as well. Every new employee takes part in a 16-hour orientation session modeled after Disney's Traditions program. About half of the orientation program is devoted to organizational culture.

After determining that turnover rates spike after 6 months of employment, Baptist leadership began a "ServU" program for employees during their fifth month with the organization. The 6-hour program is designed to inspire employees at a critical juncture and encourage them to suggest ways the organization can improve.

Leadership education has become an organizational priority. Employees are eligible to take part in ongoing leadership development programs and classes through "Baptist University," an inhouse educational program featuring best-selling authors and speakers from around the country. Baptist's 500 upper and middle managers take part in quarterly, day-long training programs through Baptist University, which evolved from the Bridges program begun by Eleanor McGee's team in 1996.

Service Rituals

As a new president, Heer began an influential ritual when he asked that a letter be delivered to the room of each new patient. The letter expresses Heer's conviction to provide outstanding care and urges patients who are dissatisfied to contact him personally. In the letter, Heer provides his direct number in the hospital and his home phone number.

"This letter changed our lives as leaders," Pierce recalls. "You can bet we didn't want our patients and colleagues calling him at home! So we got smart and started giving them *our* home numbers. 'If you need anything, anything at all, call *me*!'" she quotes herself, laughing.

Patient care rituals were some of the hardest to sell in the evolving culture. Although she now works with organizations around the country helping them learn from Baptist's transformation, Pierce was initially resistant to the new ideas herself.

In the mid-1990s, Pierce was nurse manager for a unit that was not doing very well. "Overall, the hospital had patient satisfaction scores in the 20s [percentile]," she says. "Mine was more like 11! People would quit before they would float into [work temporarily in] my unit!"

Even so, Pierce was wary of a new ritual called *rounding*, daily visits made by each nurse leader to the patients on his or her unit. "I could have come up with a hundred reasons why I could not do rounding every day," Pierce confides. But she soon realized that her unit's patient satisfaction scores began to rise when she made rounds and learned more about patients' and guests' requests. The change was especially hard to ignore considering that satisfaction scores and comparison charts were now being posted throughout the hospital.

"I started thinking, 'My [patient satisfaction] numbers are going to come up! I won't be left behind,'" Pierce remembers. "'You want a Coke?' I'd call Dietary and say, 'Send 'em a six pack!'"

Pierce was also initially doubtful about *scripting*, the practice of using carefully designed statements and questions to convey the organization's mission. "Especially nurses, we just didn't want to be told what to say," Pierce declares. "I said, 'I'm not going to script.' Now, I didn't say it to my boss. But I said it to my coworkers!"

However, as the organization started to change, Pierce felt left out. One day, she found herself tongue-tied during rounds and resorted to a script: "I'm the Nurse Leader on your unit. I want to assure you that we will do everything possible to exceed your expectations. . . ." She soon began using scripts on a regular basis. A few of the scripts used by Baptist staff members include:

"Is there anything else that I may do for you? I have the time."

"I'm glad you asked that."

"We will be asking you throughout your stay how we can do things better."

"You physician cares about you very much, so [he or she] has asked that we get a blood sample very early so the results can be posted on the chart by the time [he or she] makes rounds in the morning."

Pierce says her staff members were also dubious. "I have the time," they recited. "What if we don't? Do you want us to lie?" Pierce's answer was unequivocal: "'Absolutely!' I told them, 'When that patient needs something, you have the time. If you need to make up that time later, let me know and I'll help you. But while you're with the patient, you mean it."

Recognition Ceremonies

Baptist Health Care has adopted many mechanisms to reward outstanding performance. The organization even has its own *Rewards and Recognition Handbook*. Administrators regularly send handwritten thank-you notes to employees mentioned favorably in patient surveys and letters. Heer has been known to send letters to employees' family members thanking them for their support.

As with most changes, the effort to reward employees began gradually. Baptist leaders initially asked supervisors to reward employee efforts with "WOW" certificates. "When we first started with WOW's, we gave WOW's for smiling and showing up," Murphy says, laughing. "In fact, we had to force leaders to account for how many WOW's they gave out, because they just weren't very good at it yet."

The WOW program continues. Employees who collect five WOW certificates can redeem them for gift certificates. As the culture has changed, however, supervisors have become more accustomed to recognizing employee efforts, and the threshold has risen. Because smiling is no longer an unusual achievement, WOW's are used to reward higher-level accomplishments.

Organizational leaders have developed additional tiers of recognition as well. Employees who demonstrate exceptional behavior are honored as *Champions* and *Legends*. Champions are honored with a standing ovation by the board of directors, their pictures are posted on a board in the hospital, and they each receive a framed plaque. Legends and their guests are treated to a resort getaway via limousine. They are recognized in media releases, video tributes, and booklets describing the contributions of each Legend.

Glen Moe, a registered nurse at Baptist, was honored as a Champion for risking his life to save a 17-year-old boy caught in a riptide at the local beach. Another employee, Mari Harvey, was honored for setting up a support system for an employee undergoing treatment for breast cancer. Harvey organized employees throughout the hospital to help pay for needed supplies and provide daily meals to their coworker in need.

Parties are also a regular part of life at Baptist Health Care. When Baptist's Gulf Breeze Hospital was rated number 1 in patient satisfaction for the 76th consecutive month, every employee was awarded $76. Likewise, Baptist Hospital in Pensacola held a 1950's-style celebration when it made the 99th percentage 50 months running. Everyone was invited for a free lunch, including ice cream desserts, hoola-hoop contests, 50s music, and, for a dollar a shot, the chance to toss a pie at an administrator.

Murphy's philosophy of celebrating involves four P's: Party with a Purpose and Plan to Party. "We have a leader who puts it on his calendar: 'Time for a party,'" he says. "What have we done well? Look for the successes." Murphy encourages leaders to celebrate regularly and make it clear what milestones the group has reached. Baptist Health Care maintains a fund for celebrations so that department leaders need not use money from their own budgets.

COMMUNICATION NETWORKS

Communication networks are the mechanisms by which organizational members transmit and interpret information. Organizational goals, achievements, and failures are shared via the network, which includes formal and informal channels of communication.

"No Excuses, No Secrets" Policy

The celebrations previously mentioned are built on a careful system of setting goals and monitoring progress. Part of the Baptist credo is "no secrets, no excuses." Murphy describes the origin of Baptist's no-excuses policy: "For 24 years, we had a reasonable excuse for 30% employee turnover. The Navy base! It's a military town. People come and go." That excuse fell through, however, when turnover dropped to 13% following changes at Baptist.

"Did the military leave?" Murphy asks. "No! Now we have a saying that reminds us not to hide behind excuses. Now we joke, 'It's a Navy town!' That reminds us—we used to make excuses before. It didn't work."

The second half of the credo—no secrets—works in tandem with the first. The Baptist staff has found that members feel more accountable if they know the goals and where they stand. Thus, up-to-date information—including turnover rates, patient satisfaction scores, financial reports, market reports, and 90-day action plans—is posted on prominent "Communication Boards" in each department. Easy-to-read charts show how satisfaction scores vary over time and between departments. Employees, patients, and guests are invited to review the numbers and make suggestions.

Daily Line-Up

Another channel of regular communication is the *daily line-up*, a practice the Baptist staff borrowed from the service award-winning Ritz-Carlton hotel. At Baptist, a 10-minute daily line-up is conducted in each unit during each shift. The daily line-up includes an educational item, a supporting reference to the Pillar of the Day (based on the pillars of excellence), and an inspiring quote or story, which is often pulled from patient letters or satisfaction surveys. Pierce concludes each daily line-up with a question: "What can I do to help you do your job today?"

The 10-minute daily line-up provides a regular opportunity for two-way communication, reminds staff members of their mission, provides a means of recognizing individual and group achievements, and serves as a form of continuing education. For the majority of employees, the 10-minute sessions add up to about 40 hours per year.

Feedback Loops

Two dangers in strong cultures are that innovation will be stifled by members' eagerness to fit in and that members will resort to gossip and griping because they feel discouraged from voicing their concerns to higher-ups (Denison, 1990). Baptist has offset this danger by actively rewarding innovation and problem solving. From the first day of orientation and every day thereafter, employees are asked to contribute ideas for improvement.

"Bright Ideas" is an extensive program of collecting, reviewing, and implementing employee ideas. "This is not a suggestion box program," says Murphy. "We made a lot of mistakes when we began. We encouraged ideas, but 99% of the time, we didn't do anything with them. Then we formed a committee to review and implement ideas and we started tying Bright Ideas to performance evaluations."

Employee evaluations are based partly on how many ideas the employee has contributed and seen implemented. The expectation is two Bright Ideas, suggested and implemented, for each full-time employee and one annually for every half-time employee. Nearly 7,000 bright ideas are implemented (not just submitted) per year. Employees who submit "Bright Ideas" are given cafeteria discounts and are eligible for prizes, drawings, and departmental celebrations.

Some Bright Ideas are cost-saving measures, which are estimated to save the organization about $2.9 million annually. Others are oriented to people or service. A few years ago, Paul Fontaine, Director of Laboratory Services at Baptist, came up with the idea to provide umbrellas with the Baptist Health Care insignia to visitors caught in the rain. "It sounds funny, but now every time it rains, we're out there in it, meeting people, giving them umbrellas and telling them they can keep them," he says. Led by Fontaine, the staff has given away more than 100 of the bright blue umbrellas. A coworker says, "Every time it rains, you'll see Paul running around just soaking wet!"

Communication is also stimulated by a continued commitment to shared governance. Employees participate on teams devoted to the organization's mission. The original list of seven teams has evolved into five—Culture, Communication, Employee Loyalty, Customer Loyalty, and Physician Loyalty. The idea is the same: Involve people at all levels in defining and supporting the organization's mission.

Storytelling Rituals

Storytelling is a cherished ritual during Baptist daily line-ups and other gatherings. Letters from patients and their loved ones are circulated throughout the organization and read to employees at every level.

"We read the letters to remind us why we're here," Murphy says. "We celebrate that. We reward that. The reason we're here is to make a difference." He tells of a letter thanking a nurse who baked a red velvet cake for a cancer patient after he remarked that it was his favorite. "No one asked her to do it. No one would ever have known," Murphy says. "What do you think we do when we read that letter to every employee in the hospital? We raise the bar."

OUTCOMES

The results of the cultural transformation at Baptist Health Care have attracted international attention. Health care professionals from around the world visit Baptist Hospital in Pensacola and its affiliates, which now include four hospitals in Florida and Alabama, two medical parks, a subacute care center, an addiction treatment center, a mental health center, and a vocational enterprise staffed by persons with disabilities.

The once-discouraging statistics have risen nearly off the charts. Whereas employee satisfaction at Baptist Hospital was below the national average on 13 of 18 indicators in 1996,

1 year later, employee scores were higher than average on 17 of the 18 satisfaction indicators. Since 1999, employee satisfaction has exceeded the national average on every indicator. *Fortune* magazine consistently includes the Pensacola-based health care organization in its "100 best companies to work for" list ("The 100 Best," 2002, 2003, 2004).

Staff turnover has dropped by 50% since 1996. In an industry in which 20% annual turnover is the norm ("War of Attrition," 2002), Baptist is at 13%. This translates into money saved. "We estimate it costs us $35,000 to replace a nurse with training and everything," Bilbrey says. "Reducing turnover saved us millions of dollars."

As hoped, higher employee satisfaction was closely followed by rising patient satisfaction scores. Between 1996 and 1998, the Pensacola hospital rose from the 20th percentile to the 99th percentile in patient satisfaction scores and has stayed there ever since. The organization's Gulf Breeze Hospital has ranked number 1 in patient satisfaction among hospitals its size every month since 1995.

Baptist Health Care has earned a list of honors, including the prestigious Malcolm Baldridge National Quality Award in 2003, the Quality Cup for Service Excellence awarded by *USA Today* and the Rochester Institute of Technology, the National Leadership Award for excellence in patient care by Veterans Hospitals of America, and the Marriott Service Award.

Far from guarding their "trade secrets," Baptist leaders make their techniques and progress public. The organization has attracted so much attention from other health care agencies that it has created an inhouse Baptist Health Care Leadership Institute, whose staff organizes workshops and site visits to share their story with others. So far, more than 1,000 groups comprised of 5,000 health care professionals have visited the Pensacola location.

Even with so many advantages, challenges lie ahead. After being at the top of the charts for so long, if Baptist's scores slip even a few points members may feel they have failed. However, if scores stay high, it may be difficult to maintain a sense of attentiveness and adaptability. "It sounds simple," Murphy acknowledges. "But I was asked once, 'How much time in your day do you spend worrying about this stuff?' I thought about it. 'Every single minute!'"

RELEVANT CONCEPTS

Accountability: A sense of being responsible for one's actions and the outcomes they produce.

Communication networks: Formal and informal pathways by which organizational members transmit and interpret information.

Cultural heroes: People who inspire others by embodying the culture's core values.

Cultural villains: People who are viewed negatively for mocking or disobeying a culture's core values.

Empowerment: The freedom and ability to control significant aspects of one's environment, obtain and use key resources, and help establish the rules of interaction.

Feedback: Response from communication partners.

Organizational culture: A set of accepted behaviors and values generally upheld by members of a particular business or nonprofit enterprise.

Organizational leadership: The process of influencing people, shaping attitudes, and defining goals.

Organizational values: Deeply held convictions about what is right, just, fair, and good.

Rituals and ceremonies: Practices within a culture that uphold key values. Rituals are typically performed as part of everyday routines. Ceremonies are typically less frequent and more formal.

Storytelling: Personal narratives through which people share information, entertain others, and collaboratively interpret the events of their lives.

DISCUSSION QUESTIONS

1. How did the Baptist staff initiate change?
2. What values emerged as the organization changed? How were these values communicated and perpetuated?
3. What role did communication play in instigating change and improving satisfaction scores?
4. What factors contributed to the success of the cultural change at Baptist?
5. What challenges lie ahead for Baptist Health Care? How can the staff address these challenges?
6. Visit the Baptist Health Care website at www.ebaptisthealthcare.org. In what ways does the organization present itself as employee- and patient-focused?

LETTER FROM A PATIENT'S FAMILY

Dear Sir,

We've known Chuck for 17 years. He and his wife Claire couldn't be closer. We've helped raise each other's children, acting as surrogate aunts and uncles. We've laughed and celebrated and cried and mourned with these dear friends.

About $3^1/_2$ years ago, Chuck became ill. After many tests and specialists, a diagnosis of pancreatic cancer was determined.

Chuck served two tours of duty in Vietnam as a helicopter pilot. He was awarded two Silver Stars, a Purple Heart, and the Distinguished Flying Cross. Chuck was gentle and kind and tough as steel. He fought this unholy disease, the way he lived his life, with strength, grace, and dignity.

On Friday, February 28, Chuck was admitted to 3rd floor Oncology, Gold Coast Wing. It was apparent he was gravely ill.

Chuck had many friends, at least 30 of whom came to visit during his final days and hours. He was able to smile and speak to everyone. The sheer volume of people must have been inconvenient to the staff. They never made anyone feel unwelcome.

The staff in fact could not have been more gracious. No request was unattended. Each time the nurse call button was pressed someone appeared in seconds.

Early Tuesday morning (March 4) Chuck nearly died from respiratory distress, but the nurses kept him alive another day. Thank God for them. The next few hours of life were such a blessing.

Chuck's condition improved throughout Tuesday (in no small part as a result of the care given him by Daphne Graybeal). In the early afternoon Claire and the children were alone with Chuck. He talked with each of the children, telling them how much he loved them and how proud he was of them. They held hands and prayed.

Later in the afternoon Chuck's 3-year-old granddaughter climbed into bed beside him. She stroked his arm and said, "I love you Pappa." He found the strength to hug her for a long moment. She kissed him on the cheek, then ate the cake from the lunch tray.

During the evening Chuck's condition deteriorated. Breathing became labored and shallow. Shaz Kirsch, his nurse, was as close as a shadow, caring for Chuck, keeping him comfortable, consoling and comforting Claire.

At 3:05 Wednesday morning, Janie Quick lovingly cradled Chuck's head in her hands. Shaz's hands patted and rested on his shoulder, his wife of 26 years held his left hand. God, I'm certain, held his right hand. Chuck took two quick breaths and left this world.

It's hard to express our appreciation to the fine staff who attended Chuck, his family and friends. Their professionalism and loving compassion allowed a final goodbye that was intimate and peaceful. Our heart felt thank-you.

With Warm Regards,
Dennis and Margie Burr

P.S. This is a partial list of Chuck's caregivers: John Voight, Daphne Graybeal, Shaz Kirsch, Janie Quick, Sandy Martin, Tracey Dulac, and Luisa Palacies. It is by no means complete. It does not include dietary, respiratory, custodial or pastoral staff, all of whom were top notch.

ENDNOTE

[1] Patient satisfaction statistics in this chapter are reported by Press Ganey Associates, a firm commissioned to survey approximately 6,000 health care facilities in the United States.

REFERENCES/SUGGESTED READINGS

Deal, T. E., & Kennedy, A. A. (1982). *Corporate cultures: The rites and rituals of corporate life.* Reading, MA: Addison-Wesley.

Deal, T. E., & Kennedy, A. A. (1999). *The new corporate cultures: Revitalizing the workplace after downsizing, mergers, and reengineering.* Reading, MA: Perseus Books.

Denison, D. R. (1990). *Corporate culture and organizational effectiveness.* New York: John Wiley & Sons.

The 100 best companies to work for. (2002). *Fortune, 145*(3), 72.

The 100 best companies to work for. (2003). *Fortune, 147*(1), 127.

The 100 best companies to work for. (2004). *Fortune, 149*(1), 56.

War of attrition: Turnover rates for hospital jobs reaching crisis proportions, study warns. (2002, August 12). *Modern Healthcare,* 21.

VI

Issues in Information Dissemination

26

No, Everybody Doesn't: Changing Mistaken Notions of the Extent of Drinking on a College Campus

Linda C. Lederman
Lea P. Stewart
Rutgers University

It was Thursday night. Three college sophomores, Helen, Meg, and Laurie, had just arrived at a typical "start of the weekend" party at a dorm somewhere on campus.[1] They walked in and began to mingle. Jack, a friend from their bio lecture, saw them and tried to get them into the swing of things. Many of their other friends, men and women from classes, dorms, and frats, were there. The party had been going on for some time. Helen, Meg, and Laurie were the only ones who had not joined into the fun. The other students were partying. They were all chanting and taunting the three to join in. After they'd been there a while, they were approached by one of the guys.

"Come on," Paul, a junior who had been drinking since late Wednesday afternoon, shouted over the noise of the crowd. "Don't be nerds, get with it." He tried to hand Laurie a bottle. "Take a shot," he insisted. Laurie refused the shot. She didn't want to chug. She thought she'd had enough already and just didn't want to. But Helen did. She wanted to go for it. She joined in, wholeheartedly determined to become the life of the party. "Hey, you guys," she laughed very loud, "I came to college to get an education, and I am getting educated about how to do parties!"

Meg was torn between the two. She didn't want to get wasted like Helen who she saw was already becoming embarrassing. But she didn't want to sit on the sidelines like Laurie. She looked at Laurie and thought she looked so uncool. Meg gave in to the pressure and agreed to do the shot. But that was it. She was only going to have one, and she stuck to her decision.

The party continued on, and Meg, Laurie, and Helen all continued to do pretty much what they'd been doing. The party got louder as it got more crowded. There was music and dancing and a lot of beer and mixed drinks going down. The girls kept being offered drinks, and Helen kept drinking them. From time to time, Meg, but not Laurie, had another drink. At one point, the three friends found themselves in a huddle whispering about one of the guys at the party and what a jerk he was. Helen and Meg put down the glasses they had been drinking from and joined in to listen to the secrets being whispered.

When they turned back to the table where they'd put their drinks, there were lots of other glasses. "Damn," said Meg. "I can't tell which one was mine. I don't want to take the chance of picking up someone else's drink." "Or," added Laurie, "having one of these bozos put something into it. Just leave it. That's what I'd do." Helen laughed, "They'll be out of booze soon—I'm not leaving mine." No one did anything. She reached for a glass and gulped from it. "Fine, just fine," she murmured.

Meg didn't want to leave her drink, but she wasn't just going to gulp it down either. She picked up the glass she thought was hers. She sniffed at it and then took a sip. It seemed just like what she'd been drinking. It tasted fine. She continued to carry it around with her as she'd been doing before they all huddled to laugh about the creepy guy.

An hour or so later, the three girls met up again. They were all enjoying themselves. Helen was getting pretty high, but neither of the other girls even mentioned it. They were used to her doing that. She tried to get them to drink like she did. But Meg and Laurie had each developed her own strategy for handling Helen. She was a good friend. She just drank too much, too often, as far as Meg was concerned. Laurie and Meg saw it a bit differently. Laurie thought Helen was out of control, but she didn't want to confront her.

"What's up?" they asked each other. As they exchanged dirt about who'd been doing what for the last hour or so, their eyes all fell on Evelyn, a friend from their dorm, who was making a move on a guy. They couldn't tell who it was, but were curious, and so they walked around a bit, and then saw that it was a guy she'd been talking about the other night in the dorm. "OK," the three friends said, as they slapped each other's hands in high fives. "Go, girl, go," they joked with each other.

Their conversation had gone on to some other stuff when Helen and Meg nudged each other. Both had noticed that Evelyn was engrossed in some heavy body contact with the guy. Evelyn and the guy seemed to be downing shots pretty fast, and laughing loud, and all over each other. The friends had gotten closer to them, close enough to hear the guy, Barry, invite Evelyn back to his place. The girls exchanged looks and then in unison walked over to the couple and started chatting with them.

While Helen and Meg talked to Barry, Laurie tried to persuade Evelyn not to go by reminding her of Sarah, their friend from home, who had to take a semester off after she was date-raped. "Get a life," laughed Evelyn, "I'm not Sarah." She wasn't buying it. And Helen wasn't either. She said to Evelyn, "Just enjoy yourself. Have a good time, girl." She hoisted her beer glass and swigged down its contents, mumbling, "Here's to you, Evie baby. The night belongs to us." Helen winked at Evelyn and gave a thumbs-up sign to Barry.

Meg didn't like the looks of the situation at all. She thought that Evelyn had had way too much to drink and didn't think she should go with Barry. None of them knew him and what he was likely to do. Meg grabbed Evelyn's arm and tried to pressure her friend not to go. She stressed her concern, giving Evelyn and Barry looks of disapproval. They laughed and wandered off laughing with their arms around each other.

As the night wore on, the beer vanished and so did the mixed drinks. Tons of junk food remained and so did the punch. Helen wanted another drink or two before it was time to leave, so she grabbed a cup and had some punch. It was sweet. It was strong. She drank it down.

Meg walked over and was thinking about having a glass, too. But she didn't know what was in it. She looked around, found the guys who'd made the punch and asked. It sounded too strong to her.

Laurie had a soda and was asking the other two if they were ready to go. Even though the party was going strong, it was almost two in the morning, and the girls had come to the party with the promise that they'd leave together in time to get the last campus bus back to their dorm on the north campus.

It was now only 15 minutes until the campus bus would stop running. Meg and Laurie dragged Helen out of the room, even though she said she wasn't through drinking. "You promised," they reminded her, "Come on, come on. If we miss the bus it's a long walk, and it's cold. And none of us is riding in a car with any of these guys. They've all been partying too long."

Meg and Laurie tried but just couldn't convince Helen. She told them to go on ahead and promised she wouldn't get in a car with anyone from the party. "I'll find some of the other girls from the dorm and walk back with them. Or guys we trust," she said. "Promise, Helen," said Meg and Laurie in unison. "Promise," Helen agreed.

Reluctantly, when there just wasn't time left to try to persuade her and still catch the bus, Meg and Laurie took off. They caught the last bus just as it was about to pull out from the bus stop. Helen stayed at the party for another hour or so and then was dragged along with the last group of dorm friends who were leaving to make the long walk back.

Helen had gotten a real scare on the way back. The other girls with whom she was walking had decided to stop at a bar near campus on the way back. Helen couldn't get in because she wasn't 21 and she didn't have a fake ID. The others got lost in the crowd going into the bar, so Helen just kept walking on her own. Suddenly, she noticed she was being followed by some boys from town who made whistling calls at her. A car stopped to offer her a ride and, as she was speaking to the driver, he seemed to try to pull her into the car. Luckily Tim, one of the guys who had gone to the bar with her and the other girls from her dorm, had come out and seen what was happening. The driver was someone he knew, and Tim got him to drive off and leave Helen alone. Then Tim and Helen walked together back to the dorm.

When she got there, she realized she didn't feel very well. She'd gone to Meg's room to see when she and Laurie got back, but just as she got into the room and was whispering to Meg so as not to wake Laurie, she suddenly felt sick. Helen ran out of the room and down the hall to the bathroom. After a while Meg followed and found Helen, with her head over the toilet bowl, getting violently sick.

Laurie had woken up and followed. When she saw Helen, she got down on her knees beside her and held Helen's hair back to keep it from falling in her eyes and over her face. The sight sobered Meg up. She'd been a little high herself, even though she hadn't drunk anything like the way Helen did. Helen began to hiccup. She walked toward their room.

At the stairway, Helen fell down with a thud. Rachel, another dorm resident, heard what was going on in the hall and saw Helen and Meg. She saw that Helen was vomiting. She was worried so she called Gail, the dorm counselor, to help. By the time Gail got there, the hallway was empty. Worried, Gail notified the other dorm counselors in the building, and they came to help find the drunken woman. The dorm counselors came up to a group of women talking in the lounge where the sick woman had been seen. The counselors promised that if the students told them who and where the sick woman was, no one would get in any trouble. They said they only wanted to make sure that the sick woman was safe. No one volunteered.

Meanwhile, Meg was in the bathroom with Helen who was slumped over the toilet bowl again. Meg had heard about the offer from the counselors to help but had decided to ignore them and sit up all night with Helen to make sure she was OK. Laurie came into the room and saw what was happening. She argued with Meg that they should let the counselors help. Laurie was frightened because Helen kept vomiting and then falling asleep. She tried to tell Meg that Helen could choke, but Meg was still high enough that she thought she could handle it. She said that maybe they should just put Helen on her side and let her sleep it off.

But Helen wouldn't move. She had gotten up from sitting over the toilet seat and was now lying down in the bathtub where she had passed out. Meg got a pillow from the room and decided to sleep on the bathroom floor near Helen. Laurie sat outside the bathroom door to watch out for the others who wanted to know what has going on. It was almost 5 a.m., and she wished it were time for class so that others would be up to help.

Finally it was morning. Helen and Meg woke up with much prodding from Laurie. Helen had a hangover. The three women talked about the night before. Meg was somewhat subdued, asking if she'd done the right thing. Helen was very thirsty. She was nauseous and wanted a cold soda. Laurie was tired from sleeping in the hall. Meg thought about her behavior. She hadn't really thought she would get sick. She felt that her behavior was not as safe or as healthy as it could have been. Laurie was sorry she went to the party at all. She didn't really drink, and she liked her roommates a lot better when they were sober. She was glad they were all right but mad at them and at herself for having slept in the hallway all night. She regretted not having gone to a movie instead. Helen had no regrets. She said, "What the hell. It was a typical college experience—all in the name of fun."

Later that day, they learned that Tim, who'd walked Helen back to the dorm, had been found on the floor of his room close to death from alcohol poisoning. He had been left there to sleep it off while his roommate, Barry, walked Evelyn back to her room. Bob, a dorm counselor, had found him by chance and had an emergency rescue team take him to the health services, where he recovered.

FIRST-YEAR WOMEN AND DANGEROUS DRINKING

The story of Helen, Meg, and Laurie is typical of what happens on many college campuses and the ways in which dangerous drinking is part of the social life of some college students, especially first-year students. Unfortunately, while drinking on campus concerns college health educators, administrators, and parents, most students, like Helen, Meg, and Laurie (and even their parents) come to college thinking that drinking itself as an integral part of college life. Helen, as well as Tim and Evelyn, are among the first-year students who often do not recognize their drinking as problematic because their perception is relative to those around them. People like these three students who drink heavily tend to think that no matter how much they drink, there are others who drink more. Even Meg, who didn't drink that much, and Laurie, who didn't drink at all, are typical of moderate drinkers and abstainers who also believe that everyone drinks excessively at college.

This perception of dangerous drinking during the college years as a cultural norm is created and/or reinforced on a daily basis by the media, such as college newspapers with ads targeting students with messages like "All You Can Drink" and "Happy Hours" (Haines & Spear, 1996; Lederman, Stewart, Goodhart, & Laitman, 2003). Equally as important, the cultural image is reinforced by the students' own interpersonal experiences, such as sharing war stories about the "night before" or attending fraternity parties and other social events that encourage alcohol abuse. Helen and Meg's experiences of getting Helen through the night when she was sick in the bathroom are typical of the kind of "bonding experiences" that many students associate with a heavy drinking episode. When the emphasis in on the bonding, especially during the lonely times of adjusting to the first year at college, alcohol is seen by many of these students as a social facilitator. As one student put it, "It is social glue."

Thus, students learn about drinking by the images they receive from the media and by the talk that goes on among them about their own behaviors and their perceptions of the behaviors of others. If simply getting drunk helps students achieve their social and interpersonal goals, students can be expected to keep getting drunk. If alcohol generally is the key to some ultimate pleasure, the downside of drinking can be endured as long as it is not worse than the rewards gained.

At Rutgers University (RU), more than a decade of research into college drinking led a team of researchers to conclude that the myths about college drinking were alive and well. Random surveys of the campus, repeated periodically, indicated that the majority of Rutgers students (67%) did not drink dangerously (five or more drinks for a male student, four or more drinks for a female) when they drank and that 20% of the student population didn't drink at all. In addition, it was found that the students who tended to drink the most were first- and second-year undergraduates. In fact, the first semester of freshman year was the time when the highest percentage of students consistently reported drinking dangerously. This finding was consistent with national surveys in which first-year college students generally report drinking more than juniors and seniors.

Armed with solid data that convinced the research team that the majority of students didn't drink dangerously, but that a high proportion of first-year students did, the team decided it was important to do something to educate first-year students about the actual norms of drinking on the campus. The RU SURE Campaign, a prevention campaign to address dangerous drinking on the campus, was the solution to the problem.

ENLISTING COLLEGE SENIORS TO HELP CHANGE THE IMAGE OF DANGEROUS DRINKING AS ACCEPTABLE FOR FIRST-YEAR STUDENTS

The RU SURE Campaign was designed by a team of researchers working together with health educators and upper-level undergraduate Communication majors. This coalition called itself the Partnership for Communication and Health Issues and was eventually successful enough in its efforts that it was institutionalized at the University as the Center for Communication and Health Issues (CHI).

Working together with an undergraduate class studying health campaigns, CHI set out to create the campaign it came to call the RU SURE Campaign using a social norms approach with an emphasis on changing the misperceptions of students' beliefs about the prevalence of dangerous drinking on campus that was experientially based. The goal of the campaign was to change first-year students' misperceptions by increasing their awareness of the actual norms for college students' drinking. The basic message of the campaign was that dangerous drinking is not the norm at the university. The implementation of the campaign was preceded by collecting baseline data. Thus, actual local norms were used as a basis for all messages. The data indicated that two thirds of Rutgers students have three or fewer alcoholic drinks when they "party" and that one out of five students does not drink at all. These messages formed the basis for the norming messages disseminated throughout the campaign.

Because CHI team members were sure that students were more likely to be resistant to messages that they perceived to come from campus authorities, they decided that a more effective approach would be to involve students themselves in the campaign from the beginning. So a class of senior Communication majors was enlisted in the design and dissemination of prevention messages. The goal was to include students in the campaign as the messengers for other students. As a result, a major component of the campaign was involving college seniors in the design and dissemination of messages to first-year students, the target audience.

After working with this class of seniors, the project team focused on creating the primary messages for the campaign. The messages were that two thirds of students stopped at three or fewer drinks and that one in five didn't drink at all. CHI team members asked the senior Communication majors to work with them in creating a way to incorporate these messages into campaign materials and into their dissemination. The students came up with a campaign idea and called it the Top Ten Misperceptions at Rutgers. The Top Ten Misperceptions included three alcohol misperceptions messages as well as seven humorous statements to get students engaged in message processing, followed by a norming message to give students accurate data. All messages were pretested extensively with students in the target population and reviewed by university administrators for acceptability to authorities involved in various aspects of student life. The Top Ten Misperceptions at Rutgers were:

1. RU students don't write papers at the last minute.
2. It's easy to find a parking space on campus.
3. Everyone who parties gets wasted.*

4. FAT CAT = Fat-Free and FDA-approved. [Note: The Fat Cat is a bacon cheeseburger with french fries and mayonnaise on a bun.]
5. There's always an empty seat on the bus.
6. Everybody at RU drinks.*
7. Everybody goes to first period classes.
8. Most students at RU drink to get drunk.*
9. You don't need shower shoes for the dorms.
10. Used books are cheap.

*Two thirds of RU students stop at three or fewer drinks. Almost one in five don't drink at all.

The students suggested that T-shirts with the Top 10 Misperceptions on the back would be seen as cool by their fellow classmates. To complete the project, they designed an RU SURE logo for the front of the T-shirt. The RU SURE logo design consisted of four beer mugs with the last one containing the message "RU SURE?" and an additional line—"Yes, three or fewer. We got the stats from you!" This message was designed to reinforce that these data were obtained from students themselves and that this message reiterates the reality of college drinking.

When the messages were printed on T-shirts, they were distributed in various campus locations, including in front of the library, in dormitories, and at various student events. The students working on the project felt reinforced when they discovered how eagerly the first-year students snapped up the T-shirts and began to be observed wearing them around campus. To reinforce this behavior, the CHI team decided that students who were seen wearing the T-shirts on various occasions would be given a $5.00 certificate that could be used at the campus bookstore or food courts.

But the campaign did not stop at mediated messages alone. During the next semester, a new group of Communication majors working on the campaign focused on developing an interpersonal component to the message delivery. They designed an activity, RU SURE Bingo, in which students fill up a bingo card by finding other students who fit particular characteristics (e.g., were born in a large city, don't drink, have seen the misperceptions messages on campus, are majoring in a social science). Winners received prizes, such as candy bars (with stickers containing the Top Ten Misperceptions on them) and RU SURE T-shirts.

When the activity had been designed and field tested, the Communication majors working with CHI got permission to run it in dorms during evening hours. The purpose of these interactions was to spread the campaign messages to create new images of drinking norms for students. The students publicized the events and ran the games. They reported that they found that the activity allowed the first-year students to have fun by interacting with other students and with the upper-class students. This reinforced the message that first-year students didn't have to drink dangerously to fit in. In this way, students modeled and learned the social skills that they might otherwise have felt they needed alcohol to achieve. First-year students came together in a group to meet each other, socialize, share food, and interact with more advanced students in an alcohol-free environment that reinforced that dangerous drinking is not a prerequisite for a fulfilling social life.

EVALUATING THE IMPACT OF THE CAMPAIGN ON THE TARGET AUDIENCE

All aspects of this campaign were continuously assessed with quantitative measures, such as surveys and intercept interviews, and with qualitative measures, such as focus groups and debriefing interviews.

Because the University does not release students' phone numbers or let anyone place things under the doors in residence halls, it was decided that the most effective way to solicit information from members of the target audience was by approaching them in a random manner as they entered or exited residence halls. Thus, intercept interviews were conducted by Communication majors involved in the campaign activities to maximize the likelihood that students would participate in the survey. The survey instrument contained a short series of questions designed to assess the impact of the campaign on first-year students' drinking attitudes, perceptions, and behaviors. During one semester, a total of 190 first-year students completed the survey, and 74% of them indicated that they were aware of the RU SURE Campaign. Ninety-five percent of the respondents thought that the campaign was about alcohol, and 61% of them could accurately complete the key message that "two thirds of Rutgers students stop at three or fewer drinks." Over half of the respondents (55%) were able to report that almost one in five students don't drink at all. A large majority of students (72%) indicated that the overall message of the campaign was that "everyone at Rutgers doesn't drink dangerously, and you don't have to either."

Debriefing interviews were conducted with the Communication majors working on the campaign to ascertain the campaign's effect on them. These students (called the secondary target audience for the campaign) reported that they felt the campaign was particularly successful because the message was delivered by fellow students and not by health professionals, teachers, or parents. They also stressed that having a campaign that was not antidrinking, but antidangerous drinking helped establish a rapport with first-year students. The students felt the campaign message would help some students recognize that they are not the only ones who do not drink and, thus, prevent them from initially drinking to "fit in" with others on campus. The students were also asked to indicate the effect they felt the campaign had on them. Students indicated they felt responsible for educating and being a role model for first-year students. As one of the students noted:

> Working on this campaign has shown me that freshman year is very scary and that students will follow anyone who is nice to them. . . . I could see students' eyes "light up" when I told them I was in college, too, and I was in your shoes a couple of years back. This class has taught me how important these interpersonal relationships are.

AN UNEXPECTED OUTCOME

The fact that the students in the target audience weren't the only ones influenced by the campaign came as a surprise to the CHI team members. As noted in the previous section, students who worked on the campaign, who designed messages and disseminated them, also reported that their own attitudes, beliefs, and behaviors had been challenged. As Colleen[2] put it, "I was amazed at the way those cheezy freshmen girls drank. Then I was horrified when I realized that only three years ago I was one of them!"

Like many of the students who worked on the campaign, Colleen and her teammate, Rick, were very expressive about the campaign's impact on them. "I didn't believe any of it when I first began," Rick noted. "I was just going to work on the campaign to get the experience and for a line on my resume. I'm graduating and figured it'd look good for a job. But as I talked to kids all semester long and collected data from them and saw for myself that the data I got were like the campaign stats, I became a believer."

Many other students expressed similar reactions. Wynne told an interviewer after working on the campaign that she herself had never been a drinker, "Before the campaign, that made me feel out of it. But the campaign taught me that I was one of the '1 in 5' who didn't drink."

"I didn't drink either," said Alyssa. "But I acted like I did. Now I see I didn't have to do that." "Yeah," said Cia, "I don't have to drink. That's cool."

LESSONS LEARNED

What CHI team members learned from the RU SURE Campaign was that college drinking could best be conceptualized as socially situated experiential learning and that this reconceptualization allowed for a different approach to addressing the culture of college drinking. Rather than looking at drinking behavior in isolation, drinking needs to be looked at as part of the social interactions that naturally occur among students. If the social interaction rather than the individual is used as the focus of analysis, what becomes clear is the relational nature of college drinking for many students and how, in those relationships and in relation to one another, students are learning about the social cache of drinking. They engage in drinking behaviors because they believe everybody else does. It is behavior that allows them to feel like they belong. It is behavior that gives them something to talk about the day after, to tell war stories, to be part of what's happening. In all these ways, drinking dangerously is used as a way to meet the need to form and maintain relationships. How this is accomplished and in what ways grow out of students' own socially situated experiential learning.

For students for whom the problem is making social connections or finding and forming social relationships, the solution is about helping them to find ways in which they learn that they can meet others and become part of the college culture without drinking dangerously. Understanding college drinking as socially situated experiential learning provides new ways to think about and address what needs to be done on the college campus. At Rutgers, these insights are continuously used to create an environment in which students know that everyone doesn't have to drink to fit in and that those who choose to drink can do so moderately and be socially involved. As Carla put it, "I've learned you don't have to drink a lot to be a lot."

RELEVANT CONCEPTS

College drinking: The use of alcohol by college students that takes place during their college years. Generally associated with the image of excessive drinking on campus, although the image is often inaccurate.

College health: The area of health care that focuses on the health issues that are particularly prevalent among college students.

Dangerous drinking: The excessive use of alcohol that results in unwanted social, emotional, and/or physical consequences. Generally measured in terms of quantity and frequency of use, and their role in the resultant consequences.

Health communication: An area of study in which the role of communication is examined in relation to health issues. Health communication cuts across interpersonal, group, mediated, and organizational contexts of communication.

Health prevention campaigns: Media campaigns that are designed to educate people to inform them about a particular health issue or to persuade them to either adopt healthy attitudes or behaviors or reject unhealthy attitudes and/or behaviors.

Interpersonal communication: The area of communication that focuses on communication between people. Interpersonal communication is the term generally used to refer to one-to-one communication, usually in face-to-face interactions.

Social interaction: The ways in which people communicate with one another in face-to-face circumstances. Social interaction is a way of looking at interpersonal communication as growing out of socially created mores for interpersonal behavior.

Socially situated experiential learning: The experience-based process of acquiring and interpreting social information (and misinformation) received from peers and other sources within the context of their direct learning experiences (Stewart & Lederman, 2002).

DISCUSSION QUESTIONS

1. What is meant by the phrase, "the culture of college drinking," and how, if at all, does that concept influence the ways in which students drink?
2. What role can health educators play in changing the ways in which students think about drinking and in which they actually drink?
3. What are the lessons to be learned from creating a campaign like RU SURE for other health prevention campaigns?
4. In what ways does this case compare with the ways in which students on your campus think about drinking and any of their drinking-related behaviors?
5. How, if at all, have your own experiences on campus shaped your own drinking and drinking-related behaviors?

ACKNOWLEDGMENTS

Funding for this campaign was provided, in part, by the U.S. Department of Education Safe and Drug Free Schools Program, the New Jersey Higher Education Consortium on Alcohol and Other Drug Prevention and Education, and the Rutgers University Health Services.

ENDNOTES

[1] The story in this scenario is a composite of stories told to researchers who conducted a series of 16 focus group interviews with students willing to talk about the role of alcohol in their first-year experience.

[2] The stories of Colleen, Rick, Wynne, and others are composites of numerous stories from student campaign workers over five years of participation in the campaign.

REFERENCES/SUGGESTED READINGS

Berkowitz, A. D., & Perkins, H. W. (1986). Problem drinking among college students: A review of recent literature. *Journal of American College Health, 35,* 21–28.

Cohen, D. J., & Lederman, L. C. (1998). Navigating the freedoms of college life: Students talk about alcohol, gender and sex. In N. Roth & L. Fuller (Eds.), *Women and AIDS: Negotiating safer practices, care and representation* (pp. 101–126). Binghamton, NY: Haworth.

Haines, M. P., & Spear, S. F. (1996). Changing the perception of the norm: A strategy to decrease binge drinking among college students. *Journal of American College Health, 45,* 134–140.

Lederman, L. C., Stewart, L. P., Goodhart, F. W., & Laitman, L. (2003). A case against "binge" as the term of choice: Convincing college students to personalize messages about dangerous drinking. *Journal of Health Communication, 8,* 79–91.

Perkins, H. W. (1997). College student misperceptions of alcohol and other drug norms among peers: Exploring causes, consequences, and implications for prevention programs. In L. Grow (Ed.), *Designing alcohol and other drug prevention programs in higher education: Bringing theory into practice* (pp. 177–206). Newton, MA: Higher Education Center for Alcohol and Other Drug Prevention.

Stewart, L. P., Lederman, L. C., with Golubow, M., Cattafesta, J. L., Goodhart, F. W., Powell, R., & Laitman, L. (2002). Applying communication theories to prevent dangerous drinking among college students: The RU SURE campaign. *Communication Studies, 53,* 381–399.

27

Personal Stories and Public Activism: The Implications of Michael J. Fox's Public Health Narrative for Policy and Perspectives

Christina S. Beck
Ohio University

I had just finished the first part of my workout when I noticed the headline of *Us Weekly* on the rec center magazine rack—"Look Who's Turning Forty." Wiping off my face with the bottom of my shirt, I stepped off of the treadmill and walked over to peek at the article. Deciding that it might just distract me long enough to finish the last part of my workout, I carried the magazine back to the treadmill and started to read as the machine picked up speed. "1961 was a good year," I said to myself as I read brief bios of a few of the famous people who share my birth year—Meg Ryan, George Clooney, Ken (Barbie's friend), Heather Locklear, and of course, Michael J. Fox.

My eyes lingered on the paragraph about Fox. How incredibly odd to feel such a connection to someone whom I have never met, will likely never meet—yet, I have for years. He made me feel young by being my same age yet playing wonderfully youthful characters like Alex P. Keaton on *Family Ties* and Marty McFly in the *Back to the Future* trilogy. I identified with his energy and passion in *The American President*.

I glanced up at one of the television screens in front of my treadmill. Over the years, as I learned of Michael's marriage to Tracy Pollen and the birth of his kids, I had smiled and thought "how neat." I shook my head and returned my gaze to the picture staring up at me in the article. Wow, what a difference from the sick shock that I had felt when I found out that he has Parkinson's Disease! How could someone *our* age get Parkinson's Disease? How could someone like Michael possibly have it? How could my stomach hurt so much about a complete stranger whom I refer to by his first name?

Joshua Meyrowitz (1985) explains that technology has contributed to a blurring of boundaries between interpersonal and mediated communication contexts. Through television, we can gain an interpersonal connection with an actor or a character, despite the reality of physical and social distance. Of course, I don't really *know* Michael J. Fox, but I rejoiced at the news of his wedding and grieved over news of his health challenge. To clarify, I'm not an obsessed "nut;" I'm just a fan, similar to millions of other fans, who come to care about someone who seems deceptively near through the magical intimacy of contemporary media and popular culture.

For celebrities like Michael J. Fox, that intimacy constitutes a dual-edged sword. On the one hand, connectedness with fans fosters fame and, in the event of illness or injury, opportunity to translate stardom into public awareness and political advocacy. On the other hand, the deceptive familiarity with celebrities can hinder enactment of personal lives beyond the public sphere. In this case study, I explore the emergent public construction of Michael J. Fox's personal health narrative as well as the implications of that narrative for policies and perspectives about Parkinson's disease.

AN EMERGENT PUBLIC–PRIVATE NARRATIVE

As a performer, Michael J. Fox has played numerous characters on television and in movies, yet Fox's enactment of himself and his preferred identities also constitute ongoing performances. Through his verbal and nonverbal behaviors, through his choices to engage or not to engage in particular activities (such as movies, television shows, interviews, photo opportunities), he implicitly asserts who he is, who he wants to be, and how he hopes to be treated by others. Through their responses to Fox's actions and activities, others (such as viewers, media representatives, television and film producers and promoters, and, increasingly, politicians) communicatively affirm or negate Fox's preferred identities.

As I watched Fox on *Family Ties* and in *Back to the Future*, his performances rang true for me. I believed in (and liked) Alex and Marty. Moreover, I also grew to admire and care for Michael J. Fox as a person, based the admittedly limited interviews that I read or observed. In his work on narrative, Walter Fisher (1987) argues that humans are, by nature, narrative beings and that we come to understand and accept others based on the believability of their lives, their identities, as stories. Fisher suggests that believable narratives must be coherent or consistent and truthful. For me, the story of an energetic, ambitious, successful actor with refreshingly working class values rang true. As I reflect on Fisher's writings in terms of my relatively passing knowledge of Michael J. Fox, I realize that Fox's publicly constructed story easily met Fisher's criteria for an effective narrative. Fox's narrative seemed coherent; from what I could tell, everything that Fox revealed to the public fit together. Further, I interpreted Fox's story as truthful and reliable; no "red flags" waved as possible untruths.

With Fox's disclosure of his battle with Parkinson's disease (PD), though, he faced new challenges to the viability of his increasingly complicated narrative. How could he maintain his stature as an actor after revealing such an illness? How could such a young man have an "old person's disease"? How could he continue to insist on his privacy after placing his personal health saga so overtly in public and political domains? How could he believably voice concerns of "the" Parkinson's community as such an atypical and unlikely Parkinson's patient? How could public and private domains, concerns, and identities be blurred yet segregated in a coherent and truthful manner by and for a multiplicity of interested stakeholders, including Michael J. Fox?

Indeed, Fox has carefully and consciously worked to construct and control his identities as actor/private personas and as activist/private person with a public vocation. However, although Fox has continually asserted his agency to control his own narrative, in the end, his identities and personal health narrative emerge as public constructions, inherently shaped by media choices and responses from fans and increasingly from politicians and others with PD.

Michael J. Fox as Private Person Who Happens to Act

In his testimony before the House Committee on Judiciary on May 21, 1998, Fox emphasized his desire to distinguish between his public profession as an actor and his personal life as a husband and a father, noting that "I'd like to think of my life as my own. I strongly disagree with those who would argue that some sort of Faustian bargain has been struck whereby 'public'

figures are fair game, any time, any place, including within the confines of their own homes."
Fox recounted his efforts to preserve his privacy during his wedding, his father's funeral, and
the birth of his children in this testimony as well as in his 2002 book, *Lucky Man*.

Especially prior to his diagnosis with PD, Fox worked actively to carve a discretely private
domain in his otherwise public life, differentiating between the part of his narrative that could be
part of public discourse and the part that remained exclusive to family and close friends. After
struggling with the symptoms and receiving the diagnosis, Fox chose to guard his personal
health situation as well, telling only family members and trusted friends and colleagues. In
Lucky Man, Fox (2002) explained, "After my wedding and my father's funeral, I knew full
well how the tabloid press would run with a story like this—possess it and thereby possess a
greater part of me than I was willing to let go of."

Thus, Fox launched even more fervently into acting projects, developing strategies for concealing his condition, trying medications to negate some of the symptoms, and even undergoing
brain surgery in an effort to improve his condition. However, the outward indications of PD
became more difficult to shadow from the glistening intensity of Hollywood lights. In his first
public interview about his battle with PD, Fox told Karen Schneider and Todd Gold (1998),
reporters from *People Weekly*, about instructing his chauffeur to circle the block three times
prior to dropping him and his wife off at the Golden Globe Awards. "He probably thought I
was nuts," says Fox with a faint smile. "But I just couldn't get out of the car and let my arms
go, or mumble, or shuffle."

In addition to the medication that finally kicked in prior to the Golden Globe Awards, Fox
told Schneider and Gold that "there are a billion tricks I can do to hide [the symptoms] . . . I
can touch something and stop the tremors for about 15 seconds. Or I can move around.
I've done interviews where I've walked the entire time, and later the writer describes me
as nervous." Through such maneuvers, Fox disguised his disease, protecting his secret from
public scrutiny. Yet, as Fox disclosed to Barbara Walters during a December 4, 1998, *20/20*
interview, the hounds in the tabloid press started sniffing, suspecting something amiss. Faced
with the possibility of more vocal denials and/or someone else blasting his condition into the
public eye, Fox chose to take the lead in disclosing his illness and, importantly, controlling the
emergent health narrative and its implications for his public persona.

> *Walters:* As I look at you, there are absolutely no symptoms.
> *Fox:* Right.
> *Walters:* I mean, you did not have to publicly say that you had Parkinson's disease.
> *Fox:* Right.
> *Walters:* Why did you? Why have you now told people about this disease?
> *Fox:* I would say the first reason is that it's been such a part of my life for a long time,
> and I wanted to just chart my own path and live one day at a time, and so
> I—I kept it to myself. The other part of it was also wanting to—to destigmatize it
> in a way. . . . I found myself at 7 years not battling it, not struggling with it, not
> suffering from it, not breaking under the burden of it, but dealing with it. And
> the tiniest element would be that I knew that somewhere, sometime, possibly
> someone who I didn't want to tell everybody on my behalf would beat me to the
> punch.
> *Walters:* A tabloid might make . . .
> *Fox:* Somebody like that. So I thought, let me do it on my terms.

With this disclosure about his health, however, Michael J. Fox did more than update his fans
on a challenging personal issue. Given the nature of Parkinson's disease, he also faced the ne-
cessity of expanding the public construction of his multifaceted identities to include himself as

one of the PD community, no longer just an "every guy" who happened to be an actor with a family. Interestingly, responses from the media, fans, and members of the Parkinson's community contributed to the public discourse, shaping the emergent public health narrative as consistent and truthful in light of other aspects of who Michael J. Fox has come to be in the public eye.

Michael J. Fox as "Just One of Us"

Barbara Walters began her interview with Fox by acknowledging, "Last week, we all learned the secret. . . . The announcement made headlines all over the country. Millions were stunned." As Jane Pauley commenced her November 27, 1998, *Dateline NBC* report, she explained our public conundrum. According to Pauley, "For more than a decade, Michael J. Fox has been the very image of youthful energy and boyish charm. That's why this week's news that he's suffering from Parkinson's disease has been such a shock. How could this happen to someone so young." In that *Dateline NBC* episode, NBC Chief Medical Correspondent, Dr. Bob Arnot, continued, "It seems we've watched him grow up right before our eyes," and Lynette Rice, from the *Hollywood Reporter*, asserted that "he comes across as the boy next door. A great boyfriend, a great brother, a great buddy." As these reporters astutely observed, Fox's disclosure just didn't fit. How could such an illness befall the gutsy kid who drove the DeLorien, defying time and, well, all of the bullies and bad guys along the way? How could he be an "every guy," just like one of us, slugging Diet Pepsi, flashing a smile, and skateboarding right into our hearts, if he has some old man's disease? The two images just didn't mesh, and for Fox and his devoted public, the search for continuity and truthfulness in reconciling those identities began.

As Fox told his story to Schneider and Gold and to Barbara Walters, he highlighted how he had managed to pass as someone who did not have PD. He still had a normal life, loving family, active career. He disclosed later in his book that his doctor gave him 10 more years to work at the time of his diagnosis some 7 years earlier. Yet, he optimistically (but ambiguously) stressed to Walters that ". . . what my doctors do agree on is that I'll be able to—to work and function for many more years to come." Indeed, given Fox's goal of "getting on with his life," he needed to position himself as a working actor who planned to keep working in his beloved craft.

However, he could not simply assert that he's just an "every guy" or an actor just like he used to be anymore. For his narrative to ring true, the public construction of the narrative had to include discourse about the consistency and truthfulness of Fox as a person with PD as well as with his prior commitment to firm barriers between his public and private concerns.

In his 30s, Michael J. Fox certainly wasn't old as he heard the doctor disclose the diagnosis nor when he shared his condition in the mainstream media. In that initial public construction of his personal health narrative, Fox did little to address these inherent inconsistencies in his story, likely because his focus had been on surviving and hiding rather than on researching how his experience resembled that of other individuals with PD.

As the news spread, though, the media and other individuals with PD participated actively in shaping Fox's story, enabling it to emerge as consistent with little known information about PD and with Fox's preexisting identities as a person and performer. *USA Today* (1998) became one of several publications to pursue the story beyond "Fox as sick person;" reporters investigated the apparent inconsistencies for answers. For example, Davis (1998, November 27) found that, although the stereotypical PD patient may be elderly, Young-Onset PD strikes a smaller yet significant percentage of all persons with the disease. Indeed, as the media sought and shared more information about PD, an unprecedented public dialogue about the disease began, much to the surprise of Fox. In his book, Fox explained:

> What I dreaded most was being cast as a tragic figure, a helpless victim. . . . [However] much of the follow-up coverage centered less on me than on Parkinson's disease itself: there were long, detailed features describing the condition, interviews with doctors explaining the process of

diagnosis, the prognosis, and the variety of treatments available. A recurring topic of discussion was the heretofore little-known phenomenon of Young Onset PD.... Without intending to, I had sparked a national conversation about Parkinson's disease. (2002, p. 228)

Notably, such an orientation to the story by the media and by others with PD contributed to the inevitable consistency of Fox's narrative. He's not the only young person to endure PD in his 30s. Instead, given the rarity of the condition and the potential stigma of the illness, instances received little press until Fox's disclosure. Further, as Fox continues to stress, his participation in public conversations about PD focuses on PD, not about him as a person who has PD, thus enabling him to affirm and preserve his preference for personal privacy while engaging in public discourse.

By highlighting the PD community, and, in fact, increasingly seeking connectedness with the PD community, Fox ultimately sought to be "one of us," as a member of the PD community as well as an every guy with a wife, kids, and job. He continually reiterates that he speaks as part of a larger collection of individuals. During an interview with George Stephanopoulos for *This Week with Sam Donaldson and Cokie Roberts* that aired on July 1, 2001, he noted that "there is a coalition that is amassing forces and I've made myself available for whatever extent they need me. When I say amassing forces I mean that these are not political operatives—these are patients, and families of patients...." Fox told *TV Guide* ("A Grateful Goodbye," 2000) that "it's my mission inasmuch as it's something that I'm extremely committed to. At the risk of sounding like I'm bucking for papal recognition or something, it very quickly became not about me. It's about the whole thing. It's not a mission to save myself" (p. 26).

Although he did not disclose his illness to seek community, the PD community embraced him, as someone who could give voice to its cause, certainly, but also as "one of us," not just a celebrity or even an every guy. In its December 28, 1998, issue, *People Weekly* published the following letter to the editor:

Thank you for bringing attention to the plight of young Parkinsonians. My husband was diagnosed four years ago at the age of 36. We too have children who don't understand their daddy's problems, except that he has a shaky hand. Every piece of literature I read addresses the problems of the typical older Parkinson's population. It was inspirational reading about another couple dealing with exactly the same things we do. (Sanders, 1998, p. 1)

Although he positions public discourse about PD as not about him nor even for him, Fox unwittingly bolstered the courage and resolve of other Parkinson's patients, many of whom believe that a cure looms near if funding could be found. Another letter writer to *People Weekly* withheld his name, noting that "I have just started a new job, live alone and cannot let it be known that I have Parkinson's.... Michael, if you are willing to lobby for us, I will come out of the closet and be an activist as well" (p. 1).

Michael J. Fox as Expert Witness

As a fan and, well, someone who likes to think of herself as compassionate, I remember shaking my head and feeling aghast by Davis' December 1, 1998, article in *USA Today*. Leave the poor guy alone, I thought, as I read the following passage:

Abraham Lieberman, medical director of the National Parkinson Foundation, says he is putting in a request for Fox's help. "I would say, 'I applaud you for announcing that you have it. Now you should take the next step and help us find a cure for the disease by lending your energy and your spirit and your good ideas to us.' ... The goal is money for a cure. The greatest thing for polio was when Franklin D. Roosevelt had polio and chaired the March of Dimes," says Lieberman, who had polio in 1944. "He was the driving force." (p. D1)

Tell him to shove it, I advised Michael silently. Honestly, Lieberman seemed almost happy that Michael had this horrible affliction—certainly not a very nice reaction, I concluded, as I finished the article. On reflection, though, I realized that Lieberman's comments stemmed from a desire for the greater good, a larger piece of the federally funded research pie. As Lieberman well knew, celebrity voices were much more likely to be heard and heeded, especially in the political arena. Ebner and Derrick note that "when members of the Parkinson's Action Network (PAN) had spoken before the House Appropriations Committee, almost half the seats were empty. But when Fox appeared, the House was full" (1999, ¶4).

On September 28, 1999, Fox spoke to the Senate Subcommittee on Labor, Health, and Human Services, and Education Committee on Appropriations. In introducing Fox, Senator Arlen Spector, committee chairman, commented, "And one of the facts of life is that when someone like Michael J. Fox steps forward [he] very heavily personalizes the problem, focuses a lot of public attention on it . . . ." Fox also acknowledged, "What celebrity has given me is the opportunity to raise the visibility of Parkinson's disease and focus more attention on the desperate need for more research dollars."

In a subsequent Senate subcommittee hearing on September 14, 2000, Spector referenced Fox's status as a celebrity witness, positioning it again as part of the public good:

> . . . you have done spectacular work, and from time to time, questions are raised about celebrities appearing at congressional hearings. In fact, it's even more than questions. There's been pretty severe criticism about it. But we make no apologies, because we need public awareness of issues like stem cells, which could cure Parkinson's or amyotrophic lateral sclerosis or Alzheimer's. And when public attention is focused on Michael J. Fox because the American people know you, Michael, it is a great use of your talent and celebrity status to let people know what's going on and get public support for this kind of a measure.

Through on-record comments such as these, politicians validate the credibility of Michael J. Fox as a witness because of his celebrity status. However, as Hammonds contends, Fox artfully asserts himself as an expert witness as well. According to Hammonds (2001), "Cute is good, but so are smarts. Fox, already engrossed by the machinery of American politics, made himself an expert on the science behind Parkinson's. The result: He is a commanding, persuasive public face who knows the ropes."

Although one of the oft-cited soundbites from Fox's first congressional testimony on September 28, 1999 involved a personal plea, it exemplifies Fox's ongoing commitment to characterizing himself as part of the larger cause, the greater PD community, only one of a million experts on PD. In requesting additional funding for the National Institutes of Health and, in particular, for PD research, Fox implored: "But with your help, if we all do everything we can to eradicate this disease, in my 50s I'll be dancing at my children's weddings. And mine will be just one of millions of happy stories." Nearly a year later, during his testimony on behalf of stem cell research on September 14, 2000, Fox again situated himself as a member of the PD community while acknowledging his unique entry into the congressional hearing room:

> I didn't intend to become a professional witness. I'm not a politician, nor am I a doctor or a research scientist. You don't need me to explain embryonic stem cell research or its medical applications. So what qualifies me to be at this table? The answer is simple. I'm one of a million experts on Parkinson's disease in the U.S., battling its destructive nature as we wait for a cure. We need a rescue, and the country should know it. I'm also here because I'm a guy with PD who happens to be on TV. Because of that, many people have felt comfortable reaching out to me. By now, many of you have heard MY story. But, you haven't heard this story . . . . And you've never heard about Brenda, a 53-year-old former computer specialist. Recently her drugs failed to "kick-in" and she

found herself frozen in the bathtub with no one to help her... Her biggest regret, she now says, was that CNN was not there to provide live, up-to-the-minute coverage of her predicament. None of these people mind that I get more attention that they do. They simply say that if I get a shot in front of a microphone—I should start talking. So here I am. Again. (p. 1)

Notably, scholars who study arguments in the public sphere question the validity or usefulness of personal stories for public policy debates. They contend that emotional, intimate disclosures do little to advance logical consideration of important public concerns. Extending from their perspective, treating Fox as an "expert witness," even though he is not a doctor or a scientist, hinders optimal public dialogues and decisions. However, Fox, members of the Parkinson's community, and even politicians seem to understand that, in this era, personal advocacy, especially by celebrities, heavily influences policies (such as stem cell research) and federal funding. As Fox explained to Jane Pauley in a February 25, 2001 *Dateline NBC* interview:

I'm in this thing now, and—and I really want to—to do as much as I can do. I don't know what it means to be, 'It's a celebrity thing,' and maybe that's good and maybe that's bad. I don't know. All I know is that people have been moved by this and things are starting to change a little bit and all of a sudden, it's getting attention. And I just need to show up for it and be here for it and do the best that I can.

Michael J. Fox as an Activist Who Happens to Be an Actor and a Private Person

Fourteen months after he stunned the nation with news of his affliction with Parkinson's disease, Fox decided to retire from his hit sitcom, *Spin City*, and to devote himself to his family and his cause, finding a cure for PD as soon as possible. Fox told *TV Guide* (2000), "As we got toward Christmas, I started to think, 'I want to be with my family.' And I'd done some things in Washington, and I really started to feel a part of the Parkinson's community and to be energized by the potential for breakthroughs."

In his January 21, 2000 *Dateline NBC* report, chief NBC science correspondent, Robert Bazell, reported that "Fox's first brush with a new kind of limelight [testifying before Congress] planted the seed" for his decision to leave the show. Bazell concluded, "Fox is staying connected to Hollywood. He's the starring voice in the hit movie *Stuart Little* and has other film projects in the pipeline. But soon he will be best known for his courage in walking away from primetime TV to go from actor to activist."

As Fox told Katie Couric during an October 7, 1999 *Today* show interview, he hopes to urge Congress to allocate more money to the National Institutes of Health as well as to convince them to earmark money specifically for Parkinson's disease. Fox testified for the third time on behalf of Parkinson's research on May 22, 2002, gaining a very positive public commitment from Committee Chairman Senator Tom Harkin. Harkin vowed to Fox and the other witnesses that "... this Committee feels very strongly that we need to—not just a percentage increase, but we need to get as close as possible to the research agenda put forward by the Parkinson's Action Network—as close as possible. And you have my word, that language will be in there this year."

Moreover, by establishing the Michael J. Fox Foundation for Parkinson's Research in May, 2000, Fox continues to capitalize on his celebrity status by raising money. According to the foundation web site, "Since 2001, the Foundation has been involved in directing $15 million to scientists for research into Parkinson's." Hammonds observes, "Yawn. Another celebrity, another charity. Here's the thing though: In just over a year, the Fox foundation has become a strikingly effective organization—a force not just in fund-raising, but also in shaping the nation's research agenda for Parkinson's and, perhaps, for more than that" (¶7). Through the foundation, Fox participates in the continuing public dialogue about Parkinson's disease and the need for research and research funding.

Despite that ongoing involvement in public discourse, though, Fox carefully carves boundaries between what he wants to share and what he wants to shield. Consistent with Fox's public emphasis on PD, not on his personal life, the foundation web site clearly delineates between Fox as activist and Fox as actor or private person. The first four questions on the FAQ section of the web site focus on what can and cannot be obtained through the foundation or the web site—no revelations about Fox's health or treatment, no photos, no interactions about Fox as a celebrity.

Yet, by putting himself into the public discourse with regard to his battle with PD, Fox opens himself to the ongoing shaping of his otherwise personal health narrative by others. For example, in the February 28, 2000 issue of *People Weekly*, one reader commented that "if Michael J. Fox is planning on becoming even more of a public health-care advocate, he might want to quit smoking first. It seems fairly hypocritical that he is crusading for a cure for Parkinson's while simultaneously engaging in an activity that causes far more widespread health damage" (p. 4). Another reader agreed, noting that "although his disease is tragic, I was dismayed to find that Michael J. Fox still smokes cigarettes. Perhaps he should start raising money for lung cancer research as well as Parkinson's." This public debate about Fox's smoking practices extended until the March 20 issue of the magazine, with still another reader responding:

> On the same day that I read your reader's critical comments about Michael J. Fox's smoking, *USA Today* published an article regarding smoking and Parkinson's disease. According to new research presented by the American Association for the Advancement of Science, nicotine may help some brain disorders, including Parkinson's. Maybe your readers could use a little research of their own. (p. 8)

The commentary from these letter writers demonstrates Fox's challenge in his struggle to be activist and actor and celebrity and private person. First, the blurring of public and private spaces and concerns hinders efforts to distinguish clearly between the two domains. Borrowing from Gergen (1991), Fox's identities as activist, actor, celebrity, private person meld into each other. Although he can opt to highlight one aspect of his identity over another (activist more than actor) at a particular time, all parts of his social self linger, to some extent, in his relationships and in his (and other's) communicative choices. He can't stop being a celebrity and start being a private person like turning a faucet from hot to cold. Thus, through Fox's relationship with his fans, he gained celebrity status. That status gives him unique access to political decision makers, media resources, and money. However, Fox's mediated yet interpersonal relationship with fans dulls the edge of his preferred boundary between public and private. Do inquiring minds have a right to know and to comment? As exemplified previously, despite Fox's preferences, they will anyway.

Second, the letter writers illustrate an ongoing construction of consistency and validity in terms of Fox's public yet personal health and life narrative. For some readers, Fox's decision to smoke clashes with his pursuit of wellness—a giant red flag in his emergent health narrative. How can he really be concerned about his health if he continues to smoke? For the reader who also reviewed the *USA Today* report, the other letter writers' comments seemed more inconsistent than Fox's smoking habit—given the recent scientific data, how could those letter writers dare to challenge Fox? As participants with Fox in making public sense of his situation, each of these letter writers exhibits agency in negotiating aspects of Fox's health narrative, even though Fox's smoking decision can truly be characterized as a personal preference.

DISCUSSION

As this case study illustrates, illnesses or injuries challenge individuals, their families, and concerned others to juxtapose those afflictions within their lives, much already in progress. How do afflictions fit with how individuals define themselves? What adaptations to their identities must occur for their life narratives to become coherent once more? For a celebrity, the process of enacting a preferred social self in light of an emergent health issue becomes even more challenging.

Ultimately, Michael J. Fox chose the path of public disclosure and activism. For Fox, as someone who yearns for distinct boundaries between his public and private lives, that initial choice to share his situation stemmed in part from fear of tabloid disclosure. Given the increasingly fuzzy lines between public and private domains for celebrities and politicians, the ethics of implicitly forcing disclosure must be discussed by journalists and by fans who stress their "need to know."

Simply because more and more celebrities blur boundaries between their public and private lives, should public disclosure of personal issues become part of the celebrity job requirement? To what extent should the personal stories of the stars enable them to lobby on behalf of a pet cause? As I collected information on celebrity contributions to public dialogues about health issues for a larger study, I discovered over 125 actors, musicians, sports figures, and politicians who created foundations, made public service announcements, testified before Congress, coordinated fundraisers, and/or appeared on television programs to plug their particular affliction.

Yet, as this case study about Michael J. Fox suggests, choices about public disclosures of personal health matters remain complicated, muddied by fear of stigma or pity amid desires to "do the right thing" by fans, family, and fellow human beings. Although Michael J. Fox's inevitable public activism has generated millions for the greater good of Parkinson's patients and their families, his choices altered his multifaceted identity forever.

However, he has also changed the face of Parkinson's disease forever as well. Because of Michael J. Fox, others will likely see pamphlets of elderly patients on a beach as incomplete. For the young-Onset Parkinson's patients and for elderly individuals who want more from life than to sit on the beach, Fox offers hope. He inspires hope for a public voice that remained otherwise silent, hope for funding that would otherwise go to someone else's cause, hope for a cure that might otherwise take decades instead of a few years.

Because of Michael J. Fox, I want someone to find a cure for Parkinson's disease. Katie Couric made me care about colon cancer as did Gilda Radner about ovarian cancer. I feel passionately about a cure for amyotrophic lateral sclerosis because of Michael Zaslow, who played Roger Thorpe on *Guiding Light*. Through these people that I've never really met, diseases otherwise distant to me become real and personal. Despite the politics and ethics of competition for federal research funding, as celebrities such as Fox involve us in their health narratives, they inspire us to expand our concern and understanding beyond illnesses or injuries that touch our immediate family or friends.

RELEVANT CONCEPTS

Identity: The verbal and nonverbal enactment of self by an individual and affirmed by others with whom that individual interacts

Narratives: Socially constructed stories that emerge from and reflect life experiences

Parkinson's disease: According to the Parkinson's Disease Foundation, PD is a neurological disease that belongs to a group of conditions called movement disorders. PD is a chronic, progressive illness.

Private domain: An individual's personal region in terms of physical space, information, and interpersonal relationships

Public advocacy: Verbal and nonverbal efforts to impact public perceptions or social policy

Public domain: Shared physical space and negotiation of information that transcends the boundaries of individuals' private domains

Public policy: Official decisions about social and governmental practices (e.g., laws, budgeting by departments at local, state, or federal levels, etc.)

DISCUSSION QUESTIONS

1. To what extent should public figures be compelled to discuss personal health issues if such disclosures can benefit others?
2. To what extent should celebrity testimony impact federal funding decisions regarding medical research?
3. How do celebrity health disclosures impact awareness and understanding of public health issues?
4. How has reading about Michael J. Fox's emergent public health narrative influenced your own views on the public benefits and personal costs of celebrity participation in public dialogues about health?
5. Should public policy decisions (e.g., federal funding issues) occur based on the loudest or most visible voice? With limited resources, who gets to define the most important cause or the most reachable cure? Conversely, how do we decide which person's suffering is not important or less important?

REFERENCES/SUGGESTED READINGS

A grateful goodbye (2000, May 13). *TV Guide, 48*(20), 22–28, 74.
Calhoun, C. (Ed.). (1992). *Habermas and the public sphere.* Cambridge, MA: The MIT Press.
20/20, December 4, 1998.
Dateline NBC, November 27, 1998.
Dateline NBC, January 21, 2000.
Dateline NBC, February 25, 2001.
Davis, R. (1998, November 27). Fox one of few under 40 with Parkinson's. *USA Today*, p. 3A.
Davis, R. (1998, December 1). Actor Fox could spur Parkinson's funding. *USA Today*, p. D1.
Ebner, M., & Derrick, L. (1999, November 29). Star sickness. Retrieved November 2, 2000, from www.salon.com/health/feature/1999/11/29/celeb_disease
Fisher, W. (1987). *Human communication as narration: Toward a philosophy of reason, value, and action.* Columbia: University of South Carolina Press.
Fox, M. (2002). *Lucky man.* New York: Hyperion.
Gergen, K. (1991). *The saturated self.* New York: Basic Books.
Hammonds, K. (2001, November). Change agents. Retrieved October 6, 2004 from www.fastcompany.com/online/52/fox.html
Mailbag (Feb. 28, 2000). *People Weekly*, p. 4.
Mailbag (March 20, 2000). *People Weekly*, p. 8.
Meyrowitz, J. (1985). *No sense of place.* New York: Oxford University Press.
Sanders, T. (1998, December 28). Letter to the editor. *People Weekly*, 1.
Schneider, K., & Gold, T. (1998, December 7). After the tears. *People Weekly*, 127–136.

This Week with Som Donaldson and Cokie Robets, July 1, 2001.

Today, October 7, 1999.

U.S. Senate Subcommittee on Labor, Health, and Human Services. (Sept. 14, 2000). Proceedings from hearings. web.lexis-nexis.com/congcom5. Retrieved April 27, 2001.

U.S. Senate Subcommittee on Labor, Health, and Human Services. (Sept. 28, 1999). Proceedings from hearings. web.lexis-nexis.com/congcom. Retrieved February 5, 2003.

www.michaeljfox.org/foundation. Retrieved April 18, 2001.

28

Journey of Life: A Radio Soap Opera on Family Planning in Ethiopia

Kim Witte
Johns Hopkins University

Many health communication practitioners advocate using theory to develop their campaign messages, yet when faced with a "real" project and "real" data, often practitioners are at a loss for how to translate theory into a research study and then how to translate data collected from a research study into campaign recommendations. The purpose of this case study is to demonstrate how a fear appeal theory was used in Ethiopia to design both research and an entertainment education program. This type of research, called formative health communication research, was conducted using a well tested fear appeal theory, called the Extended Parallel Process Model. Based on theoretical guidance from this model and the data, a 26-week radio serial drama was developed to promote family planning. This case study first describes the Ethiopian context and research project, then the fear appeal theory, and then the results of the formative research.

FAMILY PLANNING IN ETHIOPIA

Ethiopia is a northeastern African country with a high total fertility rate of 5.9 children born per woman. Though contraceptive use is low at 8.1% of currently married women, unmet need for contraception is high, with 35.8% of currently married women indicating that they would like to use contraception but, for a variety of reasons, currently are not (Central Statistical Authority, Ethiopia, and ORC Macro, 2001). The most common reasons given for not using contraception are a lack of knowledge about contraception and how it works and/or perceptions that contraception causes negative side effects (Central Statistical Authority, Ethiopia, and ORC Macro, 2001).

In response to the high fertility rate, as well as the low levels of contraceptive use to prevent pregnancy, the Ethiopian Reproductive Health Communication Project (RHCP/E) was launched. The RHCP/E was a four-year information, education, and communication initiative in family planning supported by the United States Agency for International Development. The purpose of the RHCP/E project was to improve the health status of Ethiopians and to help

347

reduce the population growth rate. A steering committee with representatives from government agencies (e.g., the National Office of Population, the Ministry of Health), nongovernmental agencies (e.g., UNICEF), and local Ethiopian-based agencies was developed. Based on a needs assessment of family planning organizations in Ethiopia, it was determined that an entertainment education radio soap opera would be developed to promote modern family planning methods.

Entertainment Education

Entertainment education is "any communication presentation that delivers a pro-social educational message in an entertainment format" (JHU/CCP, 2002, p. 1). Because radios are the most common mass medium in Ethiopia, the Ethiopian steering committee decided to develop a 26-week-long radio serial. Formative health communication research was commissioned to determine the key messages for the scripts.

The Extended Parallel Process Model

The theoretical basis for the formative health communication research was a fear appeal theory called the Extended Parallel Process Model (EPPM; Witte, Meyer, & Martell, 2001), which is an integration of other behavior change models and has been tested in over 50 studies worldwide. The EPPM focuses on the relationship between threat and efficacy and their combined influence on behavioral outcomes (see Table 28.1 for definitions). Briefly, the EPPM suggests that when people feel at risk for a significant threat, they become scared and are motivated to act. The

TABLE 28.1
Key Variables in the Extended Parallel Process Model

Variable	Definition	Example
Perceived susceptibility	The degree to which one feels at risk for experiencing a health threat	"Is it likely that I'll have more children than I really want?"
Perceived severity	The magnitude of harm or negative consequences expected from the health threat	"Does having more children than I want negatively impact my life? How?"
Perceived response efficacy	The degree to which one believes that the recommended response works in averting the health threat	"Modern contraception will prevent me from getting pregnant."
Perceived self-efficacy	The degree to which one believes s/he is able to do the recommended response	"I am able to use modern contraceptive methods to prevent my getting pregnant."
Danger control responses	Responses that control the danger, such as adoption of the campaign's recommendations; typically attitude, intention, or behavior changes	"Modern contraceptive methods are good." (attitudes) "I intend to use modern contraceptives." (intentions) "I use the pill." (behaviors)
Fear control responses	Responses that control one's fear (and not the danger); typically psychological defense mechanisms such as reactance, defensive avoidance, or denial of a threat	"Modern contraceptives are just a way to destroy our people. They're a UN plot." (reactance) "I don't even want to think about my risks; it's safer to just block out scary thoughts." (defensive avoidance) "I'm not at risk for having more children than I want. God will protect me." (denial)

greater the threat perceived, the greater the motivation to act. If people believe they are able to do something to effectively avert the negative consequences of the health threat, they are motivated to control the danger and adopt the campaign's recommended responses to protect themselves. On the other hand, if people have strong threat perceptions but doubt whether or not they are able to do something to avert the health threat and/or believe the recommended response to be ineffective, then they will turn instead to controlling their fear about the health threat and engage in maladaptive actions like denial, reactance, or defensive avoidance.

Study after study has proven that the EPPM's four theoretical variables of perceived susceptibility, severity, response efficacy, and self-efficacy work together in predictable manners to predict health-related behaviors. Typically, three types of outcomes can be predicted from the theory. First, if people have low threat perceptions, they will have no reaction to a campaign. For example, if people do not feel susceptible to a health threat and/or they think the health threat is trivial, they will not process the campaign message because it's not important enough to do so or is not even relevant to them. Second, if people have strong perceptions of threat *and* strong perceptions of efficacy, they will engage in danger control actions. For example, if people felt susceptible to a severe threat and believed they were able to perform a response that would effectively avert the threat, they would change their behavior to control the danger. Third, if people have strong perceptions of threat *but* felt they were unable to perform the recommended response and/or believed the recommended response to be ineffective, they would become frightened (because they did not believe they could do anything to control the danger) and turn instead to controlling their fear through such psychological defense mechanisms as reactance, defensive avoidance, or denial. Overall, a campaign should promote strong perceptions of susceptibility, severity, response efficacy, and self-efficacy to promote the greatest degree of danger control actions and always ensure that perceptions of efficacy are sufficiently strong enough to counterbalance perceptions of threat to prevent fear control responses.

Formative Evaluation

A formative evaluation was conducted to determine key family planning messages according to the EPPM's theoretical tenets. A representative household survey elicited existing perceptions of susceptibility, severity, self-efficacy, and response efficacy, as well as current use of modern contraceptives. With the baseline knowledge provided by the surveys, the radio serial campaign designers were able to systematically develop theoretically based campaign messages that promote adaptive, life-saving actions and avoid unintended effects from campaigns that might inadvertently promote fear control actions that inhibit protective action. This unique health communication approach allowed campaign designers to systematically target audience perceptions to promote optimal levels of behavior change. According to the EPPM, campaign materials that promote high levels of perceived susceptibility, severity, response efficacy, and self-efficacy should motivate danger control actions leading to self-protective behaviors. However, if campaign materials scare people without promoting strong self-efficacy and/or response efficacy perceptions, then they are likely to backfire and cause denial, defensive avoidance, or reactance responses. Following is a brief description of our methods and results, with illustrations of the recommendations made to the scriptwriters of the radio serial drama.

METHODS

In EPPM parlance, the threat was defined as "having more children than desired" and the recommended response was "modern family planning methods" to prevent having more children than desired. The target population was 15- to 30-year-olds living urban areas across five regions in Ethiopia. A statistically representative household survey was conducted with randomly selected members of the target population in the five specified regions, with a total of 792 surveyed.

Results of the Formative Health Communication Research

Overview.   A three-step process was used in the EPPM-based research. First, the frequency distribution of each theoretical variable (i.e., susceptibility, severity, response efficacy, self-efficacy) was examined to assess if it was at high or low levels. Recall that the EPPM suggests that each of these variables should be at high levels to promote maximum behavior change. Second, the mean scores of each theoretical variable were compared with each other. The EPPM suggests that as long as perceptions of efficacy are stronger than perceptions of threat, then danger control actions would be promoted. Thus, the data were analyzed to determine if efficacy perceptions had higher mean scores than threat perceptions. Third, with the information from steps 1 and 2, a chart of belief strength was created, which tells campaign designers whether or not the theoretical variables need to be strengthened or minimized in a campaign. With this information, specific, theoretically based recommendations can be given to campaign designers about what messages should be contained in a radio serial drama.

Results for Step 1.   Figure 28.1 shows the separate frequency distributions for perceived susceptibility, severity, response efficacy, and self-efficacy. These distributions give clues as to how urban Ethiopian youths view their risks of experiencing negative outcomes, as well as how they view family planning methods. *Perceptions of susceptibility* to having more children than desired were fairly split, with about 40% of respondents believing they were at risk of having more children than they wanted but with nearly 30% of respondents failing to see themselves as at risk. Some urban youths are motivated to act (the 40% who perceive high risk), but many are not (the 30% who do not believe themselves to be at risk). In terms of *perceived severity*, urban Ethiopian youths nearly universally believed that serious negative consequences come from having more children than desired. *Perceived response efficacy* was fairly high, as most urban Ethiopian youths believed that modern family planning methods worked and that they prevented one from having too many children. However, urban Ethiopian youths were split on their *perceptions of self-efficacy* toward the pill. About 50% of urban youths strongly agreed that they were able to use the pill to prevent having more children than they wanted, but over 20% of the urban youths strongly disagreed that they were able to use the pill.

Results for Step 2.   Although the EPPM suggests that campaign designers should promote high levels of each theoretical variable, it also advises that perceptions of response efficacy and self-efficacy should always be *higher* than perceptions of severity or susceptibility to promote danger control responses and prevent fear control responses. Therefore, each theoretical variable should be between the 4 and 5 marks to represent high levels of each *and* the efficacy variables should be higher than the threat variables to promote danger control responses and prevent fear control responses. Figure 28.2 shows that only perceived severity and perceived response efficacy fall within the desired 4 to 5 range. Perceived susceptibility hovers around the neutral point of the scale and perceived self-efficacy is slightly higher. Perceived severity is higher than any of the efficacy variables, indicating a risk for fear control responses as opposed to danger control responses.

Results for Step 3.   Steps 1 and 2 allow us to create a chart of belief strength and specific campaign recommendations. In Table 28.2, an X is marked in boxes indicating high, medium, or low perceptions. This table gives a snapshot of what an intervention needs to focus on. Recall that to promote danger control actions (i.e., self-protective attitude, intention, or behavior

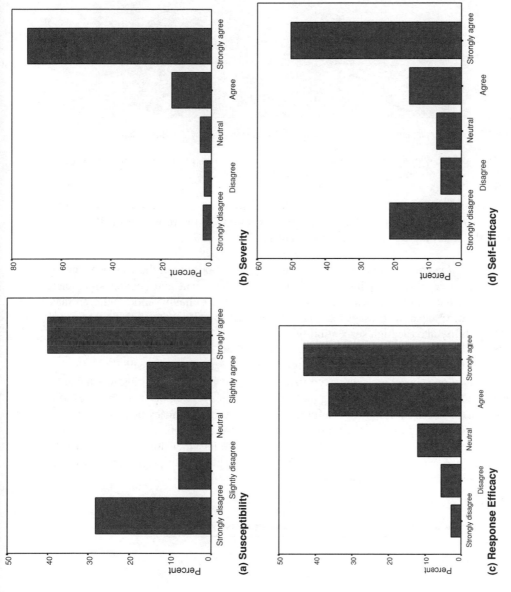

FIG. 28.1. Perceived susceptibility, severity response efficacy, and self-efficacy distributions. (a) Responses to perceived susceptibility statement (single item), "I am at risk for having more children than I want." (b) Responses to perceived severity statements, e.g., "Having more children than I want leads to serious negative consequences." (c) Responses to perceived response efficacy statements, e.g., "Using modern family planning methods work in preventing my having more children than I want." (d) Responses to perceived self-efficacy statements, e.g., "I am able to use the pill to prevent my having more children than I want."

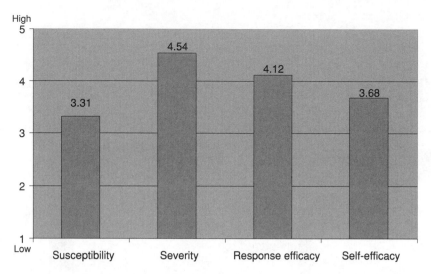

FIG. 28.2. Mean score (average) responses to each theoretical variable on a scale of 1 to 5, with 1 representing *low* and 5 representing *high*.

change) according to the EPPM, people must have high levels of perceived susceptibility, severity, response efficacy, and self-efficacy. Thus, according to the results of this formative evaluation, the following recommendations can be made:

Recommendation 1: Perceived susceptibility is split, with a portion of the youths believing they are susceptible to having more children than they want and another significant portion of the youths believing they are *not* susceptible to having more children than they want. Campaign messages should be designed to shift those with no perceived susceptibility into the high susceptibility group.

Recommendation 2: Urban youths have strong perceptions of severity toward having more children than desired. There is no need for further messages on this issue.

Recommendation 3: In general, perceived response efficacy is high in that most urban youths believe that modern family planning methods work in preventing one from having more children than desired. It may be useful to reinforce response efficacy beliefs.

Recommendation 4: Urban youths are split in their perceived self-efficacy toward using the pill to prevent having too many children. Nearly half believe they are able to use the pill, but over 20% explicitly state they are *unable* to use the pill. A campaign explicitly needs to address perceptions of self-efficacy.

TABLE 28.2
Chart of Belief Strength to Guide Campaign Message Development

Theoretical Variables	Weak or Low Belief Strength	Moderate Belief Strength	Strong or High Belief Strength
Susceptibility	×		
Severity			×
Response efficacy		×	
Self-efficacy		×	

Summary Recommendations.   The results illustrated in Figs. 28.1 and 28.2 indicate that an intervention needs to increase perceptions of susceptibility and self-efficacy and, to a lesser extent, response efficacy. However, there is no need to address the issue of perceived severity of having more children than desired because it already is at a high level. Perceived susceptibility is low enough to suggest that many urban youths are in denial about their risk of having more children than they want. Interventions need to educate them about these risks. Similarly, interventions need to think of creative ways to increase urban youths' perceived ability to use modern family planning methods like the pill. Entertainment education programs that show similar youths modeling how to use the pill, where to get it, and what its effects are is a useful strategy in increasing perceived self-efficacy. This unique health communication research demonstrates how a theory can be used to segment and analyze the audience to give specific guidance to campaign designers.

THE COMMUNICATION CAMPAIGN

The purpose of this formative research was to develop recommendations for campaign designers that were grounded in the audience's reality and were theoretically based. On completion of this formative research, a two-week-long scriptwriter's workshop was held in which the characters and main storylines for the radio serial were developed. Professional scriptwriters then fleshed out the 26 episodes, actors were hired, and production began. The radio serial was first broadcast the last week in November 2001, with the final broadcast airing June 16, 2002. Following is a brief description of the campaign.

Journey of Life

Journey of Life (JOL) was a weekly radio drama that focused on promoting family planning and preventing HIV and AIDS.[1] Based on the theoretically based formative evaluation, the scriptwriters focused on increasing perceived susceptibility with regard to overpopulation and perceived self-efficacy toward using family planning by discussing the benefits, myths, and rumors about family planning and by motivating the audience to realize that family planning is the most important way they can improve their own lives, the lives of their families, and the quality of the life throughout Ethiopia.

The main message in JOL was "Yichalal" (It is possible), meaning that it is possible for people in Ethiopia to improve their quality of life by planning their families and it is possible to control the epidemic of HIV/AIDS by taking appropriate measures to control the spread of the disease. The emotional focus of the series was to generate feelings of *hope* and *confidence* that determining one's own family size and protecting oneself from HIV/AIDS are things that can be achieved by all. Table 28.3 shows that the majority of episodes focused on family planning issues (Episodes 2, 3, 6, 7, 10, 14–18, 22–25). The synopsis is as follows:

> Askale, a female police investigator, and Bahiru, her husband, were an affectionate married couple that actively educated and taught others about health topics like family planning. They constantly tried (and eventually succeeded) in persuading their mother, the interfering and vocal Amelwork, that child-spacing was the best way to raise a healthy and economically stable family. Saba was Askale's carefree sister who went out drinking and socializing with many men. She did not heed her sister's warnings to either abstain from sex or use protection, and Saba wound up discovering that she was HIV-positive after she had infected others. Tedjic, their servant, frequently asked questions on health-related issues and adopted the use of condoms for himself as well as developed healthy beliefs regarding the benefits of child-spacing and the birth control pill.

TABLE 28.3
Content of *Journey of Life* Episodes

Episode 1:	General Introduction of Story and Characters
Episode 2:	Overpopulation and Its Consequences[a]
Episode 3:	What is Family Planning (FP) and Why Is It Important?[a]
Episode 4:	Transmission of HIV/AIDS
Episode 5:	Who is Vulnerable to HIV/AIDS?
Episode 6:	Consequence of Not Using FP[a]
Episode 7:	Cultural Barriers to Using FP[a]
Episode 8:	Technical Explanation of HIV/AIDS
Episode 9:	Need for Expert Advice
Episode 10:	Contraceptives: Condom (also for HIV)[a]
Episode 11:	General Story Development.
Episode 12:	Fear and Shame with HIV/AIDS
Episode 13:	Preventing HIV/AIDS
Episode 14:	Contraceptives: Oral Contraceptive Pills[a]
Episode 15:	Contraceptives: Injections[a]
Episode 16:	Need for Counseling and Informed Choice[a]
Episode 17:	Contraceptives: IUCD[a]
Episode 18:	Contraceptives: Norplant[a]
Episode 19:	HIV/AIDS and Marriage/Polygamy
Episode 20:	Care and Support of People with AIDS
Episode 21:	Socioeconomic Problems of HIV/AIDS
Episode 22:	Myths and Rumors with FP[a]
Episode 23:	Contraceptives: Vasectomy[a]
Episode 24:	Contraceptives: Tubal Ligation[a]
Episode 25:	Benefits of Family Planning[a]
Episode 26:	Story Conclusion

[a]Episodes with primary focus on family planning issues.

Elias, a judge, and his wife, Azeb, lived next door to Askale and Bahiru. Elias and Azeb were initially very happy in their marriage, but Azeb caused conflict, eventually destroying the marriage. Azeb had a son that she had to give up for adoption because she had been raped by an employer and needed to be childless to get a new job. She shared her concern with Askale, and they plotted to investigate, leaving Elias in the dark.

Meanwhile, another couple, Zeleke and Fikirte, agreed to take in Azeb's son and find him a family to live with. Zeleke planned to give Azeb's son to the shady character, Alemu, who cripples children and forces them to beg on the streets, extracting some of their money for profit. Fikirte caught wind of the plan and kept the boy from this fate. In order to do so, she eventually turned her husband in to Askale, and Zeleke and Alemu were sent to jail. Unfortunately, the marriage of Azeb and Elias suffered, since he was suspicious and she would not reveal what was going on. Elias succumbed to Saba's advances, contracted HIV, and infected his wife (Azeb). They both died. Saba decided to better her life and teach others to avoid her path. Intermingled in these various plots were discussions of different health-related topics like the problems of overpopulation, unwanted pregnancy, different family planning methods, ways of HIV transmission, prevention of HIV/AIDS, crimes committed against children, etc., where the character of Doctor Hailu was frequently consulted for an expert opinion.

Throughout the radio drama, self-efficacy issues were addressed by frequent role-modeling of a variety of family planning decisions and options. In addition, barriers, myths, and rumors regarding family planning were specifically countered to increase perceived efficacy. Finally, everyone's personal susceptibility (both males and females) to having more children than desired was emphasized to motivate the use of family planning. These are the variables that the formative evaluation suggested focusing on.

Impact Evaluation

The evaluation of JOL impact revealed that the targeted theoretical variables—especially perceived self-efficacy and susceptibility—were successfully influenced by the theoretically base radio drama. Specifically, almost all of the respondents (97.6%) said that JOL made them believe that they were able to use family planning methods (i.e., perceived self-efficacy). Perceived susceptibility to threat was moderately influenced, with an increase of 6% of respondents strongly agreeing that they might have more children than desired (a change from 40% to 46.6%). Overall, the impact evaluation found that about 91% of the respondents agreed or strongly agreed that JOL influenced them to use family planning.

Qualitative data from another evaluation found similarly profound effects on family planning attitudes and behaviors. For example, "Seble's" self-efficacy beliefs were influenced by modeling from Askale, "I admire her (Askale) resolve to stick to family planning in spite of her mother-in-law's constant nagging to have more children." "Belay" reported a strong desire to space his children by using family planning, "To see one's child get somewhere in life because of the care and guidance the parents gave makes one very happy. If one does not apply child-spacing, achieving this will be hard. I have learned much about family planning. Now I am better off. I feel I have to apply family planning when I get married." And a married couple ("Tigist" and "Asfaw") reconsidered their notions of an optimal family size based on JOL exposure, "I do not think that just because one has a lot of children one can consider children as wealth. Children are wealth when you have one or two and they turn out well. Having a lot of children is not advantageous."

CONCLUSION

This case study provides a step-by-step example of how a theory-based communication intervention can achieve profound attitude and behavior changes. It is an example of how practitioners, creative talent, and researchers can work together to create effective behavior change communication interventions.

This theory-research-practice model is being used around the world across a variety of theories, health topics, and populations at Johns Hopkins University's Center for Communication Programs (www.jhuccp.org). At the Center for Communication Programs, researchers work hand in hand with program development staff to help people and organizations in developing countries create interventions that work. A new initiative, the global "Health Communication Partnership" (funded by the United States Agency for International Development), plans to expand this work by focusing on different levels of analysis, such as the community and institutional level. Truly, this is an exciting time to be active in the field of international health communication.

RELEVANT CONCEPTS

Entertainment education: The use of entertaining messages and formats to educate target audiences.

Formative research: Research conducted prior to an intervention to inform the development of that intervention.

Perceived response efficacy: The degree to which one believes that the recommended response works in averting the health threat.

Perceived self-efficacy: The degree to which one believes she or he is able to do the recommended response.

Perceived severity: The magnitude of harm or negative consequences expected from the health threat.

Perceived susceptibility: The degree to which one feels at risk for experiencing a health threat.

DISCUSSION QUESTIONS

1. Define perceived susceptibility, perceived severity, perceived response efficacy, and perceived self-efficacy.
2. What combination of the above variables leads to behavior change? What inhibits behavior change?
3. How might you use the fear appeal theory discussed here (the EPPM) in other topic areas like skin cancer prevention? Occupational safety?
4. How would you counsel an HIV-negative woman in an HIV-testing clinic based on the EPPM? How about an HIV-positive woman?
5. If you were a consultant to a television drama targeted toward preventing drinking and driving among youth, what would you advise them based on the EPPM?

ACKNOWLEDGMENT

Kim Witte is a Senior Program Evaluation Officer at the Center for Communication Programs, Johns Hopkins University.

ENDNOTE

[1] This report focuses on family planning only; the HIV and AIDS results are reported elsewhere.

REFERENCES/SUGGESTED READINGS

Belete, S., Girgre, A., & Witte, K. (2003). *Summative evaluation of "Journey of Life": The Ethiopia reproductive health communication project.* Addis Ababa, Ethiopia: JHU/CCP and Ethiopia National Office of Population.

Central Statistical Authority, Ethiopia, and ORC Macro (2001). *Ethiopia Demographic and Health Survey 2000.* Addis Ababa, Ethiopia, and Calverton, MD: Central Statistical Authority and ORC Macro.

Ferrara, M., Jerato, K., & Witte, K. (2002). *A case study of "Journey of Life": A process evaluation of a radio serial drama.* Addis Ababa, Ethiopia: JHU/CCP and Ethiopia National Office of Population.

JHU/CCP (2002). *Entertainment education: What is it?* Baltimore, MD: Johns Hopkins University Center for Communication Programs.

Witte, K., Meyer, G., & Martell, D. (2001). *Effective health risk messages: A step-by-step guide.* Newbury Park, CA: Sage.

Additional Resources

http://www.jhuccp.org (full of materials, videos, survey drafts, etc.)

http://www.comminit.com/ (full of lectures, discussions, and a listserv for international health communicators)

"Scared Straight." (written, produced, and directed by Arnold Shapiro. VHS videocassettes of this program may be purchased for private home use. Please call 1-800-367-2467, ext. 306, for pricing information.)

29

Narrowing the Digital Divide to Overcome Disparities in Care

Gary L. Kreps
George Mason University

The National Cancer Institute (NCI) is a federal agency, part of the U.S. Department of Health and Human Services (DHHS). It is the largest of more than 20 major research institutes within the National Institutes of Health (NIH). The mission of the NIH is to improve the health of the American public by increasing understanding of the processes underlying human health and by developing new and relevant knowledge about prevention, detection, diagnosis, and treatment of disease. A major objective of the NCI, in particular, is to significantly reduce the national burden caused by cancers by generating new knowledge about cancer prevention and control. To achieve these goals, the NCI has developed an ambitious program of cancer research. This case study describes a unique health communication research initiative sponsored by the NCI.

The NCI is authorized by the National Cancer Act of 1971 to not only generate new scientific knowledge about cancer prevention, detection, and treatment, but to communicate relevant new knowledge learned about cancer to health care consumers, providers, researchers, policymakers, and the American public in general. In this regard, the NCI has made a large and ambitious commitment to cancer communications research and outreach. In fact, the NCI identified cancer communications as one of its priority areas for investment, an area of extraordinary opportunity. The research and development program described is part of this extraordinary opportunity in cancer communications. It was designed to learn how to communicate effectively through new communication technologies with several hard-to-reach groups of people in the United States who are most vulnerable to the lethal effects of cancer. These research projects, called the Digital Divide Pilot Projects, developed and tested new strategies for providing different poor and underserved groups of people with access to the latest and most accurate information about cancer prevention, control, and treatment.

HEALTH INFORMATION AND HEALTH DISPARITIES

Many of the people who are most at risk of dying from cancer are members of underserved populations (populations that are generally comprised of those individuals who are often of low socioeconomic status, possess low levels of literacy, are elderly, are members of ethnic minority groups, or have limited formal education.). These underserved and vulnerable populations often have limited access to relevant health information, especially information widely available over the Internet (Science Panel on Interactive Communication and Health, 1999). These vulnerable populations are also subject to serious disparities in health care and generally have much higher rates of morbidity and mortality because of serious health threats than the rest of the public, especially from cancers (Institute of Medicine, 1999). New strategies and policies need to be developed to help these underserved populations access relevant health information and to help them use such information to make informed health-related decisions about seeking appropriate health care and support, resisting avoidable and significant health risks, and promoting their health.

The pattern of limited access to relevant health information is a global issue. It occurs wherever there are pockets of poverty, illiteracy, and social disenfranchisement. Limited access to health information is a significant problem in the United States, but also is an issue in many different countries. Health and health care are universal issues that affect all people, and relevant health information is a critical resource that empowers people to make good decisions to enhance their health and well-being.

Health information is essential in health care and health promotion because it provides both direction and rationale for guiding strategic health behaviors, treatments, and decisions. The Digital Divide has been identified as a special problem in health care that can lead to significant disparities in care. Many studies show that certain minority groups, as well as low-income, low-education populations, in the United States suffer a disproportionate cancer burden and have limited access to electronic information about health (Institute of Medicine, 1999). However, too little is known about different disenfranchised groups' interests in, access to, and abilities to use health information.

NARROWING THE DIGITAL DIVIDE

The U.S. Department of Commerce and other groups have documented the Digital Divide that separates those who have access to computer technology and the vast storehouse of information available through the World Wide Web from those who lack access (National Telecommunications and Information Administration, 2000). A recent White House (U.S. White House, 2000) report indicated that the gap between people who have access to the latest Information-Age tools and those who do not is widening, and the Digital Divide is growing along racial and ethnic lines. This White House report suggested several steps they intended to implement to break down the Digital Divide. One of their goals was to make access to computers and the Internet as universal as the telephone is today. The 2010 Healthy People report for the first time has a section on health communications, with goals for access to health communication and computer-mediated health information (U.S. DHHS, 2000). The Digital Divide is a special problem in health care. Many of the characteristics that identify those on the "have not" side of the Digital Divide also characterize those who suffer the negative effects of health disparities, for example, people with less education and low income, and ethnic minorities. Although information and knowledge are not guarantees of good health care decisions and adherence to recommended health behaviors, there is ample evidence that they contribute to them. Currently, substantial barriers prevent major segments of the population from seeking and/or using online health information.

THE NCI DIGITAL DIVIDE PILOT PROJECTS

In 2001, the NCI supported development of four new demonstration research programs to examine new strategies for narrowing the Digital Divide that limits access to relevant cancer information. The NCI awarded close to $1 million to help develop these four innovative research projects to increase understanding about how to narrow the Digital Divide that exists among many underserved populations in accessing and utilizing information about cancer on the Internet. The awards were an effort of NCI's Cancer Information Service (CIS) to work collaboratively with regional cancer control groups and organizations to test new strategies designed to enhance cancer communications in underserved communities. The CIS is a national program supported by the NCI to provide the American public with answers to questions they might have about cancer. The CIS operates a national toll-free telephone network (1-800-4-CANCER), as well as an informative set of Internet-based web pages and specialized cancer information and treatment search engines available through www.cancer.gov. By working in concert with the Digital Divide Pilot Projects, the CIS hoped to learn how to better reach diverse and underserved audiences of people who need relevant health information and support.

There were several issues of concern to the NCI in engaging in these projects. Prior to these projects, many people assumed that members of low-income and minority groups would not be able to use computer equipment or understand complicated health information. The projects had to address the issues of technical competence and health literacy among the targeted populations. They had to address issues of the users' access to technology, their abilities to use computers effectively, their motivation to seek health information, and the appropriateness of the information to the users' unique interests and cultural orientations. In many ways, the Digital Divide Pilot Projects were tests of both the abilities of members of vulnerable populations to effectively use new communication technologies and about whether unique programs could be developed and implemented where these underserved consumers lived that would meet their unique needs and expectations.

The following four innovative demonstration research projects were conducted in collaboration with the CIS to identify effective new strategies for providing access to relevant cancer information to underserved populations.

The Computerized Health Education and Support System Program

A University of Wisconsin-based research group in collaboration with two NCI CIS regional offices, one in Wisconsin and the other in Detroit, developed a multiyear demonstration research project to test the feasibility of working in collaboration with the CIS network to disseminate an integrated online cancer communication system, the Computerized Health Education and Support System (CHESS), to underserved women recently diagnosed with breast cancer. The CHESS information system is a unique computer-based support program that provides users with multiple information options (cancer information, reference materials, support groups, journaling, etc.). This project is a pilot test of a new information dissemination strategy to provide underserved cancer patients with access to an Internet-based version of the CHESS system to provide them with high-quality breast cancer information and support. Results from this study will test the ability of disseminating the CHESS system broadly via the Internet and position the NCI and other organizations with cancer information services to develop innovative information dissemination strategies to effectively reduce the Digital Divide among those facing cancer. If successful, this could serve as a model for a nationwide dissemination of Internet-based cancer information and support to the underserved.

In past studies, CHESS had positive effects with high levels of utilization by test group members (Gustafson et al., 1999). However, up until now, the CHESS system software was installed as part of the computers used by respondents in previous studies. This new application uses Internet delivery of CHESS to a widely dispersed population of users to see if the system could have broader applications and dissemination potential with geographically distant audiences of potential users. A unique feature of this Digital Divide Pilot Projects study is the comparison of adoption and use of the CHESS system via Internet delivery by low-income women in rural Wisconsin and urban Detroit to better understand the unique information needs of these different underserved populations. (The Wisconsin women recruited for this study were White, and the Detroit-based women in the study were African American, providing an interesting comparison of system usage across race.) Preliminary results of this study suggest that Internet delivery of CHESS works well and results in strong adoption and system utilization, and outcome measures show the system has positive effects on user satisfaction, well-being, support, and adjustment to living with cancer. System adoption, use, and satisfaction have been strong across the Wisconsin and Detroit populations, suggesting the system works well for women from different racial and geographic backgrounds.

The Harlem Program

The New York regional CIS office and researchers at the Memorial/Sloan Kettering Cancer Research Center in New York conducted an innovative community partnership intervention program designed to teach both consumers and providers of health care in Harlem, New York, how to access relevant cancer information on the Internet. They conducted workshops teaching strategies for accessing health information online that were delivered to target populations consisting of lower-income minority (primarily African American and Latino) group members at a network of community organizations that served as both technology access sites and training centers. They also developed culturally sensitive dedicated web sites for both health care providers and consumers to enhance the relevance and appropriateness of health information delivery.

A unique feature of this study was the use of established community organizations as delivery sites for information dissemination, including nonprofit community support organizations, local government agencies, and corporations. These organizations provided easily accessible points of access for technology training and information searching. Preliminary results demonstrate increased access to and use of relevant health information among target groups. This demonstration project provides a model for how macrosocial community interventions can be used to help overcome the Digital Divide by ensuring that medically underserved populations have access to the same information and array of online tools as the rest of the population. This project also provides an opportunity to develop and test new tools for bridging the Digital Divide. The next step is to make those tools available broadly.

The LUCI Program

Researchers at the Louisiana State University Medical School, in collaboration with the Mid-South regional CIS office, developed an innovative multidimensional strategy to overcome the Digital Divide for low-literacy elderly senior center participants in Louisiana. This project uses a train-the-trainer program, a computer education program, installation of computer and

Internet resources in state-operated senior centers, and an innovative narrative-based computer-ized multimedia information translation application (interface) for improving the dissemination of cancer information. The implementation of this interface, which is called the "Low-literacy User Cancer Information Interface"(LUCI), utilizes multimedia technologies for overcoming literacy-based barriers to computer utilization and the acquisition of cancer information. To engage seniors unfamiliar with computer and Internet usage, LUCI presents information in a multimedia narrative format, similar to a televised soap opera, that does not rely on reading or computer literacy.

Preliminary results indicate the LUCI application is popular with the senior citizens and is easy for them to use. However, outcome measures have failed to demonstrate significant increases in health promotion knowledge and activity among the seniors. Perhaps longer ex-posure to the LUCI intervention is warranted. This project illustrates innovative strategies for reaching low-literacy audiences in senior centers and clinics that has the potential for broad application. The challenge is to find the best applications of this communication strategy and the most opportune sites for program delivery.

The Head Start Program

The New England regional CIS office, in collaboration with researchers from Yale University, developed an important community intervention project that established community techno-logy centers at two Head Start early-childhood education programs to provide access to health information to low-income families. In this innovative project, Head Start staff members were trained as technology coaches to deliver computer training courses to parents and other com-munity members who earned free, refurbished, Internet-ready computers to take home by completing the training program. In this project, the unique focus on the family as a unit of analysis, based on the Head Start program model, provided a rich multigenerational approach to computer skills development and utilization.

This project, like the Harlem project, provides a provocative model for using established community resources to educate underserved populations and bridge the Digital Divide in access to health information. Preliminary results suggest strong acceptance of the program within the Head Start system, as well as positive outcome influences on computer skills, health information access, and information utilization. There is great potential to develop similar technology centers in other Head Start programs, as well as in a number of different community organizations to help bridge the Digital Divide and provide underserved families with both access to and the skills needed to utilize relevant health information.

SUMMARY AND IMPLICATIONS

Each of the four Digital Divide pilot projects supported by the NCI developed provocative new community strategies for providing underserved groups of people with access to relevant computer-based information about cancer. There is great opportunity to expand and sustain these Digital Divide interventions to provide additional underserved populations with relevant health information. There may be some opportunities to combine aspects of these different projects for application in different contexts. Lessons learned from these projects can be fruit-fully applied in many other settings to narrow the Digital Divide and reduce health disparities. These funded projects attempt to increase understanding of why barriers to information and knowledge exist and use the data gleaned from these pilot projects to design programs that can lead to better health care decisions and adherence to recommended health behaviors. These pilot projects will serve as models for larger-scale efforts. Similar efforts to narrow health disparities by bridging the Digital Divide will help empower underserved health care consumers to make informed health care decisions, seek the best possible health care, and enhance their quality of life. The results of these Digital Divide Pilot Projects should be interpreted and applied to develop new programs and policies for providing relevant health information to all segments of modern society.

One of the most promising findings of the Digital Divide Pilot Projects was that poor, low-literacy, and underserved groups of people could learn to effectively use computer technologies to access health information. Evaluation data gathered in these projects illustrated high levels of user satisfaction with the programs, with their new computer skills, and with the information they were able to access. Many of the users reported using the computers for a broad range of activities, such as career development, education, and entertainment, in addition to gathering relevant health information. The users who were given computers to take home, as in the Head Start and the CHESS projects, reported using the computers to search for health information for family, friends, and neighbors, often serving as health advisors and advocates for these people. It is clear that the Digital Divide Pilot Projects had powerful and enduring influences on the lives of the people who participated in the programs. Yet, these programs touched the lives of just a small proportion of the people who need help to get access to relevant health information.

There are many other populations that suffer from both the Digital Divide and disparities in care who were not targeted by the Digital Divide Pilot Projects that need help to get access to relevant health information. Some of these groups of people who might be fruitfully targeted for future interventions include many Native Americans living on reservations, a broad range of first-generation immigrants who may have limited literacy with the English language, as well as many people living in poverty in both rural and urban settings. Unique communication strategies need to be developed to provide members of these vulnerable populations with ready access to appropriate and usable computer technologies, training in how to use these communication technologies to gather relevant health information, technical accommodations to help meet users' unique needs and abilities, as well as culturally sensitive computer programs to match users' interests and levels of literacy. Furthermore, there are many infrastructure needs for providing equipment, Internet connections, and long-term technical support to maintain equipment and connection services. There is a lot of planning needed and resources that must be provided to accomplish the dual goals of narrowing the Digital Divide and reducing disparities in care.

Providing vulnerable populations with access to health information is just one step in improving the health of the people who suffer from disparities in health outcomes. There are also important issues concerning the quality of health care that members of many vulnerable populations are able to receive. Do these individuals have the communication skills to effectively negotiate the complexities and bureaucracy of the modern health care system? How receptive are the health care delivery system and health care workers to meeting the needs of vulnerable populations? These are some of the important questions that also need to be answered to fully address the troubling issue of disparities in health outcomes.

RELEVANT CONCEPTS

Cancer Information Service: A National Cancer Institute-funded program for providing the American public with relevant information about cancer via a toll-free telephone hotline (1-800-4-CANCER) and online (www.cancer.gov).

Computer-mediated communication: The delivery and exchange of relevant information using computer-based information technologies such as e-mail and the Internet.

Digital Divide: The differential access to computer-delivered information between the most privileged and least privileged members of modern society.

Digital Divide Pilot Projects: A group of four National Cancer Institute-funded demonstration research projects testing different communication strategies for providing relevant health information via computer to underserved and vulnerable groups of people.

Disparities in health care outcomes: The differences between the health preserving outcomes of health care that often accrue to the most privileged members of society in comparison to the high levels of morbidity and mortality due to health risks suffered by those with the lowest education and socioeconomic levels in society.

Health information: Relevant data about health risks, prevention, health promotion, health care treatments, and support.

Information dissemination: Communication strategies for providing relevant health information to different groups of people.

Macrosocial community interventions: Large-scale campaign communication strategies for promoting change within targeted groups of people by involving local community organizations in delivering and sustaining campaign messages and programs.

National Cancer Institute: A U.S. federal agency, part of the National Institutes of Health, that conducts research on cancer prevention, control, and treatment to reduce the national cancer burden.

National Institutes of Health: A U.S. federal agency, part of the Department of Health and Human Services, that conducts research on health promotion, disease prevention, and health care to promote the health of the nation.

Underserved and vulnerable populations: Groups of people, often those with the lowest education and socioeconomic levels in society, who have the highest levels of morbidity and mortality due to health risks.

DISCUSSION QUESTIONS

1. Describe the relationship between the groups of people who are likely to suffer from disparities in health care outcomes and those who have limited access to computer- mediated information due to the Digital Divide. What implications does this relationship suggest for access to quality health care? Why is it an important health promotion goal to provide these people with access to computer-mediated health information?

2. Describe some of the unique health communication strategies employed by the Digital Divide Pilot Projects to increase access and utilization of relevant health information by underserved groups of people, including strategies to address the issues of technical competence and health literacy? Identify the health communication strategies you think will be most successful and explain why. Can you think of additional health communication strategies that could be implemented to reduce the Digital Divide and narrow disparities in care?

3. How could the relative success of these Digital Divide Pilot Projects be evaluated on the short-term and for the long-run? How can lessons learned from these projects be fruitfully applied in other settings to narrow the Digital Divide and reduce health disparities?

4. How transportable are each of the four Digital Divide Pilot Projects from the settings where they were developed to other settings and populations? Describe where they might work well and where they are unlikely to be effective.

5. Identify some of the at risk and vulnerable populations that were not targeted by the Digital Divide Pilot Projects. What unique communication strategies would be needed to help these groups of people access and use relevant health information available online?

6. Why is the kind of investment in health information dissemination research that the NCI made with the Digital Divide Pilot Projects important?
7. How do the unique strategies developed in these research projects help to overcome communication barriers that may limit access to and utilization of health information?

REFERENCES/SUGGESTED READINGS

Gustafson, D. H., Hawkins, R., Boberg, E., Pingree, S., Serlin, R. E., Graziano, F., & Chan, C. L. (1999). Impact of a patient-centered, computer-based health information/support system. *American Journal of Preventive Medicine, 16*(1), 1–9.

Institute of Medicine. (1999). *The unequal burden of cancer: An assessment of NIH research and programs for ethnic minorities and the medically underserved.* Washington, DC: National Academy of Sciences.

National Telecommunications and Information Administration. (2000). Americans in the Information Age: Falling through the Net II: New data on the Digital Divide, 1999. Retrieved July 22, 2004 from www.ntia.doc.gov/ntiahome/digitaldivide

Science Panel on Interactive Communication and Health. (1999). *Wired for health and well-being: The emergence of interactive health communication.* Washington, DC: U.S. Department of Health and Human Services, U.S. Government Printing Office.

U.S. Department of Health and Human Services. (2000). *Healthy People 2010: Conference edition in two volumes.* Washington, DC: U.S. Government Printing Office.

U.S. White House. (2000). White House proposal: From digital divide to digital opportunity. Retrieved February 20, 2003 from www.whitehouse.gov/WH/New/digitaldivide

Additional Resources

The National Cancer Institute's Heath Communication and Informatics Research Branch: http://dccps.nci.nih.gov/hcirb/
The National Cancer Institute's Extraordinary Opportunity in Cancer Communications: http://dccps.nci.nih.gov/eocc/
The Digital Divide Pilot Projects: http://dccps.nci.nih.gov/eocc/ddpp_awards.html
Video Highlights from the Digital Divide Pilot Projects: http://dccps.nci.nih.gov/eocc/ddpp.html

Author Index

Note: Numbers in *italics* indicate pages with complete bibliographic information.

Subject Index

375